# NURSING ETHICS IN MODERN CHINA

## Conflicting Values
## and
## Competing Role Requirements

# VIBS

Volume 140

Robert Ginsberg
**Founding Editor**

Peter A. Redpath
**Executive Editor**



a volume in
**Studies in Applied Ethics**
**SAE**
Gerhold K. Becker, Editor

# NURSING ETHICS IN MODERN CHINA

## Conflicting Values and Competing Role Requirements

Samantha Mei-che Pang

Rodopi

Amsterdam - New York, NY 2003

The paper on which this book is printed meets the requirements of "ISO 9706:1994, Information and documentation - Paper for documents - Requirements for permanence".

ISBN: 90-420-0944-6

Printed in the Netherlands

# CONTENTS

# LIST OF FIGURES AND TABLES

# FOREWORD

China is currently undergoing another revolution. Unlike the Communist revolution that led to the foundation of the People's Republic in 1949 and the notorious Cultural Revolution (1966-1976), this revolution, while no less dramatic, is economic and social, not political. China is changing, and fast. The effects of change are most obvious in the big cities and their glittering shopping malls. These beckon the newly rich with their luxury goods and make them forget the long years of hardship under stern Party rule. Evidently, not all Chinese have benefited from the country's embrace of capitalism and consumerism. The economic miracle has largely bypassed the countryside and its several hundred millions of workers, small farmers, and peasants.

Healthcare is one sector in which the ambiguities of change are felt most severely. While market forces have modernized the healthcare system and increased its efficiency, they seem at odds with the traditional values of care that have shaped Chinese medical practice for two and a half millennia.

Attention in medical ethics is usually focused on the interplay among physicians, patients, healthcare policies, and the healthcare system. The other major healthcare provider is often ignored: the nurses. Samantha Mei-che Pang's penetrating study of the value perceptions and the roles of nurses in the delivery of healthcare in contemporary China is therefore of great significance and fills an unfortunate gap in bioethical research. It represents the first major study on nursing ethics in China that draws on the rich textual resources written in Chinese and on the results of extensive field studies, through which the voices of the nurses can be heard, perhaps for the first time. The author's ability to interpret theses resources against a cultural backdrop that ranges from the Confucian classics to Mao Zedong and from Sun Simiao's concepts of jing (excellence in practice) and cheng (sincerity in the relationships with patients) to codes of practice in the Republican and Maoist eras generates remarkable insights into the long tradition of Chinese medicine and ethics.

Publication of this book is also quite timely, since the tension between traditional and modern values in the actual delivery of healthcare is of grave concern in China and the West. The author's personal and professional familiarity with nursing cultures in the West, most notably in the United States and Britain, in Hong Kong and China uniquely position her to approach the topic in a cross-cultural and comparative perspective. Her reflections about a perceived shift from a rule-based to a virtue-based ethics with its greater emphasis on the ever-changing contexts of healthcare practice, merit careful attention for anyone participating in the current ethical debate.

The author expertly combines moral theory with empirical investigation, yet she avoids sociological jargon and unnecessarily complicated terminology. Beneath the language of objectivity and sober reflection, the reader will notice another dimension of this important study: that of great appreciation of the extraordinary work of the nurses in contemporary China and of sympathy with their plight.

Gerhold K. Becker
Editor
Studies in Applied Ethics Special Series (SAE)

# ACKNOWLEDGMENTS

I am indebted to those mainland Chinese nurses who contributed to my work. Words cannot express my deep appreciation for their genuine kindness. They shared with me their joys, sorrows, hopes, and despair. Their concerns and visions still ring in my ears.

Indeed it has been a daunting task for me to maintain a clear and critical mind while undertaking this piece of scholarly work. Personally, I have had many mixed feelings about the topic. I owe my thanks to many people who in their special ways helped me to reach nurses in seven Chinese cities. My special thanks go to Professor Tim Moore, Professor Veronica Pearson, Professor Thomas Wong, Professor Gerhold Becker, and Professor Anne Davis. They have been a constant source of inspiration, knowledge, and wisdom from which I will forever benefit. They acted as valuable catalysts. They helped me to accomplish this task with their insightful comments on the numerous drafts of this book, their persistent confidence in my abilities when I had doubts, and their unfailing support in "nursing" me through the process. I am deeply indebted to Mr. Peter Luk Yiu-wang for his invaluable assistance in the various stages of the editorial process. Thanks go to the Department of Nursing and Health Sciences, The Hong Kong Polytechnic University, for provision of resources that greatly facilitated this publication.

Samantha Mei-che Pang

# One

# INTRODUCTION: IN SEARCH OF THE VOICES OF NURSES IN CHINA

Two motives launched this study to search for the voices of nurses in China. Recent reports from China and about China reveal that the country is not immune from the varieties of healthcare issues that have been arising in other parts of the world. These are issues such as active euthanasia, withholding and withdrawal of treatment, payment for organ donation, non-voluntary and involuntary use of cadavers in organ transplants, forced abortion, female infanticide, termination of the life of the mentally handicapped, surrogate motherhood and use of reproductive technologies, overcharging, unnecessary prescription of diagnostic procedures and medical treatments, and abuse of vulnerable patients. The most often reported ethical issues were uncontrolled levels of medical fees and refusal to treat patients who could not show evidence of their ability to pay. Healthcare workers were often blamed for their indifferent and inattentive attitude in dealing with these issues. Although these incidents largely happen in hospitals, hardly has any attempt to make sense of the moral experience of front-line workers, who are required to deal with these issues in their day-to-day practice. Since a majority of front-line workers are nurses, their moral experience was chosen as the vantage point of this study.

The second motive was to sustain a dialogue between nurses in China and their counterparts in other parts of the world about their views on morality. In searching through the on-line indices, while literature on nursing ethics has proliferated in other parts of the world in the past three decades, literature focusing on nursing ethics in China is scarce. The records from 1966 to 1997 for *Medline* reveal only two articles reporting nurses' views on ethical issues in China over the past thirty years.[1] Yet a review of publications on ethics in nursing within China suggests a different story. Nursing ethics has been receiving increasing attention in contemporary China. Writings on professional ethics for nurses have regularly appeared in the *Chinese Journal of Nursing* over the past eighteen years. *Chinese Medical Ethics* is another source where we can learn about nursing ethics in China. A third source is from the textbooks written by ethics scholars who teach nurses professional ethics. These writings revolve around two major themes: moral education and cultivation of desirable qualities in nurses, and fostering a sense of morality in different practice situations, such as the operating room, emergency room or pediatric ward.

In contrast to the increasing attention given to research on ethics in the international nursing community, not a single one of these writings is based on a systematic inquiry into the nurses' experience in ethically difficult situations in China. These publications primarily present a prescribed set of moral rules to follow, and qualities that a nurse should possess in fostering ethical practice, instead of giving voice to the moral concerns of practicing nurses. In this regard, I would like to see a Chinese perspective included in the study of ethics among the international nursing community, and a dialogue between nurses in China and their counterparts in other parts of the world can be sustained.

## 1. Rule-based or Virtue-based

Two conceptions of ethics or morality that differentiate each other are commonly used: in one conception rules are fundamental, and the basic issue in morality is what you ought to do; in the other conception, virtue is fundamental, and the basic issue is what you ought to be. Though any real living morality is certain to encompass both aspects, a difference is made whether rules or virtues are taken as fundamental. In an ideal world, no doubt, the two conceptions could coincide. But in the real world, they can give rise to conflicts.

To consider the two Chinese terms *lunli* (倫理) and *daode* (道德) that are used together or interchangeably to denote ethics or morality. *Dao* (道) means principles or the way of virtue, and *de* (德) refers to virtues manifested in a person's behavior. Virtues are desirable qualities that enable a person to implement principles in practice. In this sense, the Chinese meaning of virtue is similar to Alasdair MacIntyre's definition, which reads,

> [Virtue is] an acquired human quality the possession and exercise of which tends to enable us to achieve those goods which are internal to practices and the lack of which effectively prevents us from achieving any such goods.[2]

MacIntyre points out that virtue is needed to bring about a recognized good, but what is considered the good varies from place to place and periodically. He notes three quite different conceptions of virtue in Homer, Aristotle, and Benjamin Franklin. A Homeric virtue is a quality that enables an individual to discharge his or her social role. Aristotle's virtue is a quality that enables an individual to move toward the achievement of the human *telos*. Franklin's virtue is a quality that has utility in achieving earthly and heavenly success.[3]

In the Chinese sense, *daode* emphasizes putting virtues into practice, and the recognized good, which *daode* aims to achieve is indicated in the term *lunli*. *Lun* (倫) refers to the network of human relationships. *Li* (理) refers to rules, principles, or moral standards. *Lunli* means the rules, principles, and moral standards governing different kinds of human relationships, manifestation of which can bring about a harmonious and well-ordered society. *Lunli daode* (倫理道德) denote an ethical system which spells out the qualities of character that people are required to possess and rules of conduct that people are required to follow in relating to each other.[4] In this conception, the rule-based and virtue-based ethics could coincide.

But in the real world, it makes a difference whether rules or virtues are taken as fundamental. The *Analects of Confucius*, for instance, give great prominence to *li* (禮), which implies the importance of rules. On the other hand, Confucius emphasizes *ren* (仁).[5] When a conflict exists, it turns out that *ren* prevails. The etymological roots of *ren* imply two persons relating to each other in harmony. Many English translations of this term exist, ranging from benevolence and compassion to humanness, human-heartedness, good will, and love. I would say that any adequate translation of the term must include a sense of human interaction. The term must be able to convey that the focus is on people and what they can accomplish in relation to others. On this interpretation, the Confucian conception of ethics is virtue-based. Such a position is even clearer in the case of Mencius, in his account of how the "seeds" of virtues are innate.

> Whoever is devoid of the heart of compassion is not human, whoever is devoid of the heart of shame is not human, and whoever is devoid of the heart of courtesy and modesty is not human, and whoever is devoid of the heart of right and wrong is not human. The heart of compassion is the [seed] of [*ren*]; the heart of shame, of dutifulness; the heart of courtesy and modesty, of observance of the rites; the heart of right and wrong, of wisdom. Man has these four [seeds] just as he has four limbs. For a man possessing these four [seeds] to deny his own potentialities is for him to cripple himself.[6]

Mencius identified the hearts of compassion, shame, courtesy, and modesty, in addition to knowing the difference between right and wrong as the four central virtues that each person innately possesses. The question is whether people make an effort to put them into practice. Of these central virtues, Mencius prized the heart of right and wrong most. Although Mencius exhorted filial obedience as the source of all virtues, he defended for Shun, a sage king, who once committed an apparently unfilial act by choosing not to inform his father about his marriage. He argued that Shun had acted virtuously because his action showed concern and respect for what might have been the wishes of his father's inner self.[7] Tu Weiming pointed out that Mencius' justification is based on a personality ideal for guidance that transcends rules of civilized conduct.[8] Along a similar vein, the Confucian theory of moral cultivation emphasizes cultivation of an evaluating mind that can have a firm grasp of virtues to discern the right way in dealing with people.[9] This is in contrast to the doctrine of legalism, which advocates the universal standardization of behavior by explicit laws impartially applied, and through a system of rewards and punishments in regulating right conduct.[10] In surveying rules of conduct and qualities of character in the field of nursing in this book, I would keep these two conceptions of morality in mind.

## 2. Two Lines of Inquiry

I followed two lines of inquiry to make sense of nursing ethics in modern China: documentary review and empirical investigation. The first line was to examine the prescribed set of moral virtues that were required of nurses in fulfilling their role requirements in different periods of nursing development over the past century. Three essential virtues have been identified in academic writing or official documents, and in the opinions of nurses themselves. They are a sense of socialist responsibility, excellence in practice, and sincerity in relating to patients. These virtues have their roots in traditional Chinese medical ethics but are expressed within the ideological framework of "socialist humanism," in which Mao's mandate "rescue the dying and heal the wounded, serve the people wholeheartedly" is promulgated as the fundamental principle. Embedded in this mandate is an advocacy of respect for life that demands a positive duty on the part of healthcare workers to protect life and treat patients with altruistic motives. Over the past ten years, education and management measures have been instituted to foster these virtues in nurses. In reviewing contemporary issues in the healthcare system, population policies, and euthanasia movement, I argue that another set of values based on the notion of "quality of life" is promulgated by the Party leadership, which directly poses challenge to the adequacy of the mandate in informing practice.

The second line of inquiry was an empirical venture focusing on the nurses' evaluations of their ethical responsibilities in current practice. The particular viewpoints that nurses brought to their appraisal of the patient care situations where ethical practice was in question were examined. The empirical findings disclose a tension between the valuing of traditional virtues and the valuing of the virtues of the market economy. The three pairs of contrasted rankings emerging from the pattern of nurses' rankings of their multiple role responsibilities suggest that nurses in China inevitably experience moral dilemmas that emerge from three sources of conflicting values in practice situations that prevent them from taking virtues seriously. The first source derives from the emergent values that emphasize treating the patient as an individual and quality of care, but encounter the constraints posed by the value of protectiveness, which is predominant in the existing system of medical care. The second source emerges from the role requirement of having a sense of socialist responsibility in practice, but meeting with the constraints of the medical system, which is operated under the mechanism of market economy. The third source comes from nurses' emergent sense of professional care, meeting with traditional care values that emphasize family responsibility and institutional policies that require nurses to conform to rules and regulations.

To make sense of the ethical requirements of nurses in the historical-cultural context, the first two chapters examine the practice of nursing before and after China's modernization. Chapter Four examines the changes in values underpinning recent healthcare reforms, putting in question the ethical mandate's relevance to informing ethical practice. How do these changes affect the ways nurses perceive their responsibilities and the qualities that are required of them in fostering ethical practice? This question was left unanswered in the documentary review. Based on the empirical study, Chapter Five focuses on making sense of nurses' conceptualization of ethics in the context of eleven facets of nursing responsibilities. Chapter Six focuses on nurses' moral viewpoints in responding to the ethical issues they often face in practice. Drawing upon traditional ethical outlooks, international norms, and the experiences of nurses as they face ethically difficult situations, the final chapter concludes with recommendations for improving the quality of nursing in contemporary China.

# Two

# NURSING DEVELOPMENT BEFORE CHINA'S MODERNIZATION

The Crimean War and the Civil War signified the beginning of modern nursing in the United Kingdom and the United States respectively. In China, the fall of the Qing Dynasty (1644–1911), together with softening attitudes toward the control of women in the Republican period (1912–1949) provided the opportunity for nursing to become a profession for women in China. I would say that nursing in China has undergone three distinct phases of development. The first was the import of the idea of nursing as a profession that accompanied the establishment of Western-type hospitals in the late nineteenth century. The second occurred after the Communists gained power in China in 1949, inculcating the whole country with the doctrine of revolutionary humanism in their drive to realize a new China. Among radical reforms that the Communists attempted in virtually every aspect of Chinese society was a reform of medical practice that went against the professionalism of imported practices. The third came with China's era of modernization, from 1978 onwards, when China's leaders committed the country to economic reconstruction by implementing a market economy, while continuing to uphold the tenets of "socialist humanism."

This chapter examines the development of nursing before China's modernization to provide an historical background to issues in contemporary nursing. It comprises three main sections. The first section examines the traditional Chinese practices that early Western nurses encountered in their endeavor to introduce nursing as a profession for Chinese women. The second section discusses the three approaches that these pioneering nurses used to overcome the social biases that hindered their efforts to attract women to nursing. The development of nursing took a new turn after the founding of the People's Republic in 1949. Section three examines the ways in which the political ideology of revolutionary humanism redirected the development of nursing to a new course.

## 1. Traditional Caring Practices

As in other parts of the world, before the introduction of hospitals, caring for the sick in China was an affair of the private sphere, taking place only within the confines of the family.[1] The ideas of caring for the sick in institutional settings and of nursing as a profession were therefore foreign concepts when they were introduced to China.[2] When missionary nurses from the United States established the first formal nursing training programs in Shanghai and Fuzhou in 1884 and 1888 respectively, they met with difficulties in recruiting Chinese women. The first training program in Fuzhou attracted only three students.[3]

In 1907, an American nurse came to China, whose surnamed Simpson.[4] She commented in an open letter that nursing as a profession was new to China, many people misunderstood it to be servant's work. She suggested that a need existed to raise public consciousness through education, and to promote nursing as a meaningful job that could alleviate the suffering of humanity. I would contend that caring work was seen as servant's work in traditional Chinese society, but caring for the sick meant more than a bundle of tasks that could be accomplished by servants. It carried a strong notion of role responsibility and moral duty as a result of a person's relationship within the family.[5] This could be the more persuasive reason for the ambivalent view of nursing held in Chinese society. Simpson apparently failed to address the logic of care among the Chinese, which was different from the notion of shared humanity, which is the ideal of service in the Nightingalian legacy.[6] I will move to examine the logic of care that underpinned the social practices of caring for the sick.

## A. Care Responsibilities in Ancient China

A common theme in cultural studies of Chinese society is that Chinese people exist through, and are defined by, their hierarchical relationships with others. How one should behave depends on which role one is assuming at a particular moment in life.[7] The differential treatment of people based on their roles is seen as rooted in the teachings of Confucius, which cherished five cardinal relationships within which people must fulfill their role requirements. They are father and son, ruler and minister, husband and wife, elder and younger brother, and friends.[8] These role requirements are explained in the *Four Books*《四書》. The *Four Books* are the *Analects of Confucius*《論語》, *Mencius*《孟子》, *The Great Learning*《大學》, and *Doctrine of the Mean*《中庸》. They were put together with annotations by Zhu Xi in the Song Dynasty (960–1279).[9] Of the five cardinal relationships, primacy is given to that of father and son, with the relation between ruler and minister coming second. Social order is maintained when each party honors his or her requirements in the social relationship. As stated in *Mencius*, an ordered society will be achieved if affection exists between father and son, duty between ruler and minister, differentiation between husband and wife, precedence between elder and younger siblings, and faith between friends.[10] In the *Doctrine of the Mean*, how a person should act in his or her role is further elaborated as the duties of universal obligation, with the virtues required of a person varying depending on the role relationships. It reads,

> By honoring men of virtue and talents, he is preserved from errors of judgment. By showing affection to his relatives, there is no grumbling nor resentment among his uncles and brethren. By respecting the great ministers, he is kept from errors in the practice of government. By kind and considerate treatment of the whole body of officers, they are led to make the most grateful return for his courtesies. By dealing with the mass of the people as his children, they are led to exhort one another to what is good. By encouraging the resort of all classes of artisans, his resources for expenditure are rendered ample. By indulgent treatment of men from a distance, they are brought to resort to him from all quarters. And by kindly cherishing the prince of the States, the whole kingdom is brought to revere him.[11]

This notion of obligation stands in contrast to the Kantian notion of the categorical imperative, in which a universal rule is to be applied to all persons in all circumstances. Sandra Wawrytko noted this difference when she compared the notion of respect articulated in the Kantian and Confucian theories. She maintained that in the Confucian sense, respect should be paid to a person in correspondence to the dynamic social roles encompassed in the five cardinal relationships, whereas, in the Kantian sense, the imperative of respect was grounded in shared humanity justifiable by an appeal to rationality.[12] Since this Kantian notion of shared humanity is more in line with the Judeo-Christian values held by missionary nurses, we can imagine why those who failed to see humanity in a Chinese sense did not grasp the logic of care among the Chinese.

Since in China the family is considered to be the most basic social unit where a person learns the appropriate ways in relating to others, how a person treats his or her family member will be a more important indication of his or her integrity. Among all the virtues that a cultivated person needs to possess, duty to parents, or filial piety, is considered as the most crucial.[13] Filial piety, in the Confucian tradition, poses an unequal moral demand on different parties. While parents are required to be kind and loving, children are required to obey their parents, protect them, bear their burdens, and try their best to help their parents lead a good and long life. The following dialogue between Mencius and his student Tao Ying best illustrates the exemplary filial duty cherished in traditional Chinese society.

> Tao Ying: When Shun was Emperor and Kao Yao was the judge, if the Blind Man [Shun's father] killed a man, what was to be done?
>
> Mencius: The only thing to do was to apprehend him.
>
> Tao Ying: In that case, would Shun not try to stop it?
>
> Mencius: How could Shun stop it? Kao Yao had authority for what he did.

Tao Ying: Then what would Shun have done?
Mencius: Shun looked upon casting aside the Empire as no more than discarding a worn shoe. He would have secretly carried the old man on his back and fled to the edge of the Sea and lived there happily, never giving a thought to the Empire.[14]

In response to Tao Ying's challenge of the possible competing duties between compliance to the rule of law and loyalty to one's parents, Mencius gave a definite answer to the way in which a filial son should act. This example can be supported with another often cited example from the *Analects of Confucius* about covering up for a father who stole a sheep, which straightforwardly suggests that loyalty to family should have priority over justice in cases of conflict.[15] In contrast to Socrates' interrogation of Euthyphro's justification based on piety in taking his father to court because the father caused the death of a slave, the question was left open at the end of the interrogation.[16]

The kind of filial duties that are expected of a person are best represented in *Twenty-four Stories of Filial Devotion* 《二十四孝》, folk tales that pass down lessons of filial duty from generation to generation. These stories typically involve characters who, driven by devotion to their parents, act against their own interests—even to the point of sacrificing their lives.[17] For instance, the story "The scholar cleanses his mother's chamber pot" is about the well-known writer Huang Tingjian who lived during the Northern Song Dynasty (960–1127). When he became an academician of the Imperial Academy he continued his usual practice of paying respect to his mother. When his mother was ill, he personally took care of her, doing such things as making her bed, feeding her, helping her bathe, and emptying her chamber pot. When his neighbors were surprised that a person of his rank would perform these menial tasks, he replied that his duty was to see that his mother had a comfortable life. Huang's service to his mother signified that he was willing to surrender his dignity as a high official to the primacy of his mother. Other than stories of famous historical figures, tales about poor people who were willing to risk their lives or sacrifice their children's lives in order to find medical remedies for their sick parents existed.[18]

Since such importance is given to the filial duty of looking after one's parents, we can find it logical for the Chinese to regard taking care of their sick family members as a moral obligation that cannot be performed by someone who is not in the family. *Xiaoxue*《小學》, a Confucian classic compiled and annotated by Zhu Xi states as follows:

> If the parent or parent-in-law falls ill, the sons and their wives are not allowed to leave his or her side without reason. They are to prepare the

> drugs themselves, taste them in advance and administer them to the invalid. If the parents are sick, it is forbidden that their sons display carefree conduct, have any amusement, or seek pleasure. All other concerns must be given secondary importance so that they can devote themselves especially to their duty of receiving the physician, selecting formulas and preparing drugs.[19]

Any person who forfeited the filial duty of caring for his or her sick parent would be condemned as being impious, irresponsible, and bereft of proper human feelings, and not behaving as a human being should.

With the family-based relationship that forms the deep structure of a society, the phenomenon of differential treatments of in-group and out-group members could not be more pronounced among the Chinese. In many studies of Chinese culture we can see that a rigid demarcation exists between in-group family members and out-group non-family members; this, then, is where the boundary between the private sphere and public sphere of life was drawn. The family, with its friends, became a walled castle with the greatest communal co-operation and mutual help within, but coldly indifferent toward and fortified against the world outside.[20]

In their study on familial coping with mental illness, Lin Tsungyi and Lin Meichen found that the coping strategy used by immigrant Chinese families was almost exclusively intra-familial, they had minimal inclusion of some trusted outsiders in North America.[21] In the 1900s, in her study of mainland Chinese families with mentally ill members, Veronica Pearson noted that over 90% of people with schizophrenia in China lived with their families. Treatment decisions were primarily family decisions, and physicians showed no interest in examining personal problems with family dynamics as possible factors in developing schizophrenia. She contended that the reason might be more to do with inadequacy of available services and a lack of psychosocial perspective in understanding psychiatric problems.[22]

Family members to take charge of treatment decisions has been a traditional practice in China, as shown in the statements made in the Song Era (960–1279),

> Only those who understand the art of medicine can be called children who fulfill their duties toward their parents. Whoever leaves the cure of diseases to common physicians neither possesses compassion, nor does he fulfill his duties toward his parents. The knowledge of medicine is indispensable in the assistance of one's relatives.[23]

Paul Unschuld noted that the professionalization of medicine was not accepted by some Chinese practitioners because of their strongly held view that all people should have some knowledge of medicine to carry out their filial duty.[24] Ilza Veith described the practice of medical consultation that had persisted throughout the Chinese medical history. When a family member was sick, several physicians would be invited to diagnose the illness and propose a treatment regime. The family then selected the physician who had given the most agreeable answer to provide treatment for the patient.[25] In other words, family members were required to assume the major responsibility in helping their sick relatives to recover, including choosing the best possible treatment. The failure of treatment signified the failure of a person to fulfill his or her role responsibility in providing good care to the sick family member.

How a sick person is cared for is considered quite crucial in a traditional Chinese society. The oft-cited "Ten maxims for patients," written by Kung Tinghsien in 1615, spells out the importance both choosing the right physician and starting treatment at the early stage of illness, and the ways in which patients should care for themselves in different aspects of life in order to help restore their health. For instance, Kung advised his patients that "they should not have sexual intercourse," "they should guard against any excitement and should be quite careful in this respect," "they should beware of wrong thoughts and take care of themselves in peace." Regarding their daily activities, "they should eat and drink moderately," and "they should be concerned about their getting up and getting rest."[26] Undoubtedly, Kung's advice is a reflection of a common belief among the Chinese, characterized in an old Chinese saying that "30% of healing depends on curative means and 70% on nursing care."[27] Both medical remedies and ways to take care of the sick are considered as complementary in helping a person recover from illness, but how a person is cared for is more significant.

In sum, family is the first source of help, and only if the family cannot cope will people turn to others. Thus, the notion of being cared for by strangers does not sit quite easily in a traditional Chinese society. Since the expectation of assuming care responsibilities among in-group members is deep-rooted among the Chinese, seeking outside help can result in a sense of moral failure on the part of family members. Yet the nature of nurses' work is caring for sick strangers. It does not take place in the private sphere of life, but in the public sphere of hospitals. This inevitably poses a difficult issue in the development of nursing in China.

In 1914, the China Medical Commission of the Rockefeller Foundation undertook an investigation into the hospital facilities in China. The commissioners made two interesting comments that revealed their insensitivity to the logic of care among the Chinese. First, they remarked

> privacy is a thing that the Chinese value highly and they will often pay well for it, so that these [private] rooms form a considerable source of income for the hospital.[28]

Privacy in this context does not refer to paying respect to individuals' autonomy and holding in confidence their personal information, which are codes of practice upheld in the Western nursing ethics tradition.[29] The kind of privacy that the Chinese are willing to pay well for is the privilege of letting the family members stay with the patient in the same room, so that the patient's family members can continue the caring duties within their private sphere of life. The intervention by healthcare workers can also be kept to a minimum. Although the Commissioners could appreciate this Chinese sense of privacy, they did not prize it as crucial in their recommendation to improve hospital care services, as shown in the following comment.

> It is almost possible to tell whether the hospital has a foreign nurse or not by glancing into the wards. In some hospitals the wards are clean and orderly and compare very favorably with hospitals in the West. In others, where there is no foreign nurse and an inadequate native nursing staff or where the friends of the patients are allowed to camp in the wards, the general appearance is far from satisfactory.[30]

The commissioners were impressed by the effort made by the foreign nurses to implement the Nightingalian model of nursing. They noted the difficulties as expressed by most hospitals in enforcing visiting restrictions that were posted in order to maintain order and cleanliness in the wards. The Commissioners argued that only if more Chinese nurses were prepared like foreign nurses, could cleanliness and order possibly be maintained in hospitals. They believed that with an adequate number of nurses, patients' relatives and friends would not be necessary to participate in taking care of patients at the bedside.[31] Based on this assumption, the Commissioners recommended training more Chinese women by using the model of nursing practiced in the United States. The recommendations included setting up nursing schools comparable to the best Western standard, provision of scholarships for Chinese women to receive nurse training in the United States, and provision of funds for translation into Chinese of textbooks on nursing.[32]

The Commissioners, while intending to foster an optimal environment conducive to healing by replacing patients' relatives with more highly trained nurses, had overlooked the logic of care in a traditional Chinese society. A better alternative should be to allow relatives participate in taking care of the sick by having well-trained nurses teaching them such knowledge and skills. The reason to exclude relatives in hospital care might be due to the early attempts within the healthcare community in rationalizing a legitimate claim to monopolize the nurses' role in caring for the sick.

### B. Nursing as a Profession for Women

Another issue the early nurses in China met with was the introduction of nursing as a career primarily for women. As far as caring work was concerned, a wife to look after her husband, or a sister to look after her younger brother is regarded as legitimate. Hiring a maidservant to take care of the sick was also practiced. Yet only the most trustworthy servant would be assigned the duty. While the care responsibilities to be assumed were to be in proportion to the degree of closeness to the master's family, these maidservants took the most unpleasant and dirty work in view of their lower status in the family hierarchy.[33] Beyond this private realm, the notion of a woman looking after a stranger was an alien concept in ancient China.

In the thirteenth century a Yuan text recorded nine kinds of women who took part in healing work, known as the three nuns and six old women (三姑六婆, *san gu liu po*). The three kinds of nuns are: Buddhist nun (尼姑, *nigu*), Taoist nun (道姑, *daogu*), female diviner (卦姑, *guogu*). The six kinds of old women are: procuress (牙婆, *yapo*), marriage go-between (媒婆, *mapo*), woman priest (虔婆, *qianpo*), woman dispenser (藥婆, *yaopo*), woman teacher (師婆, *shipo*), and midwife (穩婆, *wenpo*).[34] Among them, the woman dispenser, woman priest, and midwife were definite healers, while the rest might take up some medical care as part of their work. In comparison with traditional medical practitioners, especially Confucian medical theoreticians, woman healers were given little credit for their work by society.[35] While the medical practitioners were respected for practicing medicine as an act of benevolence, the women healers were often portrayed as women who strolled around spreading gossip from door to door, or were accused of committing crimes, such as stealing, abortion, poisoning, or infanticide. In the classic stories describing the positive and negative examples of medical practitioners, one woman healer was recorded in *The Medical Talks* written by Kao Chang in 1189, but exemplified in a negative way. She earned her living by selling abortion herbs.[36]

Good women had to be confined to their homes, according to the Confucian teachings. A woman who worked outside the household breached the social norms, and could not be considered as a model woman. Since the Zhou Dynasty, the second century before the Common Era, a good woman was required to live according to the mandate of three obedience and four virtues (三從四德, *san cong si de*). Women were to obey their father when they were still single, their husbands when married, and their sons when widowed. The four virtues were appropriate behavior, speech, appearance, and accomplishment. The mandate was first written in *Zhou Li* 《周禮》, and further formalized in the book *Women's Commandments* 《女訓》 written in the first century. It reads,

> A virtuous woman needs not possess expert knowledge, her words should not be argumentative, her appearance should be plain but not colorful, and she has to be submissive in her work, instead of seeking for accomplishment that exceeds the others.[37]

Education for women in ancient China was largely confined to the teaching of household management and maintaining family relations. Some exceptions that daughters in better homes did learn and write and often became the first instructors of boys in the home.[38] To possess no knowledge was considered as a virtue for women. A popular belief held that a knowledgeable woman was less virtuous in conduct. They would suffer a bad fate.[39] Prejudice of this kind was pervasive in preventing women of good background from acquiring education and developing careers of their own.

The development of careers for women is a recent phenomenon in China, which came along with the gradual softening in attitudes toward women in the nineteenth century. In 1844, missionaries established the first girls' school in China. The anti foot-binding movement was launched in 1875, which was signified by the establishment of the Natural Feet Society in Shanghai. Women's education expanded rapidly since the turn of the twentieth century, and some women went abroad to study.[40] Among these women, Qiu Jin was most remembered by nurses in China. She spoke highly of nursing as a profession for women, and promoted nursing by translating nursing texts from Japanese into Chinese in the *China's Woman Bulletin*, a publication founded by Qiu to spread the ideas of woman liberation.[41]

The Communists were another force freeing women to enter into careers. The declaration of the Communist Party at the national meeting in July 1922 stated that men and women should enjoy equal rights. Mao Zedong took the liberation of women as one of his missions in the Communist revolution. In his "Report on an Investigation into the Peasant Movement of Hunan, 1927," Mao explicitly denounced the system of male superiority in China. In his words,

> A man in China is usually subjected to three systems of authority (political authority, clan authority, and religious authority). As for women, in addition to being dominated by these three authorities, they are also dominated by the men [the authority of the husband]. These four authorities—political, clan, religious, and masculine—are the embodiment of the whole feudal-patriarchal system and ideology, and

> are the four thick ropes binding the Chinese people, especially the peasants.[42]

These four thick ropes are also referred as four mountains. While men carried three mountains of feudalism, capitalism, and imperialism on their back, women also had a fourth—male supremacy. Mao stressed the importance of organizing women and saw their participation in anti-feudal struggles as part of the process of rural transformation. He proclaimed that women were a vast reserve of labor power and called on them to lift their heads and overturn these feudal barriers by committing themselves to building a socialist China.[43]

Even though some social prejudices hindering women's education and careers had been lifted, Educated women were still not willing to enter nursing. Liu Chungtung says

> not only because [caring for the sick] was traditionally a lower status woman's work, but also because it was always difficult for the Chinese to accord professional status to individuals who either performed menial duties, or touched the human body, as nurses inevitably did.[44]

If nursing work were seen as the performance in a public sphere of work normally done in the private sphere, a nurse would be seen only as maidservant who helped out with the dirty work in hospital care. The only difference from any other maidservant was that she was hired by the hospital and not by an individual master. At best, because she was not a member of the patient's in-group, she could be seen as a woman healer. Nonetheless, both maidservant and woman healer did not enjoy a high social status in Chinese culture.

Nurses inevitably had to confront Confucian social practices requiring gender segregation. A man and a woman who had no familial relation were required to keep a distance from each other. We can see this social sanction in the following much quoted dialogue between Mencius and Kun Chunyu.

| | |
|---|---|
| Kun Chunyu: | Is it prescribed by the rites that, in giving and receiving, man and woman should not touch each other? |
| Mencius: | It is. |
| Kun Chunyu: | When one's sister-in-law is drowning, does one stretch out a hand to help her? |
| Mencius: | Not to help a sister-in-law who is drowning is to be a brute. It is prescribed by the rites that, in giving and receiving, man and woman should not touch each other, but in stretching out a helping |

> hand to the drowning sister-in-law one uses one's discretion.[45]

Except in situations of emergency, any physical involvement of a woman with male strangers was forbidden.

Sexual segregation was observed in the practice of medicine. Once a practice existed in medical consultation that a male physician was required to tie a string on the wrist of a female patient to perform pulse diagnosis so as to avoid any direct contact. As far as cultivation of physicians' morality was concerned, the Chinese customarily paid great attention to sexual morality.[46] Woman healers were called to treat female patients. This made it unacceptable for a woman to take care of a male stranger. The missionary story written by Barbara Spencer was one example. The nurses working in the desert hospital were all boys whose ages ranged from nine to eighteen. They came from the poorest of peasant families, and most of them were illiterate. Patients' families assumed most of the caring work in the hospital.[47] Female patients were cared for by the family or by an untrained amah. Hospitals exclusively for male patients also existed.[48] When the old values requiring segregation of the sexes faded out, we might have expected to see some participation of men in nursing. This has not been the case. Hardly any male nurses exist in China today, so the strong affiliation between women and nursing prevails. Maybe this can be attributed to the success of the pioneers of nursing in China in promoting nursing as a profession primarily for women.[49]

## 2. The Promotion of Nursing as a Profession

With the conventional practices and ways of thinking that undermined the value of nursing work, to attract educated women to nursing was difficult. In this respect Simpson's suggestion was valid; the servant image of a nurse needed to be changed before nursing could take root in China. During the Republican period, 1912–1949, we can find that three approaches were used to raise the social standing of nursing. They were the coining of a Chinese name for nursing, promoting a professional sense of nursing, and fostering a moral sense of nursing.

### A. A Chinese Name for Nurses

Since nursing was a new profession in China imported from the West, a Chinese word was needed that could spell out what nursing was, while at the same time conveying a positive image of the nurse. The first attempt was the verb *kanhu* (看護): this derived from *kan*, to look after or guard, keep watch on, and *hu*, to take care of, to protect, or give shelter to. Thus, where in England, nursing adopted a name by analogy from the nourishment and care of children, in China it initially adopted a name meaning "to keep watch and protect." In 1914, the formal name *hushi* (護士) was adopted. The term was purposely selected after a review of the classic *Kangxi Dictionary* 《康熙字典》. The term *hu* means "to protect, maintain life, nurture, and cultivate." *Shi* is commonly used as a suffix for different professions, including intellectual ones in particular, and implies good social status. A Chinese saying reads that "those who learn to the level of excellence can be called *shi*." Thus, *hushi* became the Chinese word for nurse. Arguably, the term denotes more precisely than earlier terms the idea of nursing as a profession in a modern sense, an idea that has been promulgated since nursing entered into the Nightingale era.[50] Contrary to traditional woman healers, *hushi* acquired the healing art through formal education. The goal was to protect the vulnerable and heal the sick. *Hushi* were not "old wives." They were young ladies who were knowledgeable and compassionate in taking care of the sick. They were analogous to wingless angels instead of being one of the "three nuns and six old wives."

B. Promoting a Professional Sense of Nursing

An honorific title for nurses was not adequate in raising the social standing of nursing. The second approach was to improve the standard of nurse training and to promote a sense of professional identity among nurses. In order to increase the attractiveness of nursing, and to alter its image of servitude, the missionaries provided Chinese nurses with different educational opportunities. Most nursing programs were hospital-based, with some attached to medical colleges. As more formal programs were offered to train nurses, continuous progress was made to replace male nurses in the wards by female personnel. Wong Chimin and Wu Lienteh reported that only seven out of 189 hospitals employed female nurses to work in male wards in 1920, but this increased to 60% in 1936. Some nurses were sent abroad to further study nursing. Chinese nursing also moved quickly into the tertiary level, six years later than the United States and thirty years ahead of the United Kingdom.[51] The first undergraduate program started in Peking Union Medical College (PUMC) in 1922. PUMC was founded by the Rockefeller Foundation in 1915, with the aim of

> [creating] as good a medical college as can be found anywhere in Europe or in America with excellent staff, well-equipped laboratories, a good teaching hospital, and a nursing school.[52]

The mission of the medical college was not to address the health needs of the public at large directly, but instead of preparing professionals with a high practicable standard. Likewise, the nursing school was to meet the same standard of excellence as that of the medical school, and the emphasis was to be on education service instead.[53] The nursing program offered by the college was reported to be successful in preparing many future nurse leaders. Some of them still play a significant role in leading nursing reforms in China today.

In line with the improvement in the standard of nurses' training, effort was made to organize Chinese nurses into a recognizable professional body. The Chinese Nursing Association was formed by a group of foreign nurses in 1909. Its main functions were to plan and standardize the nursing curriculum, scrutinize certificate examinations, and issue registration certification. The first national registration examination was held in 1915. Chinese nurses began to join the association in 1914. In 1922, the association became a member of the International Council of Nurses. Such professional activities flourished in the 1920s. *Nurse Quarterly*, the first Chinese nursing journal, was first published in 1920. The first edition consisted of six articles. Foreign nurses and physicians authored four articles. Two Chinese nurses authored the other two articles. One of them was a male nurse. Numerous English nursing textbooks were translated into Chinese. In 1933, China ranked fifth in the number of publications among the member countries of the International Council of Nurses.[54]

Contrary to the experience of nurses in the United States, the foreign nurses in China did not meet with the same opposition from physicians in initiating activities to strengthen nurses' professional identity. Charles Rosenberg contends that many physicians saw in the registration of nurses a threat to their authority.[55] Elsewhere in the world this was true, apparently China's physicians were not aware of this threat, and they did not see it as a threat. Since the notion of professionalism was in its infancy in China, and the Chinese Medical Association was not formed until the second decade of the twentieth century, I would say that physicians in China did not take note of the threat. By 1930 all officers of the Association were Chinese, with the foreign nurses taking a less active role. Liu noted that this change was attributed to the anti-imperialist and anti-Christian movements in the 1920s, which created pressure for the removal of foreign influences from the association. It could also be argued that by this time nurses in China had gained their own sense of professionalism. A woman surnamed Shi, who was a physician, was appointed as the first Chinese president of the Nursing Association.[56] This suggested that physicians did not find nursing a threat because nurses were willing to remain subordinate to them. Also, nurses preferred this affiliation because physicians enjoyed a relatively high social status.

The development of nursing in China closely resembled the development of nursing in the United States. America's first three schools of nursing were founded in 1873.[57] A decade earlier than the ones founded in Shanghai and Fuzhou. The first undergraduate program started in the States six years earlier than the first such program in China. The first nursing registration law was passed in North Carolina in 1903, twelve years earlier than in China. Nurses Associations were formed in the States and in China in the early twentieth century. We can summarize that the pioneering nurses in China were successful in extending modern nursing into a territory where nursing was once an alien notion.

If we compare the ways in which modern nursing took its form in these two countries, one obvious difference can be seen. Chinese nurses played a passive role in the development of their new profession, allowing foreign nurses to lead the way. On the other hand, nurses in the States had taken an active role in defining their professional identity since the inception of modern nursing. Take the example of the activities that had been undertaken to formulate a code of ethics for nurses in the States, which took fifty-three years for its final adoption in 1950. Marsha Fowler suggests that the delay was intentional for the leaders of the nursing community of the time saw the importance of including the voices of the majority of nurses in its formulation. She quotes Isabel Robb's statement at the First Annual Convention of the Associated Alumnae of Trained Nurses of the United States and Canada held in 1898 to support her view. It reads,

> A code of ethics is the first object mentioned in the constitution. But it cannot be among the first to be realized, for such a code should be the central point of thought of the Association, reaching out in its influence and inspiration to our remote branches and toward which each individual member may look vibrant with a sense of personal responsibility toward the Association and toward the highest standard attainable by nurses. It should stand for deeds and actions, not words and form. Were we, therefore, to appoint a committee to forthwith formulate a code of ethics, we should get the words, but not the spirit. Surely, it will be better to wait until we have sufficient and better form in the matter of numbers and closer organization, to learn the mind of the greater number on what shall constitute our national code of ethics. But I would like to say, in passing, that it should be founded, not on the lines of any existing association or society, but should be formulated to meet our special needs in our own particular way.[58]

The Advisory Committee on Ethical Standards was eventually formed in 1921, and the first suggested code was presented in 1926 in the United States. Activities in reviewing and reformulating the Code for nurses continue to this day.[59] No such activities among Chinese nurses regarding the formation of Chinese Nursing Association and the introduction of registration examinations to regulate nursing practice existed. If we agree that the attributes of a profession include a sense of autonomy and professional freedom to regulate its practice, I have strong reservations about concluding that Chinese nurses had acquired even the least sense of professional identity.

### C. Fostering a Moral Sense of Nursing

The third approach used to attract more women to nursing was to lift nursing work onto a plane of moral obligation. What was considered "servant's work" was ennobled by a sense of devotion to a great cause, as Nightingale did in pioneering her new model of nursing in England. At least two measures were used in the Republican period in this regard. First, Florence Nightingale was introduced as the model nurse for Chinese young women to emulate. Second, nursing was presented as a moral discipline that was qualitatively distinctive from servant's work.

Yao Changxu, author of a nursing textbook for secondary school girls, described nursing as a lofty profession comparable to the profession of teaching, and said nursing was regarded as the most valuable kind of charity work in the West. She pointed out that many Western women from noble families became nurses, especially in wartime.[60] In a similar vein to Nightingale in *Notes on Nursing*, Yao stated that every woman should learn nursing because women are more tender and refined than men in mastering the art of taking care of sick family members. She suggested that a woman needed to acquire knowledge and competence in performing nursing tasks, and required to have a sense of morality in relating to those under her care. Wang Xiuying, author of *History of Nursing in China* described the ways in which Florence Nightingale had inspired her to stay in nursing since 1926. Her impression of Florence Nightingale was similar to Yao's view, but her call for service emphasized community instead of family needs. The following is a quotation from Wang's life story.

> In her studies she came across the story of Florence Nightingale, and was deeply impressed by the way she had rescued and cared for wounded soldiers during the Crimean War, and thus helped reduce the death rate from 50 to 2.2%. Florence was awarded a special-class medal. What was more, she wrote articles on fundamental principles [of] nursing and set up the first modern nursing school. Wang Xiuying was inspired by Florence's example and wanted to do her best to help her fellow countrymen.[61]

Wang was a model nurse of her time. She was ready to take care of critically ill patients and patients with infectious diseases. When people wondered how she could bring herself to do this, Wang replied that she just treated her patients as her family members.[62] We can note that Wang only admired the gentle and compassionate side of Florence Nightingale. The tough side of Nightingale in dealing with officials and governments in reforming hospital care was not presented. Liu remarked in her study of the early development of nursing in China that the adoption of nursing as a profession by Chinese women of whatever social class was no more than a transfer of commitment from one compelling task to another.[63] Apparently a gentle and compassionate Nightingale was more compatible with the societal expectations of women as care providers, and more likely to attract Chinese women to nursing if a qualitative distinction could be drawn between nursing work and servant's work.

In her attempt to lift nursing work to a plane of moral obligation, Yao listed the requirements of the nurse at the beginning of her book, which reads,

> A nurse should be aware of her heavy responsibility, and should always keep reminding herself of it.
> A nurse should be pure and preoccupied with a sense of morality.
> A nurse should base her practice on kindness and sincerity. She should use her knowledge to deliberate patient care. She should be determined, meticulous, and prudent, but not be rash.
> A nurse should observe her health practices, and maintain her health.
> A nurse should possess patience and courage.
> A nurse should gain a patient's trust by treating him or her with both kindness and strictness. [Kindness in relating to patients, but strictness in carrying out nursing measures.]
> A nurse should act decently, and speak no bad words.
> A nurse should keep her clothing clean and tidy.
> A nurse should obey physician's treatment orders, and carry them out faithfully.[64]

Above all, a nurse should provide a psychologically protective environment for patients, which included attending to the patient's individual needs and taking care in the use of words that might upset patient's psychological well-being. This list of requirements on the moral character of healthcare providers should not appear unfamiliar to Chinese people. A similar mandate for medical practitioners was recorded in the writings on traditional medical ethics.[65] In comparison with the "Ten maxims for physicians and ten maxims for patients," Yao's list resembles the maxims for patients more than the maxims for physicians.[66] Yao's list puts less emphasis on the requirements of excellence in practice, and more on the ways in which a nurse ought to relate to patients so as to foster healing. Seven out of the ten maxims for physicians concern practice competence, only three concerns how a physician ought to relate to patients.

In some respects this list is especially Chinese, but similarities exist between Yao's list and the list of nursing virtues Sara Parsons required student nurses to cultivate.[67] Both of them required the nurse to be subordinate to physicians and medical sciences, in the sense that the nurse could help apply but not master the knowledge of medicine. Both also emphasized the nurse's moral qualities and her ability to deal with emotions and the environment in safeguarding patient's health. Yao did not appeal to the notion of service to humanity, which was much cherished during the Nightingale movement of nursing reforms in the West. She appealed to the traditional role of a woman as care provider in a family, which I found a culturally congruent approach in helping the Chinese comprehend the qualitative distinction of nursing work. Since possessing medical knowledge in taking care of one's sick parent is regarded as a moral obligation in ancient China, this characterization of the nurse as a knowledgeable care provider for family members could attract women of high moral ideals to choose nursing as their career. The story of Chi An is a typical example.[68]

Literature on the history of nursing mainly focuses on issues related to recruitment, education, and development of professional bodies and nurses' professional identity. How nursing was carried out in clinical wards could be glimpsed through the stories told by nurses and missionaries.[69] These observations strongly suggest that nursing practice in China has followed a restricted concept of nursing. Instead of focusing on the ways of providing direct care contributory to patients' recovery, nursing is seen as primarily comprising a bundle of tasks in helping physicians implement their treatment regimens. Patients' daily care to a large extent remained in the hands of their family members, as if they were at home. We may get an impression that the path of nursing development has followed closely the Western model of nursing, but in what respect nursing has added a new dimension to taking care of the sick in practice situations has yet to be seen. Given the logic of care among the Chinese that emphasizes the responsibilities of a person in terms of his or her relationship with others, it would be interesting to know how Chinese nurses perceive their relationships with patients. How do they cross from a public sphere into the private sphere of the patient's life? But this issue was left unattended when China came under the rule of Mao in 1949, which saw nursing shift to a different course of development.

## 3. Nursing in the Maoist Era (1949–1978)

China entered a new epoch when the People's Republic was founded in 1949. Mao mandated the doctrine of revolutionary humanism in his radical reform of every aspect of Chinese society, which aimed at creating a more equal society, reducing the inequalities of China's feudalistic past—especially the differences in urban and rural areas and between the rich and poor.[70] As for healthcare services, Mao required healthcare workers to

> rescue the dying, heal the wounded, prevent illness, cure disease, practice revolutionary humanism, and maintain the health of the people wholeheartedly.

This statement is a popular slogan and appears in all Chinese textbooks on medical and nursing ethics. This mandate in many ways reflected the changing orientation in provision of medical services since 1949. Likewise, nursing underwent two major changes. First, foreign influences were stripped away and nursing in China began to chart its own course of development. Second, low emphasis was placed on nurse training during the time when China implemented a comprehensive system of medical care. In this section, I will discuss the ways in which the doctrine of revolutionary humanism and this changing orientation in healthcare provision directed nursing development.

### A. The Political Context

With the goal of constructing a truly socialist society, Mao denounced traditional practices as feudalistic, and practices imported from the West as capitalistic. He held that both practices were counter-revolutionary forces that could hinder the realization of the desired communist society. Mao strongly believed that the correct ideas necessary to overcome these obstacles came through social practices, and only through engaging people in the right kind of practice could the desired good be accomplished. In comparison with the five Confucian cardinal relationships within which a person must fulfill his or her role requirements, the doctrine of revolutionary humanism was a new way of thinking for the people of China. It made socialist responsibility the overarching principle of ethical behavior, with emphasis on contradiction and struggle, and accommodation and harmony instead. Mao reckoned this new order demanded a transformation of people's minds so they would not focus on self-, family-, or other in-group interests, but instead think in terms of the public good in making day-to-day decisions. In order to foster this sense of socialist responsibility, Mao mandated his people to uphold two main values. They were serving the people wholeheartedly and class struggle.

#### i. Serving the People

Mao's notion of serving the people is best represented by the two popular national models that the Party leadership required all Chinese to learn from. They are Norman Bethune and Lei Feng. Dr. Bethune was a Canadian surgeon who was committed to communism and had served with Mao's Eighth Route Army during the war of resistance against Japan in 1938. He died as a result of septicemia after cutting himself with a scalpel during an operation on a soldier in 1939. In Mao's essay *In Memory of Dr. Norman Bethune*, he praised Bethune in two respects. First, Mao exhorted every communist to learn from Bethune's strong sense of responsibility. In Mao's words,

> Comrade Bethune's spirit, his utter devotion to others without any thought of self, was shown in his boundless sense of responsibility in his work and his boundless warm-heartedness toward all comrades and the people.[71]

In order to demonstrate this sense of responsibility, Mao called his people to put the interests of others before their own, and be careful not to engage in irresponsible behavior. The second respect was Bethune's excellence in technical skills, especially his positive attitude toward technical work.[72]

While Bethune was the popular model in the 1950s, the movement to "learn from Lei Feng" began in 1963.[73] Lei and his family suffered many hardships in the days before the Communist Party took power. His family was overworked and maltreated by their landlord. Finally his father died and his mother, molested by the landlord and despairing of keeping the family together, committed suicide. Lei, still a young boy, was then brought up by the Party and the People's Liberation Army, who became like a family to him. Eventually he joined the Army and did many good deeds for his comrades and the people. He died at the age of twenty-two in a truck accident. He was especially praised for his virtue in his willingness to serve others even at the risk of his life, and the frugality he practiced with the aim of saving the country's resources.

Just how historically accurate the Party's representation of Bethune and Lei are is doubtful, doubt also exists as to whether Lei existed at all. Little doubt exists the Party's motives in telling these fables was to inculcate a sense of socialist responsibility in the people.[74] These virtues include "utter devotion to others without thinking of yourself," "boundless warm-heartedness in serving others," "willingness to endure hardship" and "loyalty to the Party's leadership." Gary Reed examined these socialist virtues. He contended that they bore similarity to Confucian teaching—that Lei Feng was a proletarianized version of earlier Confucian models of virtuous behavior.[75] I will leave this contention open, and will discuss how Mao's ethical mandate was rooted in traditional Chinese ethics in Chapter Four.

### ii. Class Struggle

Another task for Mao was to mobilize the people to engage in the so-called three struggles: (1) class struggle, (2) the struggle for production, and (3) scientific experiment.[76] Mao believed that the new society could only be realized by addressing the internal contradictions in society, such as the contradiction between the productive forces and the relations of production, the contradiction between classes, and the contradiction between the old and the new. He foresaw that only through struggles with these contradictions could the desired good of socialism be realized.

Of the three struggles, Mao placed much emphasis on mobilizing class struggle among the people.[77] Many policies instituted during the Maoist era reflected this emphasis on class struggle. For instance, in 1958, Mao moved against bourgeois influences in education in the Anti-rightist Campaign, advocating a new kind of school that was based on the premise of half-work and half-study. He further raised the issue of "red versus expert," placing priority on class consciousness and proletarian politics over knowledge and technical competence. Through the 1960s, emphasis on class struggle grew in intensity, reaching a peak during the Cultural Revolution.[78] Despite the tragic evidence about how this Maoist class struggle destroyed lives and hindered social progress, the advocacy of a sense of socialist responsibility was appropriate to the national condition when the Communists gained power in China.

### B. The Changing Orientation in Healthcare Provision

Promoting a sense of socialist responsibility was especially relevant in addressing the health issues of the time. Health conditions in China were notoriously poor when the Communists took power in 1949. Ravaged by political turmoil, continuous warfare, and natural disasters for almost half a century, the majority of people suffered from poor health and gross inadequacy of the availability of health care. In 1949, the infant mortality rate was about 200 per 1000 live births, and the average life expectancy was thirty-nine. Infectious disease and conditions complicated by malnutrition, such as tuberculosis, malaria, schistosomiasis (bilharzia), hookworm, and fungus diseases, were nationwide problems. Preventive medicine was almost non-existent in most parts of China, and Western-type hospital services were almost totally unavailable in the countryside. The community relied mostly on traditional healers although no medical institution was available to formalize their practice. The need to mobilize healthcare workers in constructing a socialist China through healthcare reform was obvious.[79]

In response to Mao's mandate to put the three struggles into practice, high on the agenda in healthcare reforms were extending healthcare services to address nationwide healthcare issues and fostering equity in healthcare access. In 1950, the First National Conference on Health Care was held in Beijing. All types of healthcare workers, including physicians and nurses, were represented. Under the Party's directive, they formulated four objectives in healthcare reform. First, medicine should serve the needs of the workers, peasants, and soldiers. Second, preventive medicine had to take precedence over therapeutic medicine. Third, both Chinese- and Western-types of medicine were to be practiced. Last, but not least, healthcare work had to be along the mass line. These objectives aimed to manifest the ideal of serving the people by addressing the healthcare needs of the people at large.[80]

Although much achievement was reported in mobilizing the masses in eradicating epidemic diseases through regular patriotic health campaigns and the implementation of public health measures over the 1950s, curative medical care facilities were still concentrated in cities. Even within the urban populations, David Lampton reports that access to medical care was limited to government and Communist Party personnel and workers in state-owned factories, the payment for which came entirely from the state health budget.[81] This means that a majority of people did not have access to medical facilities or could not afford to pay for such services even if they were available.

In Mao's often-quoted 26 June 1965 Directive, he criticized the Ministry of Public Health for neglecting the needs of the rural population. It reads,

> Tell the Ministry of Public Health that it only works for 15% of the population of the country and that this 15% is mainly composed of gentlemen, while the broad masses of the peasants do not get any medical treatment. First they do not have any doctors; second they do not have any medicine. The Ministry of Public Health is not a Ministry of Public Health for the people, so why not change its name to the Ministry of Urban Health, the Ministry of Gentlemen's Health, or even the Ministry of Urban Gentlemen's Health?[82]

Mao's comment was quite right to point out that whatever the budget, access to these resources should not be confined to a privileged few. But the comment reveals a more deep-seated issue over the uneasy relation between professionals and the Party leadership, and the struggle between autonomy in professional practice and political control at the dawn of the Cultural Revolution.[83] Nonetheless, Mao's directive to further extend medical care facilities to rural areas was implemented in the 1960s and 1970s. In the early years of the Cultural Revolution, provision of medical service in the countryside was limited to rotating healthcare workers in mobile medical teams from urban to rural areas. Late in 1968, the use of rudimentarily trained "barefoot doctors" as primary-care physicians in rural areas began. They worked as part of a co-operative medical system set up at the production brigade level to serve its members.[84] This was the first time in Chinese history that affordable health care became available to the rural majority.

Lampton contends that both gains and costs in the health reforms undertaken during the Maoist era existed.[85] I would see them as a mixed blessing for the rural population, but a misfortune for healthcare professionals. The gains included the formation of a comprehensive system of medical care that could reach every segment of the populace, provision of affordable medical service to rural areas through the implementation of a co-operative medical system, and above all, improvement in health profiles.

### i. A Comprehensive System of Medical Care

In the 1950s, a three-tier referral system of medical care began to take shape, with the lower levels of medical care responsible for identifying difficult and complex cases for referral up the system to better equipped hospitals and more knowledgeable physicians. Each urban area was divided into a number of districts, each responsible for providing medical care to its residents and for promoting disease control programs within its jurisdiction. Different types of health organizations, such as comprehensive hospitals, health institutes, factory health protection stations, street Red Cross stations, and group-health stations shared these tasks. In the countryside, hospitals and/or clinics were established in counties, communes, and production brigades. While county and commune hospitals were equipped with relatively modern facilities and managed by more experienced personnel, clinics and health stations were managed by healthcare workers of varied levels of training and skill.[86] This system of rationed access, as pointed out by Judith Banister, could be an inexpensive way to provide basic health care for both simple and complex medical problems.[87] In practice it did not work well. Qiu Renzong reported that high-ranking officials with medical coverage were often given special treatment, and common people had to go "through the back door" or use bribes to be treated at better-equipped healthcare facilities.[88] Lampton argues that this situation prevailed because people did not have confidence in the quality of service provided by semi-trained healthcare workers with poorly equipped facilities at the primary healthcare level. Conceivably people would seek medical care at a higher level if they could afford the cost.[89]

### ii. Medical Coverage

Provision of medical coverage was first implemented in China in the 1950s. The publicly funded medical system provided coverage for civil servants and workers in public agencies, students of universities, and disabled military officers above some rank. The funding came from general revenues. The second tier of healthcare coverage was in the form of labor insurance medical care, under which employees in state and collective enterprises and their immediate family members were entitled to full or partial benefits.

Payment was made mainly out of welfare funds of the enterprises, a portion of which was designated for medical services. The third tier of the co-operative medical scheme was practiced in rural areas. The system resembled a rudimentary medical insurance scheme in which a collective economy assisted in the provision of health facilities for the peasants. The funding came from general health and welfare fund premiums paid by the brigades and the production teams. The peasants joined the scheme on a voluntary basis by paying a nominal fee.[90] The coverage included provision of basic health clinics at the village level, immunization of children, monitoring public hygiene, and assistance in water supply. Payment of hospital fees could be included, but full coverage was not guaranteed, depending on the financial status of the scheme. This system expanded rapidly during the sixties in response to Mao's 1965 directive to meet the rural demand for medical services. The scheme was reported to be highly successful in providing medical coverage for 90% of the rural population in 1979. We can also see its decline in the same year as the quasi free-market contract responsibility system was introduced in the rural areas in 1978. This issue will be further explored in Chapter Four.

### iii. Health Profile

The third gain was improvement in health profiles. Many reports agreed that people's health had significantly improved. The World Health Organization (WHO) acknowledged China's achievement. The World Bank cited the healthcare reforms undertaken in China as a model for other developing nations.[91] The high infant mortality rate in 1949 of 200 per 1000 live births had been reduced to 34.7 per 1000 live births by 1980. The average life expectancy increased from 39 to 69 years. The prevalence of some infectious and endemic diseases had plummeted. The leading causes of death became chronic problems, such as cancer, stroke, and heart disease, similar to those in the developed countries. This changing health profile signified that China has gone through the health transition phase from being a developing country to being a developed country, with chronic non-communicable diseases the main causes of premature adult morbidity and mortality.[92] These changes inevitably cause more people to seek medical services because of aging and chronic diseases.

### iv. Deprofessionalization of Healthcare Workers

As far as healthcare workers were concerned, the Party leadership placed less emphasis on preparing experts to realize its socialist ideal. Reform in medical programs in the 1950s was modeled after the three-year program developed by the Chinese Red Army in 1931.[93] A core curriculum for all kinds of healthcare workers was nationalized and standardized by the

Ministry of Public Health. This program comprised general education, fundamentals, and specialty subjects. Different kinds of future healthcare workers, such as doctors and nurses, studied the same subjects in common before they studied their own specialty areas. To strip away outside influences, a new set of textbooks was written for the program by local experts.[94]

To further eliminate elitist tendencies and to promote a more egalitarian work relationship among different ranks of healthcare personnel, every person was addressed as "comrade" instead of honorific titles such as doctor or nurse. In the hospitals, physicians and nurses were mandated to share the menial work, such as cleaning and taking care of patents' daily needs. The people were made to believe that if everyone shared the menial work, then no one could look down on others. The previous hierarchical relationship that was the norm in the feudalistic era was believed to be able to be transformed to a more egalitarian relationship, and everyone would co-operate in accomplishing their common task to serve the people wholeheartedly.[95]

In 1960s, the anti-elitist movement further intensified. Nurse training was merged with doctor training, and medical training in general was halted for four years. Instead, more part-time health workers were trained to be primary healthcare givers: the barefoot doctors in the countryside, red medical workers in the urban neighborhoods, and worker doctors in the factories. Among them, barefoot doctors became increasingly active during the Cultural Revolution, contributing the bulk of basic medical care in the rural areas.[96] We may appreciate the ways in which the Party leadership managed to prepare an adequate number of medical personnel so that health care could be universally available on an equitable and inexpensive basis.

As Lampton points out, China had its price to pay. Many highly trained physicians left the People's Republic in the post-Cultural Revolution period. Those who stayed in China were assigned to serve in outpatient clinics or on mobile medical teams, where their advanced training was of minimal use.[97] Even worse, the mandate for class struggle profoundly jeopardized the fiduciary relationship between healthcare workers and patients.[98] Medical workers, who were supposed to cure the dying and heal the wounded, could not exercise their professional autonomy to serve the patient's best interests if the act came in conflict with the policy line. Professional oversight was supposed to be essential if medical facilities were to serve the most people in the most economical fashion. Healthcare workers could not exercise this kind of control, especially during the Cultural Revolution, for fear that others would attack them as counter-revolutionary and unwilling to serve the people.[99] I would say that healthcare workers were one of the most unfortunate groups during the Maoist era, in the sense that they gave up their professional autonomy to the manipulation in the political order.

C. Nursing from 1949 to 1978

It should not be surprising that professional activities among nurses gradually diminished after the 1950s. To strip away outside influences, the Chinese Nursing Association withdrew from the International Council of Nurses in 1949. In 1966, at the beginning of the Cultural Revolution, the association was dissolved. Journal publication and other professional activities were completely stopped in the same year. The earlier established unified national standard for registration certification of nurse training was abolished. Nursing education underwent changes as well. PUMC was closed in 1952, as was its undergraduate nursing program. Nurse training was reduced to a three-year program at the senior high school level. From 1966 to 1973, all nursing schools were closed down. Whatever textbooks were then available were burned or otherwise destroyed. Nursing schools were reopened in 1973, but the training reduced to abbreviated, two-year programs emphasizing the practical instead of theoretical.[100] Nurses' role responsibilities became diffused in the Maoist era. Some nurses were given the title of physician, and both physicians and nurses shared similar duties in hospital work. While some were sent to work in departments other than clinical wards in the hospitals, some were sent to the countryside and worked as primary healthcare workers.[101]

From the retrospective comments contained in the literature of the early 1980s, all nurses affirmed that the Cultural Revolution was a disaster for China in general.[102] A tragedy for nursing development in particular.[103] Foreign visitors found that nursing in China was frozen in the Republican period. When Kathleen Dirschel visited China in 1979, she noted that nurses functioned strictly as physicians' handmaidens in the hospitals. Physicians determined a patient's level of illness and then assigned a nurse for special care if deemed necessary.[104]

Myron Cohen and Gail Henderson reported similar observations during their stay in a hospital in China.[105] Chinese nurses made similar comments. Song Zhenying described what nurses did in the early 1980s.[106] She expressed her concern that nursing should not be reduced to a bundle of technical procedures with emphasis on merely getting the work done. She contended that other more important nursing work, such as monitoring the patients' condition, nutritional management, health education, and psychological care, were largely neglected. Wu Xingzheng further commented that patients received fragmented care in this task-orientation to work. Different nurses assigned to perform different procedures for one patient, but no one nurse was responsible for the patient. Interaction between nurse and patient was merely functional.[107]

In comparison with other parts of the world, where nursing as a profession had taken great strides, nursing in China during Mao's time was left far behind. The task-oriented nature of patient care that was used in

China was criticized in other parts of the world; primary nursing, an individualized, patient-centered approach to nursing work, was advocated instead.[108] Nurses had become dissatisfied with working under physicians' domination. To carry Nightingale's convictions forward, numerous nursing theorists worked on redefining the nature of nursing.[109] To this end, the definition of nursing formulated by Virginia Henderson was adopted by the International Council of Nurses in 1960. It reads,

> The unique function of the nurse is to assist the individual, sick or well, in the performance of those activities contributing to health or recovery (or to peaceful death) that the person would perform unaided given the necessary strength, will, or knowledge. And to do this in such a way as to help the individual gain independence as rapidly as possible.[110]

The primary focus was taking care of a patient as an individual, and helping him or her to regain independence. Many nursing theories emerged, providing a base of knowledge for independent nursing practice.[111] While nursing was experiencing a renaissance in other parts of the world, nurses in China were prohibited from any international exchange, and the training of nurses ceased. Those nurses able to make comparisons with their counterparts in other parts of the world acknowledged that the Cultural Revolution was a severe blow for the development of nursing in China.

Nursing development was further hampered by the failure of enforced egalitarianism to improve the low status of nursing. Granted, the traditional Chinese view that menial work necessitating touching the human body was viewed as low-status work was denounced as feudalistic in the new China. The masses were re-educated to believe that any kind of work was respectable as long as the person who did it aimed to serve the people wholeheartedly. Measures were initiated at the work place to reduce the differences between menial and mental workers. I would contend that these arrangements did not help to change the social prejudice against nursing work. They only encouraged a rudimentary concept of equality: everyone should have a same share of the work that no one liked to do. Nursing in China was persistently regarded as a low-status job, which people looked down upon.

Two positive dimensions in this period of nursing development in China can be seen. First, the notion of service to others as a role requirement of comradeship was a new form of role relationship that had not existed in traditional Chinese society. This sense of socialist responsibility characterized by Norman Bethune and Lei Feng enlarges a person's scope of responsibilities beyond the confines of the Confucian five cardinal relationships. We may expect to find that the moral sense of nursing would be expanded to include this socialist sense of service. Second, nursing responsibilities were extended to the provision of primary health care. While nursing in the Republican period was primarily practiced in hospitals, and nursing work was limited to helping physicians in their work, many nurses had extended their concerns to people's health, through participating in nationwide primary healthcare projects as a result of Mao's reforms.

## 4. Summary

Nursing underwent two different courses of development before China's modernization. The missionary nurses introduced the Nightingalian model of nursing to China in the nineteenth century. Confronted by social practices that were antithetical to women entering nursing, three approaches were used to raise the social standing of nursing. First, a Chinese name for nursing that had the positive connotations of "knowledgeable care provider" was coined. Second, a professional sense of nursing was promoted by raising the quality of nurses' training and the organization of professional activities among Chinese nurses. Third, a moral sense of nursing was fostered by using Florence Nightingale as a model, and by proposing a qualitative distinction between the ethical requirements of the nurse and the traditional care provider. Remarkable progress was made in the Republican era in terms of the numbers of Chinese women who were attracted to the nursing profession. Since China did not have a legacy of nursing in the Western sense, the early foreign medical theorists and trainers in China largely ignored traditional Chinese caring practices. How nurses in China fulfilled their role requirements in taking care of patients when, traditionally, care responsibilities were largely the responsibility of patients' relatives is an interesting question which remains unanswered in the literature on the history of nursing in China.

When the Communists gained power in 1949, nursing was cut off from outside influences and took a new direction. The professional attributes that nurses had acquired were stripped away. Nurses were included in efforts to implement healthcare reforms instituted by the Party leadership, guided by the doctrine of revolutionary humanism. While nurses were called to serve the people wholeheartedly, nurse training received less emphasis and came to a total halt during the Cultural Revolution. Those nurses able to make a comparison with their counterparts in other parts of the world acknowledge that this period dealt a severe blow to the development of nursing in China. A time before 1949 existed when the development of nursing education was only a few years behind the States, and might reasonably have been expected to catch up if 1949 had not intervened. China entered its era of modernization in 1978, when the Party leadership advocated reform and opening to the outside world. This provided nurses in China new opportunities for professional exchange with their counterparts in other parts of the world. The development of nursing shifted toward identifying a style of nursing with Chinese characteristics. Chapter Three will continue the discussion of the development of nursing in the reform era.

# Three

# NURSING IN THE ERA OF CHINA'S MODERNIZATION

In a reversal of the Maoist policy of destroying all professions, the professional identity that nurses had acquired before the founding of the People's Republic was reaffirmed by the Party leadership beginning in 1978. Even though the social prejudices against Chinese women developing their careers might have been lifted, the traditional view that caring for the sick is a low-status work still prevails in China. In line with the Party's policy of reform and opening to the outside world, measures were undertaken to strengthen the image of nurses and to make nursing a more attractive career for women. This chapter comprises three sections. The first section discusses the political context of nursing reform in China. Section two examines the reforms that have been undertaken to reconstruct a professional sense of nursing. Section three discusses the ethical requirements of nurses in light of the education and management measures instituted by the Ministry of Public Health to strengthen morality in hospital practice.

## 1. The Political Context

In 1978, the opening of the Third Plenary Session of the Eleventh Central Committee signified that China was entering another era of reform. First, it spelt out the Party leadership's determination to modernize China's economy. Second, it signified that Deng Xiaoping, an advocate of reform and modernization, had consolidated his power in leading China toward the realization of "socialism with Chinese characteristics."[1] To address the problems left over by the radical policies characterizing the Cultural Revolution, Deng reaffirmed Mao Zedong's idea that "gaining a clear understanding of the nature of Chinese society, namely, China's national conditions, is the prerequisite for gaining a clear understanding of all the issues concerning the revolution."[2] He reckoned that a socialist state had already been established in China, but only in a primary stage and in want of economic development.[3]

Contrary to Mao's policy, Deng reasoned that a market economy was especially suited to China in its current backward state. He felt that a period of market economic conditions could be applied to a socialist state in order to increase productivity.[4] Instead of striving for radical egalitarianism, Deng recognized that the level of development in different parts of China varied so much. Adopting one single model for production was thus not practical. Following other countries' examples were also not sensible.[5] Deng insisted on finding solutions appropriate to China's particular conditions. To this end, the Party leadership mandated that the people to participate in "one central task and two basic points of departure." The central task was to modernize China while "holding high the great banner of Mao Zedong Thought."[6] Two basic points of departure were: to be persistent in reform and opening-up, and to adhere to the Four Cardinal Principles, which were:

> We must keep to the socialist road.
> We must uphold the dictatorship of the proletariat.
> We must uphold the leadership of the Communist Party.
> We must uphold Marxism-Leninism and Mao Zedong Thought.[7]

Though Mao Zedong Thought continues to be upheld by the Party, the two core values of serving the people and class struggle promoted by Mao have undergone substantial reshaping in the era of reform. Mao Zedong Thought was reinterpreted to include the writings by Mao himself, and the accumulation of wisdom and understanding gained through the whole of the Chinese revolution. This revised posture toward Mao Zedong Thought is reflected in the collection of essays, *The Literature on Humanism*.[8] In this collection the section on Chinese Marxist ideology is arranged by theme instead of author, so Mao shares more or less equal billing with his Marxist comrades Zhou Enlai, Deng Xiaoping, Chen Yun, Zhu De, and Liu Shaoqi. The theme that comprises the largest section of collective writings is serving the people. This is further divided into four sub-themes: (1) humanity is the only motivational force in world history; (2) the desired good can only be realized if every person identifies with the mass line and is willing to serve the people wholeheartedly; (3) persistent training and self-cultivation is necessary to put the ideal into practice; and (4) the purpose of the state is to nurture a socialist new person who possesses correct ideals, and is moral, civilized, and disciplined.

The notion of humanism as portrayed in this collection largely reflects Mao's doctrine of revolutionary humanism. The emphasis is on serving others and not dwelling on one's interests, virtues modeled by Norman Bethune and Lei Feng. This collection of essays does not include class struggle as a means to serve the people. This is the aspect of Mao's philosophy that has received the least attention in the reform era. Deng called on the people to build socialism with Chinese characteristics by promising them political stability and unity. The Party leadership apparently was convinced that class struggle in terms of drawing a well-defined boundary between the capitalist way and the socialist way, suppressing elitist tendencies, undermining material incentives and eliminating wage differences had not made China into a modern socialist state. What was more important was to provide a stable environment to facilitate economic growth. Differences between rich and poor were accepted as a national condition. Deng believed that to let part of China become prosperous first was necessary in order that common prosperity could be reached.[9]

Since 1978, two aspects of change in the economic system were most prominent. First, the gradual transfer of decision-making powers from the central government to the producers of goods and services, and second, the gradual move to a market economy. Collective agricultural production gave way to the contract responsibility system, and the state-owned and state-managed concerns began to give way to private, free enterprise ownership. Along with all these changes came the introduction of material incentives and worker initiative to improve production, methods that had once been denounced by Mao.[10] Similar reforms were instituted in the healthcare system. Much skepticism was expressed in later days that such market reforms in the healthcare system would be incompatible with the Party's mandate that everyone should have equal access to medical care.

Another major difference between the revised version of Mao Zedong Thought and Mao's own views concerns attitudes toward China's cultural traditions. Instead of denouncing China's cultural traditions as undesirable remnants of a feudalistic past, the Party in the era of reform affirms that China has a proud cultural tradition in spite of its negative elements. The negative elements included focusing on agriculture to the neglect of trade, authoritarianism, rigid hierarchy, patriarchy, and personality cults. Hard work and simple living, unyielding pursuit in life, tolerance of others and seeking harmony, patriotism were some examples of "the cream of traditional Chinese culture."[11] As Deng maintained

> socialism with Chinese characteristics integrates the cream of both traditional Chinese culture and foreign cultures and further enhances it, thus turning itself into a modern and new type of Chinese culture. It has ushered Chinese culture into a new stage of development with a splendid future ahead.[12]

This optimistic claim has yet to be vindicated. To what extent the introduction of a market economy can bring forth economic progress without challenging the dominant political ideology of the Party, and at the same time be congruent with the Chinese cultural tradition is debatable. In 1981, the "Five Standards and the Four Beauties" movement was promoted among Chinese youth. The goal of this movement was to reinforce a code of morality, civility, and courtesy in line with Communist ideals.[13] In 1983, a nationwide ideological campaign against "spiritual pollution" with the aim of reaffirming the Party's leadership by guarding the people from the "corrosive influence of decadent bourgeois ideology and remnant feudal ideas" was initiated by the Second Plenum of the Twelfth Central Committee. In the late 1980s, a continuing series of student demonstrations demanding further social reform, brutally suppressed in 1989, reveal competing undercurrents produced by increasing competition from alternative ideological influences. These posed potential challenges to the stability of society and the control of the Party in promoting China's modernization. Against this backdrop, hardly surprising that nursing in China has undergone substantial changes over the past two decades.

What follows is a review of literature around the theme of recent nursing developments in China. In tracing these developments, the remarkable progress nurses in China have made to catch up with international nursing developments, and to strengthen the training and management necessary for preparing quality nurses and assuring quality services was impressive.

## 2. Reform and Opening-up

In 1978, the Chinese Nursing Association, in collaboration with the Medical Administration of the Ministry of Public Health, conducted a national survey to gain an understanding of nursing conditions in different parts of China. The Ministry of Public Health subsequently made seven recommendations. (1) The doctrine of revolutionary humanism had to be fostered among nurses as the fundamental principle for practice; (2) the quality of nursing had to be improved through strengthening in-service training and professional activities at different levels; (3) the job descriptions of nurses had to be defined. Nurses were only to be assigned appropriate nursing duties; other work had to be left to healthcare assistants. And more nurses were needed in view of shortages all over China; (4) working conditions for nurses, especially experienced nurses, should be improved, in order to keep them in the profession; (5) a vigorous reform of nursing education was considered imperative, and university-level training was recommended; (6) role responsibilities for the different grades of nurses had to be defined, and a system of career advancement should be set up; and (7) nursing management had to be strengthened.[14]

The Ministry of Public Health showed its explicit intention to redefine the once diffused role of nursing, and to recover the professional identity of nursing that had been undermined during the Cultural Revolution. In the following years, the Party leadership used these seven recommendations as a blueprint for nursing reform. What follows is an examination of three major aspects of nursing reform. They are educational reform, management reform, and the reconstruction of nursing's professional identity.

### A. Education Reform

#### i. Nurse Training Programs

One of the most important nursing issues in the early 1980s was the serious nurse shortage in China. In 1985, the nurse to population ratio was 1:1600. Wang Xiuying estimated that a further two million nurses were needed if a ratio of 1:430 between nurses and the general population were to be reached.[15] The Ministry of Public Health saw an urgent need to institute educational reforms to improve the quality of nurses and increase the supply. In the 1980s, the number of nursing schools was increased, and they began to offer different levels of programs with flexible modes of attendance.

In 1984, the Ministry of Public Health and the Ministry of Education organized the First National Education Conference, where the direction of nursing education reform was formulated. The Conference again affirmed that nurse preparation needed to be adapted to China's particular conditions; China required nurses who know how to assess people's health needs and to provide them preventive and curative care in the particular areas where they served. To this end, a three-year nursing program for junior high school entrants and a two-year program for senior high school entrants offered by colleges or hospitals was recommended. In the early 1980s, most nursing schools reopened three-year programs at the junior high school entrance level. In 1990, these three-year programs were extended to four years. According to an official source, in 1994, 500 nursing schools for junior high school entrants, and twenty-three nursing schools for senior high school entrants existed. The number of nurses has increased remarkably over the past two decades. In 1980, only 17,000 nurses with senior high school entrant qualification existed. The number increased to 674,000 in 1996. Of the total number of healthcare workers, the percent of nurses increased from 13.1 in 1980 to 21.5% in 1996. The physician-nurse ratio was improved as well, from 2:1 in 1980 to 1:0.74 in 1996.[16] The nurse-to-population ratio has improved from 1:1600 in 1985 to 1:1000 in 1995. The target of 1:430 has yet to be reached.

As far as higher education is concerned, in 1983, a five-year baccalaureate-nursing program was started in Tianjin.[17] In the 1984 Education Conference, the Ministry of Public Heath decided to extend this program to other universities because graduate study was affirmed as crucial to advance nursing science and to prepare future nursing leaders. By 1996, eighteen universities offered baccalaureate-nursing programs and four with nursing programs at the master's level. The first three-year master's program started at Beijing Medical University in 1994. The first class of master's nursing students graduated from the China Medical Board-funded program offered by Xian University and Chiang Mai University (Thailand) in 1996. In addition to full-time programs, part-time and distance learning programs are offered so that every nurse would have an opportunity to further her or his study.

In 1993, national examination for nurses' registration was re-introduced to monitor the standard of nurses graduating from different training programmes.[18] Appendix 1 is the translated version of "Nurses' Registration Ordinance of the People's Republic." The stipulations are written in Chapter Two of the Nursing Ordinance, which reads

> Those who apply for practice should pass a national examination conducted by the Ministry of Public Health and obtain a certificate titled "Practice Certificate for Nurses in the People's Republic of China"[19]

Nurses who pass the examination are licensed to practice. Exemption is only granted to those who receive their nursing education at college level, or who have graduated from nursing schools accredited by the Health Administrative Department at the provincial level or above. In sum, formal education for nurses has expanded steadily over the past two decades, although the number of nurses is still short of the target of having enough nurses to serve all strata of the population.

### ii. Nursing Curriculum

One major feature of educational reform was the move of nursing away from medical sciences and toward establishing nursing as an independent discipline. The nursing curriculum, which was primarily based on a medical model, has been under review in the reform era. Growing acçeptance exists among nurses that nursing as an applied science, which is built on medical sciences, and on the humanities and social sciences.[20] Subjects such as psychology and cultural studies were introduced to the curriculum. Initiatives to include new developments from North America, such as the nursing process and primary nursing, in nursing curricula, and innovative teaching methods have been undertaken to introduce these new concepts to students.[21]

In 1996, the Peking Medical Union College (PUMC) took the radical step of changing its curriculum to a four-year program based on a human needs model. Compared with the conventional program, this new curriculum, as shown in Appendix 2, has three obvious differences. First, humanistic sciences and medical sciences are emphasized in the foundation subjects, with a health focus instead of disease focus. Second, subjects on communication and interaction are especially emphasized in the first two years of the program. A course called "Communication" is offered in year one, and "Nursing Therapeutics Related to Social Interaction" is offered in year two. Third, critical thinking and problem-solving skills are emphasized throughout the four years of study. "Inquiry and Logical Reasoning" is offered in year one, and subjects related to research skills, such as "Data Management," "Problem Solving Skills and Strategies," and "Clinical Nursing Project" are offered from year two onwards. This initiative can be seen as a positive sign that nursing in China has been gaining increasing recognition as an independent discipline.

As nursing education is expanding into the tertiary sector, the major issue today is the provision of qualified nurse teachers. Since higher education for nurses had stopped for thirty years, and all nursing schools were closed down from 1966 to 1976, conceivably the number of qualified nurse teachers was not sufficient to meet demand in the 1980s. Physicians were allocated to serve as nurse trainers, especially in university level nursing programs. By having medically trained lecturers to teach nursing, we may wonder the extent to which nursing is taught as an independent discipline with a substantial distinction from medicine. Chen Lingyan, a medically trained nurse teacher, believes that medical knowledge alone is not enough to teach a student how to take care of patients. She says she had to study nursing, in theory and in clinical practice, before she knew how to teach nursing. She contends that only when nursing is taught by qualified nurse practitioners can nursing education be improved.[22] The issue of moving nursing education away from its strong medical dominance is still high on the agenda of nursing education reform today.

### B. Management Reform

The Ministry of Public Health has played a major role in initiating management reforms within the healthcare system over the past two decades. In the 1980s, the focus was on setting standards for different job responsibilities, the introduction of a system of job titles, and career advancement.[23] As the market economy began to have a significant effect on the healthcare system in the late 1980s, policies were instituted to address the problems of uncontrolled care standards and questionable staff quality. The main issue was to improve the quality of care with less reliance on government revenue. In the Maoist era, healthcare facilities were owned by the state. The costs of service were fully reimbursed by the government. Since the decision-making power was centralized, many healthcare facilities nurtured an inclination of "waiting, depending, and requesting" to gain funds from the central government. This practice largely compromised healthcare workers' motivation to increase productivity and responsiveness to the healthcare needs of the community that they are supposed to serve.

Similar to the reforms implemented in the countryside, the Party leadership began to enact a responsibility system in healthcare and medical institutions in the early 1980s.[24] Sun Guangde reports that the essence of this system was the "five fixed quotas," in which the staffing, job responsibilities of each staff category, their professional standards, the number of hospital beds, and budget subsidies were standardized.[25] This was to allow hospital administrators more autonomy in allocating resources and in controlling the quality of their services on the one hand, and to be more independent in the generation of income to cover their operating costs on the other. In other words, hospitals were required to operate within the mechanisms of a market economy, where patients were seen as consumers and medicine was seen as a commodity. This then required hospitals to improve their service in order to attract more patients, and hospital staffs were required to be quality and cost conscious in order to receive bonuses.

Sun noted that this system of linking work performance with monetary rewards would make for more motivated healthcare workers. This in turn might lead to better utilization of health facilities, shorten patients' waiting time, and make healthcare services more responsive to patients' needs. With these positive features of healthcare reform came problems of overcharging and abuses in medical insurance. Issues related to the commodification of medical services became increasingly serious.[26] Further hospital reforms were instituted in the late 1980s, to foster a moral sense of practice on the personal level, and to control the quality of service on the institutional level.

In 1989 the Ministry of Public Health launched reforms in hospital management by introducing grading standards and measures to evaluate hospital services. Two documents were issued in the same year, *The Grading Measures in Hospital Management* and *The Grading Standards of General Hospital Management*. Zhang Zhikuan summarized the four aims of grading assessment, as follows:

1. It will benefit regional medical programs and primary health care.
2. It will strengthen management of hospitals, rectify medical service structure, and improve disorderly conditions.
3. It will improve service attitudes and quality of treatment, and strengthen scientific management.
4. It will perfect hospital functions and raise the comprehensive levels of hospitals ... so as to meet social needs and promote the progress of medical science.[27]

Each hospital is assessed on the basis of its functions, tasks, technical levels, facilities, qualities of medical services, and levels of scientific management. Three levels exist, and each level has three grades. For instance, a level-three, Grade A hospital is required to demonstrate excellent quality in four basic functions and three tasks. The four functions are treatment, prevention, acute-care, and rehabilitation. Three tasks are medical treatment, education, and scientific research. If a hospital fails to demonstrate the relevant qualities, it will receive a penalty of degradation and reduction in fund allocation. Zhang reported that the pilot phase was completed in 1991, and the first phase of implementation was to be completed by the end of 1995. Along this policy line come corresponding reforms in nursing over the past two decades.

i. Job Responsibilities and Professional Titles

Since 1979, professional titles, such as senior nurse, vice chief nurse, and chief nurse, have been given based on different criteria. For instance, a senior nurse is required to be at least a diploma holder and to be engaged in clinical research. A chief nurse is required to demonstrate extensive understanding of the international trends and developments in his or her area of expertise, have extensive nursing experience and be able to make a significant contribution in research.[28] To be promoted, nurses must be assessed in their professional knowledge, management skills, education level, and experience. More importantly, they must fulfill come political criteria:

> He or she must support the leadership of the Communist Party, love socialism, diligently study Marxism and Mao Zedong Thought, have a high sense of political awareness, be red and expert, serve the people wholeheartedly, and endeavor to perfect his or her skills and make a contribution to society.[29]

This is to make sure that those who may get promoted into senior positions are loyal to the Party and are ready to identify their personal desires with the common goal of serving the people. Conceivably a conflict between these political requirements and the work can arise, especially in patient-care situations where the professional judgment does not go along with the directive from the Party leadership.

Reflecting on the Chinese nursing publications over the past years, this system of career advancement has had its positive effect. Nurses are being motivated to continuously upgrade their professional qualification, initiate patient care improvement projects, and share their clinical expertise with the nursing community at large through conference presentation and publications. The professional community also provides a facilitative environment for nurses to develop professionally. For instance, the Chinese Nursing Association established an award for technological advances in nursing in 1991. A total of 123 projects were given the award in the past six years.[30]

Clinical research activities have also proliferated in recent years. A survey on the utilization of research findings published between 1991 and 1993 in the *Chinese Journal of Nursing* revealed that of the 207 returned questionnaires (response rate was 52.54%), 62.8% reported that they had used some research findings to improve patient care quality.[31] A survey was conducted on 288 nurses working in large teaching hospitals in 1996. The findings showed that 4.5% had their works published, over 30% had participated in research activities, and over 60% intended to conduct research. Only 24.7% reported that they did not get support from managers, and 28.1% found their colleagues not co-operative.[32] These reports also pointed out that nurses' research knowledge was generally insufficient, and the quality of their research work is still not always of a high standard. Nonetheless, it gives an impression that a forum for professional exchange has been established, facilitating the initiative and creativity of clinical nurses in the advancement of their professional knowledge and skills.

### ii. The Responsible Nursing System

In the early 1980s, the organization of nursing work in Chinese hospitals was basically functional. As noted by Gail Henderson and Myron Cohen during their stay in a Wuhan hospital in 1980, nursing tasks were allocated in three shifts. They were the nursing shift, the treatment shift, and the chief shift. Nurses were assigned to these shifts in rotation, so every one would have an equal opportunity to work in different shifts. The duties of the nursing shift were delivery of direct patient care, such as keeping the ward clean and tidy, feeding helpless patients, monitoring the condition of critically ill patients. The treatment shift nurse was responsible for administering medication, intravenous therapy, carrying out treatment according to physicians' orders, and maintaining the ward equipment. The duties of the chief shift nurse were to make sure that physicians' orders were carried out by the treatment nurses, to update patients' medication cards, to order supplies for ward use, and to communicate with other departments about admission, discharge and other patient appointments.[33] While this mode of nursing work organization is still predominant in hospitals in China, nurses' voices in support of implementing a more holistic approach in delivering patient care began to be heard in the early 1980s.

The notion of the responsible nursing system comes from primary nursing. Numerous studies have been carried out since the 1970s in different parts of the world to investigate its implementation in different care settings.[34] In brief, primary nursing is an approach to patient care management based on a professional organizational principle of autonomous practice in the context of a one-to-one relationship between nurse and patient. Marie Manthey stated the four guiding principles in its implementation: (1) allocation and acceptance of individual responsibility for decision-making in respect of a particular patient as one individual; (2) assignment of daily care by case method; (3) direct person-to-person communication; and (4) one person being operationally responsible for the quality of care administered to a patient twenty-four-hours-a-day, seven-days-a-week.[35] Using a patient-centered approach to allocate nursing work, the primary nursing system requires qualified nurses to accept professional responsibility in taking care of a group of patients from their admission to discharge. They have to exercise professional judgment to assess patient problems, implement nursing intervention, and evaluate care outcomes.

In the early 1980s, primary nursing and the nursing process were introduced to the Chinese nursing community through international professional exchange.[36] While primary nursing emphasizes the individual responsibility of the nurse in taking charge of patient care, the nursing process demands the nurse to exercise professional judgment in identifying the patient's problems and to take initiative in helping the patient resolve his or her problems. These ideas are attractive to the Chinese nurses who would like to widen their scope of responsibilities from a task orientation to a total patient care orientation, and to promote a sense of personal responsibility.[37] This emphasis on nursing responsibility is reflected in the Chinese name given to primary nursing, which means "responsible nursing system" (責任制護理 *zeren zhi huli*), and the Chinese name for the primary nurse is "responsible nurse" (責任護士 *zeren hushi*).[38]

Considerable effort was made to implement the responsible nursing system in the 1980s. The earliest report on this appeared in the *Chinese Journal of Nursing* in 1984, written by a clinical nurse of a teaching hospital in Shanghai.[39] A national seminar was held in 1987 to discuss further implementation of the responsible nursing system in hospitals at all levels.[40] Discussion of how to apply the nursing process in clinical settings began to appear in the nursing literature in 1985.[41] These publications remained anecdotal or prescriptive, and the first evaluative study on the new system was reported in 1989. In this report, five aspects of patient satisfaction were explored. They were: (1) planning and implementation of patient care, (2) nurse-patient relations, (3) health teaching, (4) psychological care, and (5) instruction on discharge. The findings revealed that except for the aspect of psychological care, a significant improvement of patient satisfaction occurred after the implementation of the new system of nursing.[42]

In 1992, the Administration and Management Committee of the Chinese Nursing Association held a national conference on the responsible nursing system. 135 delegates from twenty-nine provinces attended the conference, with seventy-four papers presented.[43] This indicates that the responsible nursing system as an alternative method of allocating nursing work had been publicized and attempted in different clinical settings in different parts of China. Standards were also set to facilitate its implementation. For instance, only nurses holding the professional title of senior nurse or above are eligible to take sole charge of patients, while nurses and nursing aids are assigned to patients under supervision. A new system of nursing documentation based on the nursing process has been introduced to record and evaluate patient care, with emphasis on psychological care and health teaching.[44]

The introduction of the responsible nursing system inevitably challenges conventional nursing practice in which management of patient care is accorded to a set of routine standards with emphasis on collective responsibility instead of individual responsibility. Nurses are required to establish a close relationship with the patients who are under their care. This includes establishing a therapeutic relationship with the patients, negotiating with patients the best ways to take care of them, delivering direct patient care, and continuously monitoring patients' progress.

We have noted that traditionally in China, taking care of the sick is regarded as a requirement of family members. How a patient should be cared for is also a family affair. One characteristic of this tradition is that, though the tasks related to taking care of the sick may be seen as low-status work, care responsibilities toward a sick family member is regarded as a moral obligation that cannot be taken over by persons outside the family. Introducing the responsible nursing system signifies that nurses do not want to confine their duty to routine nursing tasks, but to extend their duty to include taking charge of the care responsibilities. This requires nurses to cross the boundary from the public sphere to patients' private sphere of life. Since the notion of caring by strangers is not compatible with traditional practices, the issue of how a nurse should relate to patients and their family members must be resolved before the responsible nursing system can be fully implemented.

### iii. The Systematic Approach to Holistic Nursing Care

In the 1990s, the responsible nursing system has been further modified, leading to an all-embracing nursing care delivery system called "the systematic approach to holistic nursing care." This care approach is defined as a patient-centered system of care using the nursing process as the framework to systematically link the different facets of clinical practice and nursing management. This care delivery system has three levels of implementation. The first level refers to the patient-centered approach to nursing that addresses the patient as a bio-psycho-social being. The second level refers to building a quality control system to monitor and evaluate patient care. The third level refers to the implementation of nursing services to uphold hospital objectives and policies so that quality service can be improved as a whole.[45] This move from the responsible nursing system to the systematic approach to holistic nursing can be seen as nursing's response to the hospital management reform implemented by the Ministry of Public Health beginning in 1989. Scientific management concepts such as quality assurance, standard measures, nursing audit, and continuous quality improvement have been introduced. In 1994, several hospitals in Beijing and Wuhan received funds from the World Health Organization to set up model wards to experiment with this mode of care.[46] Evaluation on its implementation is in progress, hoping that a nursing system with Chinese characteristics can come from these projects.

In tracing these recent developments in nursing, the remarkable progress nurses in China have made to catch up with international nursing developments was impressive. Beginning in the late 1970s, activities were undertaken to reconstruct the professional identity of nurses. The Chinese Nursing Association was re-established in 1977. The *Chinese Journal of Nursing* resumed publication in 1980 and distribution outside China began in 1981. Conferences and seminars at the national and provincial levels are now regularly organized to keep nurses in different parts of China informed of the latest nursing developments. Reports on exchange programs and collaborative projects between nurses in China and their counterparts in other parts of the world become more frequent. One obvious impression gathered from these reports is that nurses in China are receptive to new ideas and are enthusiastic to translate them into practice. They share a sense of urgency to lead Chinese nursing back to the international scene and to catch up with nursing developments in other parts of the world. Curriculum reform and the establishment of model wards to experiment with the systematic approach to holistic nursing care are reforms instituted with funds and expert consultation from abroad. They represent the cream of nursing development in China only. Strong evidence exists to indicate nursing remains an unattractive profession in China.[47]

### C. The Reconstruction of Nursing's Professional Identity

In order to strengthen nurses' professional identity, activities were also undertaken to promote nurses' self-esteem. Deng Yingchao, the widow of Zhou Enlai, acted as honorary president of the Chinese Nursing Association in 1981. Her inscription "Respect Nurses and Love Nurses," which was dedicated to nurses, was widely publicized in the media.[48] In 1982, *Health Bulletin*, a national newspaper on health issues, in association with Chinese Nursing Association, jointly organized a singing contest for nurses in different parts of China to promote a positive nursing image. In the same year, 301 nurses were selected as model nurses. Their contributions to nursing and society were published and distributed nationwide. In 1983, the nineteenth annual meeting of the Chinese Nursing Association was held. At this meeting nurses all over China were asked to affirm nursing as an independent discipline, and to make their central task fostering the quality of nursing and to strengthen nurses' sense of professional morality. In 1983, of the 295 women who were awarded the title of advanced workers, ninety-seven were nurses. In 1985, *Health Bulletin* started a special column on nursing with an intention of raising the public's consciousness with respect to nurses.[49]

Among other measures, model nurses, representing an ideal image of nursing, were publicized to encourage emulation by young nurses. The model nurses who were given nationwide attention had received nurse training in the Republican period.[50] This is significant in the sense that nursing as was practiced in the Republican period was being revitalized in the 1980s. Wang Xiuying, a winner of the Red Cross International's Nightingale award, received nurse training in 1926. Her life story was also collected in *Women of China*.[51] The Grandmother-Nurse whom Renee Fox and Judith Swazey met in Tianjin is another example. She was She Yunzhu, who started her nursing career in 1925. Fox and Swazey described her as a good exemplar of ethical practice.

> [She] personifies the indissoluble bond that she believes exists between the observance of certain ethical principles, virtues, and rules, and the achievement of greater technical excellence, humanity, and commitment to service, in nursing and in medicine.[52]

Another example is Madam Wang Meide. She is recognized as a virtuous model because of her life commitment to nursing. Her life and work is recorded in *The 110th Anniversary Album of the First Affiliated Hospital to Suzhou Medical College*,

> In her youth, she studied and worked very hard, determined to devote herself to the country's cause of nursing. In the 40-odd years with clinical teaching and research in nursing, she has passed all her knowledge to the younger generation. Referring to Nightingale's saying "A nurse is a wingless angel who brings people sincere sympathy and selfless devotion," she often encourages younger nurses to qualify themselves with a lofty ideal to serve the people.[53]

The celebrated qualities shared by Wang Xiuying, She Yunzhu and Wang Meide manifested the virtues of Norman Bethune and Lei Feng in terms of their selfless devotion to serving the people wholeheartedly, and virtues in the nursing tradition of Florence Nightingale—purity, sincerity, and compassion.

In addition to these celebrated nurses receiving nationwide attention, ordinary nurses were also identified as virtuous exemplars. For instance, Liu Xudong praised a young nurse, Bu Fan, who worked long hours and did not mind doing such dirty work as cleaning patients and handling their secretions and excretion. She also kept a systematic diary of her work and tried her best to improve her skills.[54] Liu Ying praised the nurses who nursed wounded soldiers back to health during the border clashes between China and Vietnam.[55] Huang Xuehua and Ou Qing urged the nurses to learn from Lei Feng's sense of responsibility and altruistic sentiment in serving the people.[56] Huang Dongfei identified fourteen model nurses to illustrate the commendable attributes of an "angel" nurse. These nurses were pure and compassionate, willing to treat patients as their own family members, and gentle but prudent and strict in performing their duties. They also had a sense of self-sacrifice, were responsive to patients' needs and did not fear doing the dirty work of nursing, did not avoid hard work, were willing to learn, and were diligent in improving their skills and knowledge. Above all, they carried the spirit of Norman Bethune and Lei Feng.[57] This list of attributes manifested by an angelic nurse is similar to those described in the list of nurses' ethical requirements compiled by Yao Changxu in 1939.[58] The only major difference is that, in this case, these attributes are presented against the background of the doctrine of socialist humanism; the model nurses were presented as Lei Feng in the guise of "wingless angels," or socialist humanist Florence Nightingales.

Over the last two decades, this angelic image has been used commonly in Chinese nursing literature. Wang Tong maintained that the angel was a symbol of happiness, warmth, and compassion, which were the central attributes of an ideal nurse. Zhang Jingru described nurses as wingless angels who took care of patients meticulously in every aspect and treated patients better than they did their family members.[59] Wei Guifang described a nurse as God's messenger who brought life to the dying, a goddess who saved people's lives and an angel who brought blessings to the sick.[60] Wang Sanhu summarized six nurse images. They are (1) mother, (2) servant, (3) religious person, (4) handmaiden, (5) angel, and (6) hero. Among these six images, Wang found the angel image most representative of a nurse. In her description, an angel nurse was optimistic, genuine, knowledgeable, kind, gentle, careful, diligent, skilful, not afraid of hard work, ready to help others, and put others' interests before herself.[61] These are qualities worthy of respect, but I wonder whether these are realistic expectations for "human" nurses dealing with the reality of nursing practice.

Concerns have been raised by nurses that, regardless of the efforts that have been made to affirm the professional identity of nursing, social prejudices that make taking care of the sick seem to be servant's work are still prevalent in China. They assert that the predominant view of "looking up on medicine and looking down on nursing" is so deeply rooted in the minds of the people that changes in such attitudes are still far away. Pan Shashan found that most nurses had relatively low self-esteem because they did not receive the respect due them from the public.[62] Fu Aimin contended that nursing was not reckoned as an independent practice. Nursing was also not given adequate opportunity to develop as a profession.[63] Duan Jiangli pointed out that the public's prejudiced view of nursing as low-status work caused feelings of inferiority on the part of nurses.[64] Huang and Ou noted that most nurses did not respect their profession and held an indifferent attitude at work because nursing was perceived as a difficult, but unappreciated job.[65] I share this concern that presenting this angelic image will do little to foster a sense of professional identity among nurses if they are still seen as doing servant's work.

### 3. Fostering Morality in Practice

Among the major concerns of the Ministry of Public Health is the strengthening of morality among healthcare workers. The Ministry developed a set of rules of conduct in 1981 and revised it substantially in 1988. A review of these two sets of rules shows that the moral requirements for healthcare workers promulgated by the Party have shifted over the past decade. This change is reflected in recent issues of the *Chinese Journal of Nursing* and *Chinese Medical Ethics*. Professional ethics for nurses have been receiving increasing attention since the early 1990s, although the number of publications is not impressive. More importantly to note that most of the authors of these articles are teachers of nursing ethics, instead of nurses. These writings revolve around two major themes: moral education and cultivation of desirable qualities in nurses, and fostering a sense of morality in different practice situations. The following section will examine the rules of conduct articulated by the Ministry of Public Health, and the ways in which the nursing community has responded to these ethical requirements.

#### A. The 1981 Rules of Conduct for Healthcare Personnel

In line with the Party policy of upholding the four fundamental principles in constructing a socialist China, Mao's mandate to "rescue the dying and heal the wounded, serve the people wholeheartedly" is affirmed as the fundamental principle for healthcare workers in China's era of modernization. A set of rules of conduct was developed by the Ministry of Public Health in 1981 to foster its implementation. It reads

1. Love the motherland, love the Communist Party, love socialism, and uphold Marxism and Mao Zedong Thought.
2. Study politics diligently, endeavor to perfect your professional skills and be both red and expert.
3. Develop revolutionary humanism in healing the wounded and rescuing the dying, have sympathy and respect for patients, and serve the patients wholeheartedly.
4. Carry out national law and implement regulations.
5. Obey superior political bodies, be concerned with the collective, help each other, criticize and self-criticize.
6. Be extremely responsible in work, strictly carry out regulations and rules.
7. Be honest in performing official duties, be reliable in performing assigned duties, and be against unhealthy tendencies.

8. Develop a civilized society and common courtesy, actively participate in patriotic health campaigns, and make the environment beautiful, keep the hospital clean, tidy and quiet.[66]

Beyond the general intention of restoring effective management within the hospital organization, these rules reflected the Party's determination to continue the implementation of socialist morality as defined in the 1950s. The "five loves" formed the core of this morality, with priority given to the goals of the collective. The five loves are (1) love for the motherland; (2) love for the people; (3) love of labor; (4) love of science; and (5) protection of public property.[67] In the 1980s the emphasis of moral cultivation shifted from class struggle to building "socialism with Chinese characteristics." Likewise, the boundary between professional ethics and political ideology remained vaguely defined. Both were often seen as complementary, serving similar purposes by preparing nurses who would uphold the four cardinal principles, be willing to serve the people, and be perseverant in improving their knowledge and attitude at work.[68] The secretaries of the Party committee are given the duty of educating their units' staff on correct political thinking and professional behavior, and they are often assigned to teach ethics in schools as well. This further blurred the boundary between medical ethics and political education.

In the 1980s, the slogan, "be a red and expert people's nurse," was propagated as nurses' role requirements.[69] While to be expert demands nurses to be committed to advances in nursing sciences contributory to China's modernization, to be red demands that nurses uphold Mao's mandate in practice, to serve those in illness and wholeheartedly help them be restored to health. Embedded in this slogan is the requirement that nurses manifest a sense of socialist responsibility in practice. First, a people's nurse needs to put the interests of the collective before herself—to be an angelic Lei Feng, or a socialist humanist Florence Nightingale. Second, nurses are required to assume role responsibilities, which are defined within an organizational context, and in a political-ideological context where an individual has to be responsible to the Party leadership. In Mao's words,

> Our point of departure is to serve the people wholeheartedly and never for a moment divorce ourselves from the masses, to proceed in all cases from the interests of the people and not from one's self-interests, or from the interests of a small group, and to identify our responsibility to the people with our responsibility to the leading organs of the Party.[70] Since the Party claims to represent the interests of the people, a person having a sense of socialist responsibility needs to carry out what is mandated as ethical practice as passed down by Party officials through the chain of command.

> (1) The individual is subordinate to the organization; (2) the minority is subordinate to the majority; (3) the lower level is subordinate to the higher level; and (4) the entire membership is subordinate to the Central Committee. Whoever violates these articles of discipline disrupts Party unity.[71]

Statement 5 of the Rules of Conduct has this requirement stated. This practice may encourage nurses to consider ethical practice as equivalent to what is officially defined in terms of rules and regulations. Strong control by government bodies inevitably undermines the development of a sense of professional autonomy, which, arguably, is more important for healthcare workers to internalize ethical standards and establish a fiduciary relationship with patients. This inevitably breeds indifferent attitudes on the part of nurses if they have no sense of control in improving practice when the existing rules and regulations fail to address the issues they face in clinical practice.

### B. The 1988 Criteria for Medical Ethics

Along with the hospital management reforms that were launched in 1989, the Ministry of Public Health replaced the 1981 Rules of Conduct by issuing a directive titled *Regulations on Criteria for Medical Ethics and Their Implementation* in December 1988.[72] Article 3 of the directive states the criteria for medical ethics. It reads,

> 1. Heal the wounded, rescue the dying, and practice socialist humanism. Keep the interests of the patient in mind and try every means possible to relieve the patient's suffering.
> 2. Show respect for the patient's dignity and rights and treat all patients alike, whatever their nationality, race, sex, occupation, social position or economic status.
> 3. Service should be provided in a civil, dignified, amiable, sympathetic, kindhearted and courteous way.
> 4. Be honest in performing medical practice and conscientious in observing medical discipline and law. Do not seek personal benefits through medical practice.
> 5. Keep the information related to the patient's illness confidential and practice protective healthcare. In no case is one allowed to reveal the patient's health secret or compromise his or her privacy.
> 6. Learn from other doctors and work together co-operatively. Handle professional relations between colleagues correctly.
> 7. Be rigorous in learning and practicing medicine and work hard to improve your knowledge, ability, skills and service.

In comparison with the 1981 Rules of Conduct, the 1988 Criteria for Medical Ethics (the 1988 Code) continues to uphold "rescue the dying and heal the wounded" as the ethical mandate. The way in which serving the people should be realized is interpreted quite differently. To my mind, these two codes have at least four differences. First, the term "revolutionary humanism" is replaced by "socialist humanism" in the 1988 Code. The focus is more on patient-healthcare worker relationships than the country and community instead. Second, phrases with strong political overtones, such as "study politics diligently," "obey upper political bodies, be concerned with the collective, help each other, criticize and self-criticize" did not appear in the 1988 Code. Third, the requirements of healthcare workers in relating to patients and co-workers are more explicitly stated in the new Code. Emphasis is on respect and co-operation instead of obedience and control by rules and regulations. Fourth, the concept of patient rights is officially addressed for the first time, although the practice of protective medical care is maintained, with the scope of patient rights limited to the right of fair treatment, and the right of privacy and confidentiality.

While the Ministry of Public Health aims to improve hospital service at management level through implementing *The Grading Measures in the Hospital Management* and *The Grading Standards of General Hospital Management.*[73] The *Regulations on Criteria for Medical Ethics and Their Implementation* aims to improve hospital service quality at the individual level.[74] As stated in Article 11, the same criteria for medical ethics are applied to all healthcare workers regardless of their job titles. The ruling Party believed that strengthening a sense of professional morality through education and management is crucial to counteracting the undesirable practices brought by the introduction of market factors to health care in China.[75] These practices include overcharging patients, demanding or accepting bribes for treatment, indifferent attitudes at work and grumbling over poor working conditions and low salaries.

The formulation of the 1988 Code signifies that medical ethics has begun to be differentiated from political education and has emerged to be an independent subject of inquiry. In the same year, the Medical Ethics Association was established under the auspices of the Chinese Medical Association. A bimonthly journal, *Chinese Medical Ethics*, published under the direction of the Ministry of Public Health, was also inaugurated. Formal channels for healthcare workers to exchange viewpoints on ethical issues have been formed. In 1989, the National Educational Committee directed that moral education be strengthened in schools.[76] Most textbooks on medical and nursing ethics were published around the early 1990s. The subject is no longer solely taught by Party secretaries; instead, social scientists and medical doctors with a genuine interest in ethics have begun to take up the teaching of ethics.

### C. Ethics Education for Nurses

Ye Shujun reported how nursing ethics was introduced to nursing students in Shandong Province. In 1991, in response to the directive of the Ministry of the Public Health, standardized teaching materials on professional ethics for nurses were developed there.[77] While the subject began to be offered in nursing schools, Ye suggested that all nurses should re-take ethics as an in-service course. First, he believed that a systematic study of medical ethics could help strengthen the sense of morality of nurses in dealing with the undesirable effects market reforms have had on their work. Second, Ye found that nurses were required to deal with increasingly complex relationships at work as modern nursing moved from a disease-focus to person-focus. This shift demanded that nurses be aware of all factors influencing patients' recovery, and that they harmonize the relationships between physicians and patients to provide the best possible care to patients. He suggested that nursing ethics could prepare nurses for the role.

An examination paper of nursing ethics at the diploma level published in 1992 reveals that the subject matter offered in ethics course evolved around the criteria for medical ethics articulated by the Ministry of Public Health. The examination paper contained items on medical ethical concepts, virtuous models such as Nightingale, Qiu Jin, and traditional Chinese medical practitioners, desirable nursing qualities, attitudes, and customary ethical practices. The ways in which the questions were asked revealed that teaching approach emphasized students' comprehension instead of critical analytical skills.[78]

I doubt whether the issues raised by Ye can be resolved merely by strengthening nurses' sense of morality. Definitely Ye's suggestions served to materialize the directive issued by the Ministry of Public Health, which stipulated that staff at all levels are required to receive ethics education and appraisal of their ethical performance.[79] This can explain why recent publications have tended to focus on two major themes: cultivating nurses' qualities and role requirements in various practice settings.

Over the past ten years, hospital measures to implement the 1988 Regulations have included organizing in-service programs for all grades of nursing staff, initiating activities to learn from models, appraisal of individual performance, identifying model workers, and setting up a promotion system that rewards good performance and punishes misconduct. Hou Lin and Zhu Youming report that they had successfully improved staff quality in a comprehensive hospital in Jiangsu Province by using such measures.[80] They claimed that three aspects of nurses' quality were improved. They were a sense of socialist responsibility, skill competence and compassion in relating to patients—in the sense that nurses treated patients as their family members. We may say that Hou and Zhu were successful in fostering emulation of a socialist humanist Florence Nightingale or an angelic Lei Feng among the nurses.

Presumably these ethical standards were defined by the hospital administration and imposed onto the nurses from above. I doubt just how effective these ethics-inducing measures were, and whether the nurses would continue to emulate such contrived models without pressure from above. These standards imposed on the nurses are quite unrealistic and fail to adequately address the issues they face in day-to-day practice; the opinions and experiences of the nurses themselves have not been considered in formulating these ethical standards. Recent literature on nursing morality in China focuses on the virtues nurses should possess in manifesting this mandate.[81] But the implementation of market factors in healthcare reform has already brought emergent values and practices that threaten the relevance of this mandate in informing practice. If this is the case, the ethical requirements articulated in 1988 will need further modifications.

## 4. Summary

Nurses in the modern era in China have revitalized their professional identity, renewing much of the promise that nursing had lost after the founding of the People's Republic. Measures have been taken to foster a sense of professionalism among nurses. These include promoting an angelic image of nurses, giving public recognition to nurses who perform well, and encouraging professional activities and exchange programs at the national and international levels. Over the past two decades, numerous nursing reforms have been undertaken with the intention to strengthen nursing as a profession and to improve the quality of nurses. Such measures include the provision of higher education opportunities, accreditation of job titles, initiatives to develop nursing into an independent discipline through curriculum reform and implementation of the responsible nursing system and the systematic approach to holistic nursing care.

In this era of reform, nurses' role responsibilities are changing in two respects. First, the recent reforms in ways nursing care is delivered demand that nurses take greater responsibility for patient care and use a holistic approach. Nurses are required to demonstrate competence in performing their traditional nursing tasks, and in taking charge of total patient care. Taking care of the sick was regarded as a role for family members, and decisions regarding a patient's care were also considered a family affair in traditional Chinese society. This emergent notion of professional care in China will increasingly give rise to ethical issues concerning patients and patient families that nurses must face in their day-to-day practice. Second, among the reforms that aim to improve the quality of nurses is an attempt to strengthen a sense of professional morality in nursing. A comparison of the 1981 Rules of Conduct and the 1988 Criteria for Medical Ethics reveals that the orientation for ethical practice has undergone substantial modifications with China's modernization. Education and management measures have been undertaken to cultivate the ethical requirements as stated in the Criteria for Medical Ethics. These measures foster external compliance instead of ethical reflection on the part of nurses. The aim was to cultivate a socialist Nightingale or angelic Lei Feng model for emulation.

I doubt the effectiveness of these measures in preparing nurses to ethically address the issues they must face. "Rescue the dying and heal the wounded" is upheld as the fundamental principle of health care, making it the basis on which these ethical requirements are formulated. Emergent values and practices that have come along with the implementation of market factors in the reform of healthcare compete with the values upheld in this mandate. This consequently jeopardizes their relevance in informing practice.

# Four

# THE ETHICAL MANDATE IN QUESTION

In 1988, the Ministry of Public Health announced new criteria for medical ethics, by which healthcare workers' ethical performance was to be evaluated. Mao Zedong's mandate to "rescue the dying, heal the wounded" continues to be upheld as the fundamental principle. Hospitals are required to institute educational and management measures to foster implementation of these ethical criteria for counteracting problems such as indifferent attitudes, bribery, and overcharging that have emerged since the introduction of market mechanisms into hospital care. The values upheld in this mandate are apparently out of step with the changing values of Chinese society, which, ironically, makes it a competing instead of overriding principle for ethical practice. To illustrate this contention, three contemporary issues that put this mandate in question will be examined. The three issues are healthcare access, population control policy, and the movement in support of legalizing euthanasia as a medical measure. This chapter comprises two sections. First, the values upheld in Mao's mandate will be explored in light of the Chinese medical ethics tradition. The second section discusses how this ethical mandate fails to address the three major Chinese healthcare issues.

## 1. Rescue the Dying and Heal the Wounded

"Rescue the dying and heal the wounded" has been promulgated as the fundamental principle for healthcare since Mao undertook leadership of the Communist Party, even before the founding of the People's Republic. This mandate was relevant for the time, when the combined effects of a disintegrating social structure, poverty, famine, and almost non-existent public hygiene, with epidemic and endemic parasitic and infectious diseases plagued the whole country.[1] Underpinning this mandate is an advocacy of respect for life that demands both negative and positive duty on the part of healthcare workers to protect life. Respect for life has always been a highly regarded value in medical ethics, but whether it implies a positive duty to protect life is arguable.[2]

In the Hippocratic tradition, physicians should not do anything intentionally that may harm a person's life. As written in the Hippocratic Oath,

> I [physician] will give no deadly medicine to anyone if asked, nor suggest any such counsel; and in like manner I will not give a woman a pessary to produce abortion. With purity and with holiness I will pass my life and practice my art. I will not cut persons laboring under the

> stone, but will leave this to be done by men who are practitioners of this work.[3]

Nurses, too, uphold this tradition. In the Nightingale reform era, nurses were required to make the following pledge,

> I will abstain from whatever is deleterious and mischievous and will not take or knowingly administer any harmful drug.[4]

The Code for Nurses adopted by the International Council of Nurses in 1973 (ICN Code) affirms that "inherent in nursing is respect for life, dignity and rights of man."[5] The same statement is found in the Code of Professional Conduct for Nurses in Hong Kong, which was formulated by the Nursing Board of Hong Kong in 1986.[6] These codes state a moral obligation not to do any harm that may take a person's life, and the fundamental responsibility of the nurse is to promote health, to prevent illness, to restore health, and to alleviate suffering. The duty of healthcare workers to save life at all cost, as implied in Mao's mandate, is not overtly stated.

## A. Medical Ethics in the Chinese Tradition

Mao's mandate is not incompatible with the Chinese medical ethics tradition. This notion of having a positive duty to protect life is a predominant theme in the writings on medical ethics in ancient China. The first medical book, *The Yellow Emperor's Classic of Internal Medicine*, written in the Period of the Warring States (400–240 BC), contemplates the ways in which a person can live a long life and enjoy good health. It reckons that healthcare workers are morally obligated to prolong human life to the best of their ability, and to regard pursuing medical knowledge as a continuous endeavor. In the discourse of therapeutic regimes, the Yellow Emperor demonstrated openness and modesty in seeking advice from his subordinates.[7] Obligations of this kind were sustained in ancient China. In the seventh century, Sun Simiao (581–673 AD) wrote a treatise entitled *On the Absolute Sincerity of Great Physicians*, which is also known as the Chinese Hippocratic Oath. Sun is one of the highly regarded thinkers in contemporary China. His biography is collected in the *Critical Biography Series of Chinese Thinkers*.[8] To further extend what has been upheld in *The Yellow Emperor's Classic of Internal Medicine*, this treatise affirms respect for all forms of life. It reads,

> From the early times famous persons frequently used certain living creatures for the treatment of diseases, in order to thus help others in situations of need. To be sure, it is said: "Little esteem for the beast and high esteem for man," but when love of life is concerned, man and animal are equal. If one's cattle are mistreated, no use can be expected

> from it; object and sentiments suffer equally. How much more applicable is this to man.[9]

Grounded in this notion of the sanctity of life, Sun maintained that a physician is obligated to "commit oneself firmly to the willingness to take the effort to save every living creature," and condemned using living creatures as medicine. He justified his stance that "whoever destroys life in order to save life places life at an even greater distance."[10] To fulfill a physician's obligation, the person is required not to "ponder one's fortune or misfortune," but to "preserve life and have compassion for it" even at one's cost. As the treatise states,

> Neither dangerous mountain passes nor the time of day, neither weather conditions nor hunger, thirst nor fatigue should keep him from helping wholeheartedly. Whoever acts in this manner is a great physician for the living. Whoever acts contrary to these demands is a great thief for those who still have their spirits![11]

To this end, Sun mandated that a great physician should possess "absolute sincerity." Gan Zuwang suggests that "absolute sincerity" (精誠) connotes the two core virtues and five criteria for ethical practice. The two core virtues are *jing* (精) in technical competence and *cheng* (誠) in relating to patients.[12] To maintain *jing*, or refinement in practice, medical practitioners are required to devote themselves to medicine, and be diligent in work and study. They need to constantly update their knowledge and refine their skills. The common English translation of the word *cheng* is sincerity.[13] The meaning of *cheng* as embedded in a Chinese cultural context may be commensurate with the meaning of sincerity, but is not identical. While sincerity means freedom from deceit or falseness, honesty, trustworthiness, and truthfulness, the character *cheng* is made up of two Chinese words, one means "speech, talk, or words," the other means "finish, complete, or accomplish." The meaning of *cheng* can be illustrated by a Chinese idiom, which reads, "What is said must be done, and what is done must be brought to fruition." This notion of *cheng* has a strong moral connotation—people should keep their word and demonstrate good intention in their deeds, *cheng* is a fundamental principle, which should guide all human actions. As the *Doctrine of the Mean* explains,

> Sincerity [*cheng*] is that whereby self-completion is effected, and its way is that by which man must direct himself. Sincerity is the end and beginning of things, without sincerity there would be nothing. On this account, the superior man regards the attainment of sincerity as the most excellent thing. The possessor of sincerity does not merely accomplish the self-completion of himself. With this quality he

> completes other men and things also. The completing himself shows his perfect virtue. The completing other men and things shows his knowledge. Both these are virtues belonging to nature, and this is the way by which a union is effected of the external and internal. Therefore, whenever he—the entirely sincere man—employs them, —that is, these virtues, —their action will be right.[14]

A person who possesses the virtue of *cheng* understands the nature of things, self, and other people. This enables the person to see into others, to foresee the good and the evil in things, and to acquire the right ways in relating to others. In this regard, the five criteria for medical ethics require healthcare workers who possess "absolute sincerity" to demonstrate understanding of the patients under their care, and be compassionate to the patients' suffering. They can master the necessary skills in treating the patients so as to help them restore from illness, and have a high sense of responsibility. Instead of obtaining a profit for themselves, sincere medical practitioners treat all patients equally, as they would treat their family members. This is represented in the popular Chinese saying, "a person who professes medicine should have the parent heart." This point is not in Paul Unschuld's translation. He translated the sentence as "he should always act as if he were thinking of himself." The original meaning should be "he should always act as if he were thinking of his significant others."[15]

This moral imperative of respect for life and treating patients with parental love is further elaborated with a sense of urgency, as if one were rescuing someone from a deadly crisis. Lu Chih's (754–805 AD) treatise on medical ethics maintains

> When someone suffers from a disease and seeks a cure, this is no less crucial than if someone facing death by fire or by drowning calls for help. Physicians are advised to practice humaneness and compassion. Without dwelling on [externals such as] tresses and a cap that fits, they have to hasten to the relief of him [who asks for it]. This is the proper thing to do. Otherwise accidents such as burning or drowning take place.[16]

Likewise, medical practices that go against the sanctity of life would be denounced as misconduct.[17]

Mao's ethical mandate can be seen as a continuation of medical values passed down from traditional Chinese medical ethics, but expressed within the ideological framework of socialist humanism. The doctrine of socialist humanism requires people to assume a sense of socialist responsibility by upholding the values of equality and the collective good instead of acting for one's self-interests or for the interests of one's family. Thus, comradeship and serving the people wholeheartedly, with loyalty to the masses and the

Party leadership are cherished as core moral virtues. These values apparently challenge the Confucian ethical system, which defines a person's role requirements within a network of hierarchical relationships and with filial piety as the most important virtue.

The notions of equality and not acting in one's self-interests are values also advocated in the Chinese medical ethics tradition, grounded in a belief of the existential equality of humanity. Texts to illustrate this contention are numerous. For instance, in Sun's treatise, a passage reads,

> If someone seeks help because of illness or on the ground of another difficulty, a [great physician] should not pay attention to status, wealth or age, neither should he question whether the particular person is attractive or unattractive, whether he is an enemy or friend, whether he is Chinese or foreigner, or finally, whether he is educated or uneducated. He should meet everyone on equal ground.[18]

Since everyone has to be treated equally, including those who cannot afford to pay, physicians are required not to make a profit for themselves. One of the maxims for physicians is as follows:

> They should not esteem profits too high, but instead cultivate humaneness and righteousness. Although we distinguish between the poor and the rich, only one kind of medicine exists.[19]

Negative examples of physicians who overcharged patients but later suffered heavenly punishment at their end of life were used to warn physicians about committing such wrongs. In sum, the values upheld in Mao's mandate for healthcare workers were firmly rooted in the Chinese medical ethics tradition.

### B. Protective Medical Care

In this tradition where healthcare workers are required to possess technical competence, parental love, and a sense of socialist responsibility in serving the sick, we can see the logic why protective healthcare is advocated in the 1988 Criteria for Medical Ethics.[20] As far as nursing is concerned, protective care has been practiced since its early development in Republican China. In Yao Changxu's list of role requirements for nurses, she put much emphasis on the nurse's duty to protect the patient from harmful effects by all means, including protecting the patient from unpleasant messages, and using kind words to cultivate hope of recovery.[21] The philosophy of protective medicine holds that the psychological link between the patient and his or her disease is so significant that patients should be protected from all unpleasant stimuli that might retard the healing process. The duty of healthcare workers is to mobilize all the strengths of the patient to fight the disease—including helping the patient develop a positive outlook.[22] Maintaining patients' confidence in therapeutic regimens and hope in recovery is one of the most important ethical obligations for healthcare workers in contemporary medical care.

The Ministry of Public Health's 1988 criteria for medical ethics include statements such as "respect the patient's personality and his or her rights," "treat everyone equally without discrimination," and "respect the patient's privacy and keep his or her personal information in confidence." The scope of patient rights is confined to the right to fair treatment and the right to privacy. These are implied rights in both the Hippocratic and Chinese ethical traditions. Nonetheless, keeping patients' personal information in confidence carries two meanings in the Code. Other than the common understanding that healthcare workers should not disclose patients' personal information to others, Li Benfu, Ding Huisun and Li Chuanjun state that it also means that one should not disclose medical information to vulnerable patients who may not benefit from knowing their conditions.[23] Hence, information disclosure is neither regarded as a patient's right, nor is to be determined by the patient's level of competence in understanding the information and making rational decisions. The consideration of protecting a patient from possible psychological harm after learning about his or her critical condition precedes all other considerations.[24]

This practice of information disclosure is contrary to mainstream ethical thinking in the Western world. Protecting the interests of vulnerable patients in terms of the disclosure of information has attracted much discussion recently. The most debatable issues are how to identify which patients are vulnerable and need to have decisions made for them, and who can legitimately represent patients' best interests in making treatment decisions. The patients' competency in exercising their autonomy and self-determination is seen as the most important consideration in identifying the vulnerable group who require protection on the part of healthcare workers.[25] But the institutionalization of protective care is obvious in China. All textbooks on medical and nursing ethics advocate this approach to patient care.[26]

In 1994, a hospital in Hangzhou formulated a patient charter, comprising six rights and six obligations for patients as listed in Appendix 4.[27] Although it states that patients have the right to information, the right is limited to those who are "suitable to hear the truth directly." For those who may not benefit from learning the truth, healthcare workers have to inform their family members. In other words, family members' right to information takes precedence. In Chapter One, I discussed how traditional practice in China requires that family members assume primary responsibility in taking care of the sick. Hence, this system of protective medical care can be seen as a continuation of what has been practiced in ancient China.

Isolated discussion of patients' right to informed consent has recently appeared in the literature in China.[28] An article written by Li Jimin suggests that patients' rights should include the right to choose, the right to informed consent and the right to give comments. He speculates that informed consent is beneficial even to terminally ill patients, basing his argument on recent research findings in other parts of the world. He further suggests that promoting patient rights helps to protect patients' interests in view of the recent commodification of healthcare.[29] But these ideas have not gained much acceptance. Presumably the patient's right to informed consent and right to self-determination in treatment decisions are still not part of the ethical mandate in contemporary Chinese society.

So far, I have attempted to make sense of the mandate that has been upheld as the fundamental principle for medical ethics since the Maoist era. The question that follows is whether the values embodied in the mandate are realistic in the sense that they can be put into practice. In view of the competing values emerging from the contemporary issues that healthcare workers have to deal with, I will proceed to examine three major issues that put the mandate in question. They are healthcare access on a fee-for-service basis, population control policies that represent the Party's intention to foster "superior quality of birth and superior quality of child rearing," and changing views of society on legalizing active euthanasia as a medical measure.

## 2. Access to Healthcare Services

The Party's efforts to "serve the people" through provision of medical care to every strata of the populace are well documented. It does not necessarily follow that people have free access to healthcare services, nor has it ever been the intention of the Government to provide universal medical care free of charge.[30] Since China began its reforms, the issue of unequal access has become more marked, both at the macro- and micro-levels. At the macro-level, differences between urban and rural areas persist—people in the countryside are more disadvantaged in getting access to medical care. In the cities, changes in hospital funding have biased provision of medical services toward those who can afford to pay. At the micro-level, tensions inevitably emerge in meeting the healthcare needs of those who are not able to afford it. In the following I will examine in more depth these issues of healthcare access and funding in China.

### A. Healthcare Profile

Many claims exist about the achievements of China's reforms. The comprehensive healthcare system that began to develop in the 1960s became more formalized in the 1980s. Today the system is characterized by a three-tier system of organization and referral in both rural and urban areas. The three tiers are primary, secondary, and tertiary care at the village, township, and county levels in rural areas, and street, district, and city levels in urban areas. Health institutions, such as epidemic prevention stations, maternity, and child care centers, and epidemic prevention teams are responsible for preventive care. The lower levels of organization are supposed to deal with minor illnesses, with more complicated cases referred to the next higher level. In reality, this system does not work as intended because medical care is primarily offered on a fee-for-service basis. This encourages those who can afford it to go directly to better-equipped facilities.[31]

Another claim is that healthcare facilities in China have improved as a result of market reforms. The State Statistical Bureau reported that the number of hospitals increased, from 2.02 hospital beds per thousand people to 2.39 beds in 1995.[32] Counting all healthcare workers trained at different levels, 1.62 physicians and 0.95 nurses per thousand people existed in 1995.[33] The *People's Republic of China (PRC) Yearbook 1996* also cheerfully reported that more investment had been placed on developing advanced medical science and technology. Sixty-seven Chinese institutes collaborating with the World Health Organization in different parts of China in 1995. These collaborative centers provide training for healthcare workers, funds for equipment, and exchange of scientific information. Research projects that had reached advanced international standards were undertaken. These included innovative methods on prevention and treatment of hepatitis B, cancer, cardiovascular, and cerebrovascular diseases, new contraceptive methods, reproductive technology such as in-vitro fertilization, partial liver transplants from living donors, the manufacturing of new drugs, medical instruments, and traditional Chinese remedies.[34] The availability of more advanced facilities implies a corresponding rise in healthcare costs.[35] This further complicates the issue of how to ration limited medical resources and who should benefit from these advances in medical care.

Another achievement often heralded is that the mortality and morbidity profile in China has become similar to that of developed countries. Cerebrovascular disease, malignant tumors, and heart trouble in urban areas and respiratory disease, cerebrovascular disease, and malignant tumors in rural areas were the first three major causes of death in 1996. Significant differences in the urban and rural areas are noted. Infectious disease and pulmonary tuberculosis remain problems of considerable concern in rural areas.[36] Official statistics reveal that the percentage of infectious diseases has declined over the past decades, but the difference between urban and rural areas remains significant. While 5.59% of diseases in urban areas were infectious or parasitic diseases, the percentage in rural areas was 7.52% in 1996.[37] On the other hand, the changing health profile indicates that more people suffer from chronic diseases. One of the characteristics of chronic disease is its pattern of recurrent remission and exacerbation, with no promise of a complete cure. For instance, people with diabetes mellitus must constantly monitor their blood glucose levels, together with taking precautions to prevent complications. Patients with cerebrovascular diseases most probably suffer from some degree of functional and cognitive impairment that renders them dependent, and those who are in a persistent vegetative state or irreversible coma demand total dependent care. As for patients with malignant tumors, pain, degenerative changes, and impending death are some particular features of their illness trajectory. These patients require long term care, which inevitably increase the demands on healthcare services.

### B. Medical Coverage

The *PRC Yearbook 1996* reported that patients are required to pay an average of 39.9 yuan for each outpatient consultation, and 1668 yuan for one hospitalization at an average stay of 14.7 days in government supported hospitals.[38] Since an average household expenditure per month ranges from 300 yuan to 1000 yuan, we can see that a majority of Chinese people cannot afford to pay their medical fees unless they got some kind of insurance coverage. In today's China, differences in opportunities for medical coverage between urban and rural areas are marked.

#### i. Rural Dwellers

People living in rural areas generally are not covered by public funds, but instead have to rely on co-operative medical funding schemes. Agricultural reforms, such as the introduction of the contract responsibility system, undermined the financial basis for rural health insurance as it did away with collectively organized finances at the commune and brigade levels. In the 1980s, these schemes largely collapsed. The villages with a co-operative medical scheme fell from about 84.5% in 1975 to about 5% in 1989.[39] This is an alarming figure. Since over 70% of China's populace lives in the countryside, this means that a sizeable majority has no medical insurance coverage.[40]

In the 1990s, experiments with co-operative healthcare schemes began. These are local, non-profit making, social security schemes responsible for organizing and financing rural health services on a collective basis. The objective of these schemes is to ensure access at low cost to essential health services to even their poorest members. They combine some insurance principles with practices of the old co-operative medical schemes, such as strict budgeting and risk sharing. Funding is generated from different sources, including households, collectives, and the local government, and is used to reimburse participants for part of their medical expenses. Management and ownership of these schemes take different forms. They can be owned or managed at either the village or township levels. These new schemes accounted for 13% of all healthcare schemes in 1991. They are becoming county-wide or even province-wide in some provinces, such as Jiangsu, Sichuan, and Shanxi. Feng Xueshan and associates contend that the problem of healthcare funding has not been solved in the poorer areas of China.[41] Since co-operative healthcare schemes only provide essential coverage, people need to pay non-essential medical expenses by themselves. Thus, those who lack the financial means still cannot gain access to medical services at a tertiary level regardless of the severity of their illnesses.

### ii. Urban Dwellers

People who have medical insurance are obviously a privileged class in the existing healthcare system. The government funds public insurance programs for employees working in state agencies, and worker insurance is provided to all permanent workers in state-owned enterprises and to some workers in collectively owned enterprises.[42] Chiu Waisang and Wong Cheongwing reported that in 1989 43.5% of the healthcare funds were spent on insurance for this group comprising only 10% of the population.[43] Veronica Pearson also noted that in 1994 approximately 200 million people—less than 20% of the population—were covered by the government and labor insurance schemes, yet they consumed nearly 60% of healthcare spending.[44] Not all city dwellers have medical insurance.

A survey conducted by Gail Henderson and associates affirmed that only the privileged group mentioned above had insurance coverage. In capital cities, over 50% of those interviewed were covered. At the county level, about 30% were covered. Only 7.4% had insurance coverage in rural villages. They investigated factors related to the distribution of medical insurance coverage in eight Chinese provinces in 1989. They found that the people more likely to have coverage were men who lived in more developed urban areas, had the capacity to work, had a higher level of education, had a higher per capita household income, and were either professionals or managers. Only 3.8% of subjects reporting farming as their primary occupation had insurance coverage.[45] The findings also revealed a striking difference between different employment sectors. While 86.3% of those working in state-owned work units had insurance coverage, only 8.7% of the sample were workers in the private, non-business sector. The percentage was even less in the private, agricultural sector, of only 3.4%.[46] This severely compromises the principle of equity in healthcare access, especially at the level of micro-allocation.[47]

C. Medical Costs

Since the introduction of market mechanisms to the healthcare system, ownership of healthcare facilities has become decentralized, with management going from the central government to the individual facilities, and with cost recovery as the foundation of their financing system. Government subsidies to hospitals have been reduced to basic salaries and minimal administrative costs including procurement and repairs of some expensive items.[48] In 1995, Ma Xu, a hospital administrator in Shanghai expressed his concern that the government was not investing enough in healthcare. He based his argument on the right of the people to have access to healthcare.[49] He contended that hospitals received less than 10% of public funding throughout the country. In some developed areas, such as Jiangsu Province, government subsidy had been reduced to less than 5%. He further pointed out that the public funds spent on healthcare were decreasing, from 3.1% in 1965, to 2.3% in 1975 and 2.4% in 1993, which is well below the standard 5% as recommended by the World Health Organization for developing countries. Ironically, he found that in 1993 the amount of public funds spent on entertainment was the same as that spent on healthcare.[50]

Ma characterized current healthcare financing as perverted, with insufficient funding and overspending of public money happening simultaneously.[51] Since healthcare facilities need to recover operational costs from user fees, one of the most often used strategies is to arbitrarily charge those with public medical insurance a higher fee. For instance, figures in 1991 showed that the hospital stay of patients with insurance coverage was longer than that of self-financed patients, with 147% more for patients suffering from viral hepatitis and 69% more for those with lobar pneumonia.[52] Another common strategy used to recover operational costs is to mark up drug charges. For instance, in 1978, the percentage of the total retail value of drugs in the country sold by healthcare facilities was 37.3%. By the end of 1988 this share rose to 57.19%. The reason was healthcare facilities over-prescribed drugs to generate revenue.[53] Since both medical consultation fees and hospital fees are fixed as stipulated by the Ministry of Public Health, healthcare facilities have to resort to other means to recover costs. These include increasing the utilization of sophisticated medical tests and selling high-priced drugs. Presumably this practice can help healthcare facilities to be guaranteed some amount of income from public money, without asking those patients who are self-financed to pay more.

In recent years, measures have been implemented to control insurance costs. Deductibles or caps have been added to reimbursement policies, or rebates to individuals who did not spend beyond some level for healthcare.[54] This may help to cut down unnecessary expenses by those who have insurance coverage. Yet the vulnerable groups, such as children, the older persons, and individuals with chronic diseases become more disadvantaged in gaining access to medical services.

Undoubtedly, this perverted system has affected healthcare workers' ability to do their duties in accordance with the ethical mandate of serving the people wholeheartedly. Qiu Renzong believes this system of healthcare finance greatly compromises the fiduciary relationship between healthcare workers and patients. In his words,

> Although this [leasing-contract-responsibility] program lessens the financial expenditures of the central government, it poses a heavy burden upon the factory or institute where a patient is working. As a result of this program, a kind of crisis of trust in the relationship between physicians and patients exists. If the physician makes an all-out effort in treatment, the patient or relatives wonder if the physician only wants to get money from the treatment. If the physician's treatment is rather conservative, the patient and relatives wonder if the physician or hospital manager wants to save scarce resources for officials of high rank or other privileged patients.[55]

Qiu's concern is that problems such as overcharging may not be resolved merely by having healthcare workers' sense of morality fortified with the ideal of respect for life and serving the people wholeheartedly; the system itself is the source of the problem.

D. Utilization of Medical Services

Surveys on health service utilization reveal that one of the crucial determinants for a person to seek medical service is whether he or she gets insurance coverage.[56] A study was conducted in 1992 to investigate the reasons why terminally ill patients with insurance coverage had sought medical treatment. The findings revealed that, other than seeking a chançe for a cure and for relief of pain, the main reason was that they had insurance coverage (32 out of 35 patients). Of the three who expressed that they would seek medical care regardless of insurance coverage, two patients were more realistic about their incurable illnesses and eventually requested to return home.[57] Another survey conducted in Shanghai revealed that 24.5% of self-financed patients did not seek medical attention within two weeks of falling ill, whereas the percentage of patients who had insurance coverage was only 7.7%.[58]

Discrepancies in the utilization of medical services between urban and rural areas are marked as well. A national survey on the reasons why patients did not seek medical advice when they fell ill was conducted. In Twenty percent of patients from the countryside reported that they had financial difficulties, which stopped them from seeking medical advice.

Only 2% of city dwellers reported that they had similar difficulties. A survey conducted in Jilin Province in 1985 revealed that the hospitalization rate in cities was about 55%, but less than 35% in rural areas. The discrepancy in Shaanxi province was even more marked, varying from 60% to 25% in urban and rural areas respectively.[59] These surveys affirm the contention that ability to pay is one of the crucial determinants for people in seeking medical treatment, especially those living in the countryside.

### E. Practice of Treatment Withdrawal

Liu Yong investigated the phenomenon of forgoing treatments in China, and suggested two reasons why this practice prevails, especially in the countryside.[60] One reason is attributed to some cultural beliefs that if people die elsewhere, their souls cannot return home. Hence, often the wish of patients and families exists to take the sick home at their terminal stage of illness. The second reason noted by Liu is financial. It has been a practice that people are not willing to spend money on medical treatments without an assurance of complete cure. A popular folk saying among the Chinese exists, "be careful not to end up with futile treatment and wasting all your money." Liu contends that since 88% of the population has no insurance coverage, this traditional practice will continue in modern China. Decisions to forgo or continue treatment are usually made by patients' families, with or without patients' participation. Physicians provide information about patients' disease condition, treatment options and prognosis, but are excluded from the final decisions. When family members have decided that treatment should be withdrawn, they are required to sign a statement to the effect that was their voluntary decision to discontinue treatment, and that they will bear responsibility for the decision.

Liu further classifies withdrawal of treatment into active and passive withdrawal. In the first situation, patients' explicit wishes are taken into account. In the second situation, patient's consent is not sought because he or she is in a state of clouded consciousness. Liu argues that both practices are ethical as long as withdrawal of treatment is in accordance to patients' implied or expressed wishes. He justifies his stance by pointing out that the decision can relieve patients' families from the burden of unnecessary medical expenses, and medical resources can also be better utilized. He warns that these practices will be unethical if patients' families refuse treatment even though a good chance of recovery exists. Yet he is confident that deeply rooted Chinese family values such as filial piety and humaneness and the fear of public opprobrium are sufficient to maintain acceptable ethical practices in the community.[61] What is left unexplored by Liu is how to distinguish between patients whose conditions rendered medical intervention futile and patients whose conditions could be benefited from medical care. If relieving the burden of medical bills justifies the family's decision to forgo treatment, then the rule of cost-benefit based on utilitarian grounds is observed, instead of making a decision based on a clinical judgment that the patient is in an incurable stage of an illness.

Zhang Zanning compared the practices of treatment withdrawal in China and that of the Western countries and concluded that "passive euthanasia" was more liberally practiced in China. Zhang sees the common practice of withdrawing treatment, and taking terminal patients home as a kind of passive euthanasia. He noted that legal matters that had raised heated debates in the West, such the case of Nancy Cruzan and Baby Doe, were not seen as issues with legal consequences in China.[62] In China, the decisions of patients' families can always override physicians' preferences for treatment, without ending up in court, as happened to the Cruzan family. He shared some of his experiences as a village physician to illustrate his point. Once he took care of a feverish patient with renal failure. The patient was delirious and confused during her hospital stay. At the time, the patient showed some positive signs of recovery of renal function, but her family members concluded that no chance of recovery existed, and decided to take the patient back home. Zhang disagreed, but could not convince the family, and nothing he could do but accept the family's decision. He later visited the patient at home so that treatment could be continued, and fortunately the patient eventually recovered. Zhang argues that passive euthanasia in terms of withdrawal of treatments have always been an accepted practice in China. As for the ethical justification, instead of upholding clinical evidence of futility in treatment, or respect for patients' rights to informed consent, the wish of patients' families is paramount. He feels, though, that this does not imply that Chinese people lack concepts of humanism and medical morality, but they are more pragmatic in evaluating the medical costs and possible benefits in treatment decisions.[63]

In sum, a majority of people in China cannot afford medical services unless they have some kind of coverage, and the current system of healthcare finance and medical insurance schemes provide coverage only to a privileged few. Survey findings reveal that the main determinant for people in utilizing medical services is whether they are financially covered. The practice of forgoing treatment is common especially in the countryside. This can be due to the traditional cultural view that the terminally ill to die at home is the best. Ample evidence exists that financial considerations are also a crucial factor in the continuation of this practice. In other words, treatment is often withdrawn from patients who may not be in a state of illness that renders medical treatment futile. Further reform to make healthcare services more equitably accessible to those who are in need is needed. Presumably, healthcare workers will experience moral tensions if they are mandated to uphold values respecting life within a context with inequitable and discriminatory healthcare access.

### 3. Superior Quality of Birth

In contrast to the ethical mandate to respect all life, the Party uses the slogan "quality of life" to promote its population control policies. The "one-child" family policy was proclaimed in 1979, with legislation intended to enhance superior quality of birth enacted along with its implementation. These include the 1988 law enacted in Gansu Province that prohibits reproduction by mentally-retarded persons, and the 1995 Maternal and Infant Law mandating premarital screening for different hereditary, reproductive and mental disorders. The socio-economic considerations in implementing such stringent population control policies are clear. In 1971, China instituted its first national family planning program by propagating the slogan "one is not too few, two are just right, three too many." This policy was found to be successful in bringing the birth rate down from 33.43 to 18.21 per thousand between 1970 and 1980 and the fertility rate down from 5.7% in the 1950s to 2.5% in 1980.[64] The target of slowing down population growth was still difficult to reach because of improvements in average life expectancy. The death rate decreased from 17 per thousand in 1952 to 6.34 per thousand in 1980, while the average life expectancy reached 69 years in 1980. China's population grew from 575 million in 1952 to 963 million in 1975, and had already reached 1.2 billion in 1996. Chinese officials are worried that the demands of this alarmingly huge population will soon outstrip China's natural and economic resources. Restricting population growth is seen as crucial to achieving the central task of China's modernization, and fostering economic growth and improving the people's quality of life.[65]

#### A. Issues Regarding the One-child Family Policy

Over the past two decades, China's population control policies have elicited ambivalent responses from the international community. Measures need to be undertaken to curb China's population growth, but many cannot agree with the way in which China implements its control policies.[66] Reliable sources report that coercion has been substantially used to meet the pre-set quota of new births, which violates the basic human right of freedom of choice. This goes against United Nation's recommendations. According to the World Population Plan of Action 1974, all countries are required to "respect and ensure, regardless of their overall demographic goals, the right of persons to determine, in a free, informed and responsible manner, the number and spacing of their children."[67] Abortion has been carried out so liberally that it has disturbed those who are pro-life, and those who advocate reproductive rights.[68]

Another disturbing issue is female infanticide, which practice became more serious in the 1980s. This issue was first officially addressed by absolving the government of any responsibility, but blaming the people for their lingering feudal attitudes in wanting a son to carry on the family line.[69] The government did take steps to lessen the problem. In the countryside, some places allow a couple to try for a second child after a five-year gap if the first child is a girl, while some areas permit a second child irrespective of the sex of the first child. In the cities, the policy is stricter. Yet some places allow a couple to try a second child in either one of the following conditions: (1) the first child has a birth defect; (2) in the case of remarriage, if one partner has no child from the previous marriage; (3) they hold some undesirable or dangerous occupations, such as mine workers; or (4) both partners are themselves from one-child families. The last condition implies that the policy will apply for only one generation.[70]

Since the establishment of the one-child policy, the changing population demography has shown some worrying signs. In particular, the ratio of male to female children is becoming increasingly unbalanced, and, the ratio of dependant elderly and children to the adults they are dependent on is changing. The 1990 Census revealed that China had kept the rate of population growth relatively constant, with a population of 1.143 billion, and a birth rate of 21.06 per thousand. Compared with the 1982 Census, the population had increased by 12.45%, the birth rate by 0.07%, and the natural growth rate by 0.15%, with a decrease in the death rate of 0.08%.[71] Changes in the population structure were more alarming. Significantly more men than women existed, with the ratio increased by 0.3% in 1990 census. Therese Hesketh and Zhu Weixing reported that the ratio of males to females in reported births was as high as 115:100 in rural Hebei and 116:100 in Shaanxi in the early 1980s. The 1995 population survey reported average ratios of around 108:100 in rural areas.[72] The number of elderly people also increased markedly. The number of people over sixty or above will increase dramatically in the coming decades, from 7.6% of total population in 1982 to 14.7% by 2000, and 28.7% by 2032.[73]

Jing Qicheng notes that this aging trend in the population will eventually change the profile of the urban population from a pyramid to an inverted pyramid in fifty years time, with the rural population structure remaining a pyramid until 2040 due to less successful family planning programs in rural areas. Jing postulates that urban China will be having a working force of less than one half of the total population supporting more than one half of the total population, consisting of the quite young and the quite old. Traditionally, socialization of the interdependent roles within the Chinese family first takes place in the form of children's dependence on parents. Later, when the parents become elderly, they rely on their adult children to care for them. Children are taught from a young age that their filial duty exists to look after their parents when they grow old. Jing points out that changes in intergenerational patterns of population distribution will inevitably upset the traditional values that place importance on interdependence in the family. He worries that these changes in intergenerational patterns may cause dilemmas for adults to whom they should invest their resources, their children or their elderly parents.[74] Because the phenomenon of concentrated devotion to children to the neglect of the aged has already emerged. A 1991 study conducted by Liu Xian and associates in Wuhan revealed that elderly people in China were under strong pressure to provide more social support, instrumental support in particular, to their children and other relatives, while they received less.[75]

Tu Ping expresses similar worries in his analysis of population aging in China. He found that China's population is aging at an unprecedented rate, faster than developed countries like Japan, Sweden, Germany, and the United Kingdom. Looking at it in terms of the balance between population age and economic development, China is aging faster, with less economic development, than has been the experience of other countries. The country has to face the problems of having an aged population before it has had sufficient time or resources to establish an adequate security system for the elderly. Tu notes that the reduction in the number of dependent children in the family often leads to an increase in the level of current consumption, instead of a significant increase in productive investment or long term savings for care in old age. The increased dependency burden due to the growth of the aged population poses bigger demands on emerging social security systems and services for the elderly. He further argues that presently it might be more prudent to enact a two-child instead of one-child family policy. This could balance the restricted population growth and reduce the burden the current generation of adults will place on the next generation.[76]

Judith Banister arrived at similar conclusions in her study of China's changing population. She contends that a two-child or voluntary family alternative would enhance instead of diminishing people's quality of life. She made two justifications, which I found quite valid. First, in the interests of the majority, many prefer to choose two or more children and to accept a lower per capita consumption over the alternative of one child with higher per capita consumption. More importantly, this helps to preserve the Chinese values that place high importance on love and devotion between generations in a family. Second, the proposed alternatives would improve the quality of life by reducing the strong incentive for female infanticide, and women would have their life quality improved by the restoration of reproductive freedom if mandatory birth restriction is lifted.[77]

## B. Eugenic Laws

Along with the implementation of the one-child policy, maternal and child health policies are instituted with the intention of ensuring that children are born healthy and improving the quality of life of the entire population. While the international community often describes these as eugenic laws and has reservations about the ethics of these policies, debating on the extent communal control of reproduction to ensure "the best babies" is ever justifiable.[78] Chinese officials take a defensive stance, rationalizing that eugenics in a Chinese sense means *you sheng you yue* (優生優養), as "better birth, better care" and does not have the negative overtones of illuminating an unwanted race as what the Nazi did.[79] As far as prenatal care is concerned, Chinese authorities defend these laws as being solely for the purpose of prioritizing resources and improving the quality of services. Such activities largely involve publicity about healthier and better births and more encouraging premarital healthcare. Healthcare workers are required to offer advice on better prenatal care and provide prenatal diagnosis, treatment of genetic diseases, and fetal monitoring.[80]

Reasons exist to worry over these so-called eugenic laws. Along with some positive measures to improve prenatal health also come measures to eliminate the incidence of children with birth defects. In 1988, Gansu Province passed the first law in China prohibiting mentally-retarded people from having children. Women diagnosed as being mentally retarded must be sterilized before getting married or they must have their pregnancies terminated. Following Gansu's example, many provinces drafted similar regulations for mandatory sterilization of mentally-retarded persons.[81] Two major controversies are raised. First, evidence exists that mental retardation is often due to dietary deficiency and environmental factors instead of defective genes. This means that the problem should be dealt with by improving nutrition and living conditions instead of mandatory sterilization.[82] Second, the implementation of these laws are mandatory, which contain no provisions which could be described as either guidance, or as accommodating, or ensuring individual choice. As Linda Johnson pointed out, they reflect a national policy that desires a perfected race by resorting to science as a means to eradicate the unfit, by a justification based upon practical social benefits that largely undermines the concern for human life and respect for personal rights.[83]

New controversies emerged when China passed the Maternal and Infant Law in June 1995. This law supports the systematic implementation of premarital medical check-ups in order to detect whether one of the couple suffers from serious hereditary, venereal, or reproductive disorders, and relevant mental disorders or legally contagious diseases. Those deemed unsuitable for reproduction should undergo sterilization, abortion, or remain celibate in order to prevent inferior birth.[84] Although the law explicitly points to voluntary sterilization and individual choice, we may wonder just how much freedom an at-risk couple has when they are mandated not to have a defective child. One of the worrying signs of this law is that it promotes the concept of "superior birth," without making clear exactly how to tell "normal" birth from "inferior" birth.[85] Pro-life humanists are especially worried that, with these regulations, the practice of infanticide will become more common in China.

To summarize, the government places much emphasis on controlling the population growth through its policies promoting the birth of healthy, "normal" children. While emphasis is placed on producing healthy children, these policies do discriminate against "defective" or "abnormal" children, in essence making some lives more worthy of respect than others. Obviously, this quality orientation challenges the ethical basis of the mandate for healthcare workers, who are required to respect human life through positive actions to rescue the dying and heal the wounded. These population policies and the subsequently changed population composition inevitably create tensions for healthcare workers in meeting their role responsibilities. Healthcare workers are the ones who have to implement these birth policies. Since they need to put the interests of the country before individual interests, conflicts inevitable emerge when dealing with persons who are reluctant to comply. This undoubtedly hinders healthcare workers in establishing fiduciary relationships with their patients.[86] On the other hand, greater demand for healthcare by the elderly is inevitable. The issue of taking care of the elderly within the existing system of healthcare, where access depends on a person's ability to pay, has to be addressed. Chinese medical ethics that emphasize the duty to take positive action to save life and cure disease may not be able to address the healthcare needs of the elderly, who are highly likely to be suffering from chronic ailments instead of acute illnesses.

## 4. Euthanasia as a Medical Measure

While the government promotes superior quality of birth and quality of life, voices in support of quality of dying are also emerging. Concepts of brain death and euthanasia were officially criticized as products of capitalist society before 1978. A passage representing this stance reads

> Some Western bourgeois doctors engaged in organ transplantation run counter to science, and even go so far as to inhumanly and brutally pose a deceitful, absurd theory—"brain death"—in order to unscrupulously open up the source of grafts for organ transplantation from the dying patients.[87]

Euthanasia was seen as a perverted product of Western society that was not congruent with the principle of "revolutionary humanism."[88] Changes in attitude toward death and dying are noticeable in the 1980s. In 1980, a journal, *Medicine and Philosophy*, was inaugurated by the Academy of Social Sciences in Beijing. This provides an open forum for Chinese scholars to share their views regarding contemporary bioethical issues. In 1988, physicians and medical scientists voted their support for adopting brain death criteria to define death. In 1992, a draft of the criteria for brain death to be used as a legal definition in China was proposed in the Sino-American Symposium on Heart Transplantation. In 1990, legislation to legalize active euthanasia was first proposed. With a claim of public support, a draft of legislation legalizing euthanasia as a medical measure was proposed in the National People's Congress in 1995.[89] Although relevant laws have not yet been enacted, the euthanasia movement over the past decade signifies that life and death values have been changing in modern China. This in turn raises issues over the relevance of the traditional mandate in defining the ethical requirements of healthcare workers. In the following I will review the debate among Chinese scholars over the definitions of euthanasia, the values inherent in these definitions, and the ways in which the public's views are presented in support of legalizing euthanasia.

### A. The Euthanasia Movement

In 1980, publication of Qiu's paper entitled *Concepts of Death and Euthanasia* marked the Party leadership's change to a more tolerant attitude toward brain death and euthanasia issues.[90] Since then, considerable effort has been made to examine the conceptual, medical, ethical, and legal aspects of euthanasia.[91] The Greek word means "good death" etymologically. Its more specialized meaning in some Western languages is quite recent.[92] Here are two possible Chinese translations of the term "euthanasia": *anlesi* (安樂死), which means peaceful and happy death; the other is *wutong zhisi* (無痛致死), which means end a life without causing any pain.[93] Feng Xinyun summarized discussion of the definitions of euthanasia over the past decade, and found that a consensus has not yet reached.[94] Although the first translation is more widely accepted, debate is still open for conceptualizing euthanasia as a cause of death or a state of dying. While the concept of *wutong zhisi* is more preferred by people holding the view that euthanasia is a medical measure to end a life in a painless way, *anlesi* is more preferred by people who attempt to comprehend the meaning of euthanasia within the context of Chinese cultural practices.

### B. Definitions of Euthanasia

Those who define euthanasia as a cause of death claim that euthanasia is a kind of clinical management. But different views exist on the ethics of using euthanasia as a medical measure. Lin Yiegang claims that the definition of euthanasia should not include passive euthanasia since forgoing treatments of the terminally ill with the intention of letting the person die in peace has been a traditional practice in China and is permissible by law. This view may be justifiable if one is interested in a purely legalistic definition of euthanasia. Zhang Zanning, a lawyer, responded to Lin's suggestion. He argues that both active and passive medical measures in clinical management can cause a person's death, and situations exist where "not doing anything" may cause more suffering and pain prior to death than "doing something" to bring an end to life. He further states that even though euthanasia in the form of forgoing treatment is not considered a crime under existing Chinese law, it still should be recognized as a kind of euthanasia.[95]

The dialogue between Lin and Zhang reflects that the distinction between letting someone die and killing, which hotly debated in the West, is only gently addressed in China. The major concern is how to justify the legalization euthanasia as a form of clinical management. Arguments are raised whether euthanasia is a special type of death distinguishable from suicide, assisted suicide, natural death from disease, homicide, and entrusted homicide. To differentiate euthanasia from other forms of death, Zhang suggests that justifications of euthanasia have to be grounded in ethical principles. After summarizing the euthanasia debates of his time, Zhang formulated a definition that he claims is adaptable to China's cultural conditions. He defines euthanasia as

> a medical measure administered to patients by healthcare workers on compassionate ground to hasten or end their lives in a painless state. The decision is based on the clinical evidence that patients are suffering from an incurable disease, are in intractable pain, and the decision is not contrary to their wishes.[96]

Ending the life of seriously defective newborns and quite low birth-weight infants would not fit Zhang's definition of euthanasia. This definition limits candidates for justifiable euthanasia to the comatose and the terminally ill.

Zhang claims three ethical principles in his definition. They are "do no harm," "inflict no pain," and "do not go against the patient's will." No harm will be done because the patient's death is already imminent. Any measures to prolong life will only prolong dying. Although Zhang states that patients' wishes have to be respected, he is cautious not to state it as a positive statement such as "in accordance with the patient's voluntary consent." He purposely avoids the terms "upon voluntary request of the patient" or "request by the patient's family" to leave open the possibility that the patient may choose someone from outside the family to act as his or her proxy in making decisions regarding euthanasia.[97]

In Zhang's definition, three conditions need to be met to justify euthanasia. They involve the intention of the persons involved in deciding the act, the clinical status of the patient, and the means to end the person's life. The distinction between active and passive euthanasia, voluntary and non-voluntary euthanasia is not defined in this case. This may reflect the cultural conditions of China, where forgoing treatment for the terminally ill has been practiced for generations, and protective medical care instead of patient's right to informed consent takes precedence in current practice. In 1993, Qiu Renzong and Jin Dajie cited Zuo X-Q's definition that further limits the scope of euthanasia as

> an action that ends in advance or does not prolong a patient's life, performed from motives of compassion to the terminally ill in respect of her or his right to death with dignity and upon his or her request.[98]

In comparison with Zhang's definition, this definition affirms patients' right to choose death and emphasizes patients' expressed consent. A justifiable euthanasia act is confined to conscious patients in their terminal stage of illness. Both active and passive means to end a patient's life are included.

Apparently, Zuo's definition is more acceptable to the medical community. In 1995, draft legislation on euthanasia was forwarded to China's National People's Congress by 30 deputies. This draft proposes that euthanasia be legally carried out only in technically advanced hospitals in urban areas. The patients' relatives must give their consent in a certified letter, and the application for euthanasia must be approved by at least two medical experts. The purpose is said to alleviate suffering by patients and their relatives and to safeguard the dignity of life.[99] The proposed legislation includes safeguards against the abuse of euthanasia, the ethically questionable act of ending the lives of patients in irreversible coma, severely defective newborns, or quite low birth weight infants are not ruled out. The popular view holds that justification for these acts lies somewhere else. Yao Xuange and Yu Dehua contended that patients in irreversible coma are already dead by brain-death criteria, so ending their life is merely a matter of formal pronouncement of death, instead of a euthanasia act proper.[100] Ending the lives of severely handicapped infants belongs to the realm of "superior quality of birth," and therefore should not be considered under the scope of euthanasia.[101]

Another view holds that euthanasia is more than just a clinical problem, a societal issue also exists. Shi Dapu argues that the Chinese translation *anlesi* (安樂死), which means dying in peace and happiness, is congruent with Chinese cultural norms. He points out that the Chinese believe in two major life events that deserve celebration. One is the day of birth and the other is the day of death. A celebrated death is characterized by "passing away smilingly," or "ending the life in one's bed during sleep after a good meal."[102] Since dying in peace and happiness is a desirable form of death, euthanasia appears to provide a way for those suffering from unrelieved pain in their terminal state of illness, or irreversible coma, to die in peace.

Feng suggests that a good death in such conditions can be attained by two means. One is by controlling pain and suffering, and the second is by directly ending a patient's intractable pain. Both means share the same purpose of improving the quality of life in its final stage and in fostering a superior quality of death. People supporting this view do not believe that a death from euthanasia is any different from a natural death due to disease, or a sudden death due to accident. Neither can it be considered similar to suicide or homicide. They claim that euthanasia only fosters a better state of dying, and is therefore "scientific and civilized," demonstrating mankind's advances in the quality of life.[103]

This view of euthanasia as a form of good death opens debate on what kind of life is worth living, and what kind of life is so unlivable that death is deemed justified. More importantly, upon whose standard and under what criteria can a person's quality of life be evaluated? In line with the population control policies that propagate "superior quality of birth, superior quality of child rearing and better life quality," it has been suggested that a fourth should be added, which may be called "superior quality of death." The ultimate goal of such discussion is to improve the nation's quality of life.[104] It has been officially proposed that a person has lived a worthwhile life if he or she made a contribution to mankind for his or her entire life. The emphasis is placed on one's entire life, thus that the contributions would continue right unto death. We can see that this set of values is consistent with the virtue of "having a sense of socialist responsibility" propagated in Mao's teachings,

> All men must die, but death can vary in its significance. The ancient Chinese writer Chien Szuma said, "Though death befalls all men alike, it may be heavier than Mount Tai or lighter than a feather." To die for the people is heavier than Mount Tai, but to work for the fascists and die for the exploiters and oppressors is lighter than a feather.[105]

One obvious difference exists. The life values promoted today do not emphasize a distinction between the people and class enemies such as fascists and exploiters whom one should not serve. Instead emphasis is placed on relationship between the individual and the common good of the nation. In this respect, life quality is to be evaluated primarily by a person's social worth, which is narrowly defined as social utility. To follow the logic of this argument, if a person becomes a burden to society, his or her value diminishes, and so does his or her quality of life. In such a situation, a person can only demonstrate social worth by accepting a positive duty to die.[106]

Yao and Yu suggest an ethical justification for voluntary and non-voluntary euthanasia using this social-worth-equals-quality-of-life argument.[107] They summarize two kinds of justifiable requests for voluntary euthanasia. The act is most praiseworthy if a person makes a "living will" stipulating the conditions under which the person should be euthanasized and stipulating that his or her organs should be donated for transplant. This shows that the person does not want to become a burden to others and to society, and he or she is willing to make his or her death more meaningful to others by donating his or her organs after death. The act is also acceptable if a patient is in unbearable and intractable pain and asks his or her relatives and physician to end his or her life. This act is justifiable because the outcome of this act causes no burden, but benefits society and other people in the sense that medical resources will not be wasted to prolong life. On the other hand, Yao and Yu suggest two kinds of acts that are not praiseworthy. The first one is when people kill themselves because they want to make others regret perceived past injustices—as an act of revenge. The second kind is when people ask for expensive medicine in order to prolong their lives without considering the burdens that this can cause their families or the community. To justify euthanasia for comatose patients, Yao and Yu maintain that families' requests should be considered ethical if their intention is to relieve the patients of mental and physical suffering. Likewise, to spend medical resources on patients whose chance of recovery is minimal is equally not ethical.[108]

In sum, two different views exist in defining euthanasia in China. One focuses on euthanasia as a cause of death, and the second as a state of death. Both views appeal to different ethical justifications. The first appeals to ethical principles such as "do no harm" and "respect the patient's wishes." The second focuses on quality of life, but bases its argument on social worth, such as social utility and avoiding financial burdens. Most Chinese scholars appear to be unwilling to debate with each other to challenge the limitations of these viewpoints. Both views coexist, and in their particular ways shape the euthanasia movement in China. The first leads to the proposal of legalizing active euthanasia, and the second represents an increasing awareness of improving end-of-life care with an aim of promoting quality of death.

One unique feature is that the fine line between voluntary and non-voluntary euthanasia, and active and passive euthanasia blurs in the main stream of argument in support of euthanasia. Feng considers euthanasia justifiable if it can promote a good death without causing a burden to others, regardless of the means. He suggests setting up a special institute for handling patients who request active euthanasia, while patients asking for passive euthanasia can be taken care of by a specialist, a "good death therapist" in the existing healthcare facilities.[109] Coming with the movement to legalize euthanasia, hospice care has begun to develop in some large cities in China, beginning in 1988. The first hospice care research center was set up in Tianjin in 1988. A free-standing hospice was founded in Shanghai in the same year.[110] People who advocate hospice care are generally not uncomfortable with the idea of using euthanasia as a medical measure to end a life at the terminal stage of illness. Wang Yanxiong and Bai Hongmei suggest that promotion of hospice service is appropriate for China's national conditions because the demand for care of the aged and the dying is increasing. While they state the aim of hospice care is to foster a good death, they do not exclude the possibility of using euthanasia as a medical measure to promote it. Ma Mingzhi expresses this stance more explicitly in his attempt to clarify the concept between hospice care and euthanasia. He argues that euthanasia belongs to the realm of hospice care, since both serve the same purpose of promoting a good death.[111] This phenomenon is unfamiliar to Hong Kong. People in Hong Kong who advocate hospice care tend to hold a firm stance against legalization of active euthanasia.[112]

### C. Public Views on Euthanasia

Discussion of euthanasia is not confined to the academic arena. Bioethicists and other interested parties have been conducting surveys to evaluate the public's acceptance of euthanasia. In 1985, Qiu conducted the first survey about people's choice of options in four different medical conditions. They were: a newborn with serious congenital heart disease, a one month old female baby with microencephaly, an irreversibly comatose patient, and a person with terminal cancer in intractable pain. Responses were elicited from a convenience sample of students, professionals and healthcare workers. Farmers and workers were not surveyed. Findings revealed that more than half of the respondents (62.4%) favored active euthanasia for the microencephalic baby. Agreement varied from 14.7% to 39.4% in the other three cases.[113]

In 1988, Hu Peicheng conducted a similar survey in Hubei Province. Four hundred people's views were gathered, including workers, peasants, white-collar workers, and healthcare workers. Findings revealed that healthcare workers showed the most support for active euthanasia in at least one of the four cases (84.38%), and peasants the least (27.27%). Respondents with higher education showed a higher percentage of support than that of the illiterate (87% versus 36.36%). This survey showed that healthcare workers were more in favor of active euthanasia than were lay people. Most probably new concepts of this kind are first discussed within the circle of healthcare workers, and then spread to intellectuals and students. Hu suggests that only if people change their values so as not to consider longevity to be the equivalent of a good quality of life, will they accept euthanasia as an ethical practice.[114]

Discussion of euthanasia in the mass media began when the first documented legal case of active euthanasia was reported in Shanxi province in 1986 that the deceased's son, youngest daughter, and the physician were arrested and persecuted for murder. The deceased was a fifty-nine years old woman who had suffered from cirrhosis with acites, coma, and liver-kidney syndrome, and serious bedsores. The physician gave an injection of chlorpromazine upon the request of her son and youngest daughter that resulted in the death of the patient. The deceased's two other daughters brought the case to court.[115] A special column on euthanasia in the magazine *Public Health* was started. Most people spoke favorably of the idea of *anlesi* (安樂死), but not especially in support of active euthanasia. These respondents included Deng Yingchao, the widow of Zhou Enlai, who expressed her support for *anlesi*, and claimed that the idea was in line with dialectical materialism. She indicated that she had already written her living will that she did not want any emergency treatment when her life was near its end.[116] Deng's words should not be taken as just one among many responses from the public, but as a representative voice of the Party leadership. Her message is in line with the life values promulgated by the Party leadership since the 1990s. Of all articles on euthanasia that appeared in *Chinese Medical Ethics*, the journal issued by the Ministry of Public Health since 1988, they were basically in support of euthanasia.

The defendants in the Shanxi case were eventually found not guilty after a five-year's trial. The final ruling stated that the act of injecting the drug had caused a hastening of death of the woman, but the dose was within the limits of normal use, and did not directly cause the defendant's death. The act was considered willful in that it deprived a citizen of life, but the ruling also held that this act was not significantly serious, and no grave harm had been done.[117] This ruling obviously signifies the Chinese government's permissiveness toward active euthanasia. People who support legalization of euthanasia welcomed the ruling since it established a precedent for active euthanasia in China.[118]

In the 1990s, two voices regarding end-of-life care were heard in China, one spoke for legalizing active euthanasia, the second spoke for developing hospice care services for the terminally ill. In 1991, a nationwide exploratory study was conducted to learn about peoples' attitudes toward end-of-life care. Opinions were gathered from 454 respondents by means of random sampling. Findings revealed that 65% of the sample accepted not to maintain the life of a patient who is in a persistent vegetative state, and 45.6% felt the same way concerning severely handicapped infants. Only 27.5% supported active euthanasia for terminally ill patients, and less than half agreed with palliative care or withholding artificial nutrition. Younger respondents with higher education showed more support for euthanasia-type medical management. Han Junde, He Lixin, and Hou Shuangqi note that the traditional concept of the sanctity of life is undergoing a transformation to a quality of life orientation, especially among intellectuals and the younger generations. Since a majority still does not accept active euthanasia, a further expansion of hospice service would appear to be a more appropriate option for China at present. When they were asked about their life values, most respondents regarded contributing to the welfare of mankind from life to death as their life goal (71.1%). Only 25% were willing to donate their organs after their death. Eighty-one percent of elderly people surveyed said they were psycho-logically prepared for their death, and 69.2% indicated that they wanted a painless death even if their life had to be shortened.[119] These findings suggest that many people may have adopted the life values propagated by the Party, but only a few people would accept organ donation as an expression of their last possible contribution to society.

This distinct contrast indicates either that people only pay lip service to the life values propagated by the Party, or the findings reflect that traditional life values are still more prevalent. I believe the second view to be correct. Organ procurement has been a problem in the Chinese communities, and in countries like Japan where family values precede individual values. One explanation is that people may be willing to help family members, whom they identify as in-group, but are not willing or able to have the same concern for people whom they see as outsiders. Hence, live instead of cadaver transplants by blood-bond relative donors are more acceptable in Eastern cultures. The second reason may be due to the deeply rooted belief that a good death requires the whole body. This is based on the Confucian teaching that hair and skin should not be damaged since they are inherited from one's parents. According to this principle, all invasive procedures should be prohibited because they could constitute impious acts.[120]

Further surveys were conducted in different parts of China in the 1990s. The questions were more focused than those in the earlier surveys from the 1980s. They mainly aimed at gathering people's opinion on whether active euthanasia was an acceptable means to end the life of a patient who had an incurable illness, suffered from intractable pain, and voluntarily requested a painless death. Guo Qingxiu and associates reported that about 70% of people in Tianjin would support a euthanasia request of this kind. In Shanghai, over 90% of respondents showed their support, with 89.45% of people over sixty years old indicating their support. Over 90% of respondents expressed the view that legalization of active euthanasia was needed.[121]

These euthanasia opinion surveys were conducted in large cities where medical services are more accessible and most people have insurance coverage. They are freer than rural dwellers to make treatment choices in situations of impending death. Taking into account the logic of care responsibilities in traditional Chinese society, people are obligated to take care of their sick family members, but at the same time they would not want to become a burden on others. Hence, people are more easy to accept ending their lives if they were suffering from intractable pain and already in a state of terminal illness. This situation would be viewed quite differently by persons living in the countryside. Access to medical care is a serious issue for these people; they are forced to forgo treatment if they are not able to pay. Hence, they tend to be more concerned with how to survive hardship instead of having the luxury of thinking about whether euthanasia is justifiable.

These survey findings are used to back-up the voices in support of active euthanasia. Positive signals are emerging, demonstrating that the time to legalize euthanasia in China could be near. First, surveys show that most people support administering active euthanasia for people with an incurable disease and with intractable pain, hence legalization of active euthanasia is in accordance with the wish of the masses. Second, social and moral values are in a state of flux. Advocating a good death is in line with the government policies of "superior quality of birth, superior quality of child rearing, and better quality of life." Third, legal cases regarding active euthanasia have raised public concern of what kind of punishment should be due to the defendants of such cases. Regarding these defendants as murderers appears unjust to most people. An obvious need exists for new legislation that both legalizes and regulates such cases.[122] Fourth, the practice of euthanasia can allow for more rational allocation of medical resources, leaving means for the development of hospice care and high-tech medicine in accordance to the needs of the people.[123]

Although the proposed legislation did not pass in 1995, continuous efforts in pursuit of the legalization of euthanasia are underway. One of the latest surveys, reported by Yang Yulan and Lei Yanhong in the Eighth National Conference held by the Middle Youth Committee of the Chinese Medical Ethics Association in 1997, reveals that out of a sample of 3302, 94.8% indicated their support for voluntary active euthanasia. This survey can be seen as another attempt to affirm that the legalization of euthanasia is adaptable to China's conditions.[124]

Voices in support of legalizing euthanasia are apparently becoming stronger. Amongst these voices we can hear some worries being expressed. Vera Rich pointed that, even though the proposed legislation might have been inspired by the highest of humanitarian motives, it cannot help but to also carry considerable economic overtones.[125] A majority of the people have to pay their own way in accessing medical care; as yet no social security system exists for those who do not have the ability to pay; and the number of dependent elderly is also increasing. We may wonder to what extent those vulnerable patients would be allowed to make such choices if euthanasia were legalized. With an official policy imposing life values that cherish social worth, a logic will follows, with those who are a burden on society to have a duty to end their lives. This leads to an even more chilling consideration: does this also imply a duty of healthcare workers to identify those who have become a burden on society, those who are no longer worthy of living? This view is obviously not in accordance with the notion of respect for life. Undoubtedly, value changes are already underway. In 1995, the Chinese Medical Ethics Association reviewed the goals of medicine in its Eighth Annual Conference, entitled "Medical goals, quality of life, and medical ethics."[126]A position statement was drafted stating that the renewed medical goals should be

> To treat disease, maintain life, lower the mortality rate, prevent illnesses, decrease the morbidity rate, improve the quality of life, cultivate a better living environment, and foster mental and physical health.[127]

These developments signify that the ethical mandate has undergone further evolution, with the concept of quality of life as guiding principle. How these changes change nurses' views on their role requirements within the clinical context is a question that I will explore in the empirical study reported in the following chapters.

## 5. Summary

I have attempted to make sense of the mandate in the Chinese medical ethics tradition that requires healthcare workers to respect life, take positive action to save life, cure disease, and treat patients with altruistic motives. Unprecedented changes that have taken place in China over the past two decades directly challenge the ethical basis of this mandate.

Three major issues have been discussed. The first issue is related to provision of healthcare. Although much has been claimed about improvements in health, and advances in healthcare facilities, healthcare access in China has become increasingly restrictive with the implementation of market mechanisms in hospital management. Free medical coverage is only available to a privileged group comprising less than 20% of the population. Those who cannot pay are not able to get adequate medical attention. Forgoing treatment is a common practice, especially in the countryside. We may argue that limited healthcare access is a common phenomenon in other countries that do not provide free medical services, but I would argue that China's situation is more acute. This is because China has yet to establish a social security system to help those in desperate need, and has yet to set up a medical insurance scheme to ease the financial difficulty of those who do not have medical coverage provided by public funds. How can healthcare workers serve the people wholeheartedly if they are unable to serve those who require medical attention but cannot afford to pay the fee?

The second issue is China's population control policies, which promote the national goal of constructing a socialist China through fostering "superior quality of birth and superior quality of child rearing." While emphasis is placed on improving birth quality, it also implies that some lives may not reach minimum standards of quality thus be without value. Obviously, this quality orientation challenges the ethical basis of the mandate for healthcare workers, who are required to respect human life by taking positive action to save lives and cure disease.

The third issue is euthanasia. Reflecting on the euthanasia movement in China, we find that the Party intends to promote a set of life values with a strong quality orientation. In this view, an individual's quality of life is determined by whether one is able to make a contribution to society until the end of one's life. Instead of pursuing longevity as a life goal, the quality orientation argues that a superior quality of death is more important. In other words, a person who fails to maintain quality of life in the sense contributing to society, one may be duty-bound to end one's life. Not becoming a burden on other people or society could be considered as the person's last contribution to society. Obviously, people who express their support for the legalization of euthanasia as a medical measure hold these views. Reflecting on opinion surveys regarding people's views on euthanasia over the past decade, voices in support of legalizing euthanasia are apparently becoming stronger. Among these voices, worries are expressed that people who are identified as lacking value are not allowed an alternative to death. Furthermore, if a person's value is totally dependent on his social worth, it would then be logical to consider those who are a burden to society to have a duty to end their lives, or to have their lives ended by others. This vulnerable group could include low birth weight babies, handicapped children, and people in a persistent vegetative state, but also could include people who are not able to afford the medical expenses. This view is obviously not in accordance with notions of respect for life.

In summary, while the ethical mandate represents the values upheld in the Chinese medical ethics tradition, the emerging values that come along with China's socio-economic reforms inevitably change the orientation of medical care to an emphasis on cost containment and quality consciousness. These two sets of values co-exist in shaping healthcare practice. How these changes shape the ways nurses perceive their role requirements in fostering ethical practice within the clinical context is the issue that I would further examine in Chapters Five and Six, based on the empirical findings that I elicited from nurses in different parts of China.

# Five

# MULTIPLE ROLE RESPONSIBILITIES

As discussed in the previous three chapters, the ethical requirements of nurses in China were imported percepts that came along with the introduction of the Nightingale model of nursing, or political ideology propagated by the Party leadership. Recent literature on nursing morality in China focuses on the qualities of character nurses should possess in manifesting these rules of conduct, but nurses' voice was apparently ignored in formulating these codes for professional regulation. The objective here is to make sense of nurses' moral experience in practice contexts, the different situations encountered by nurses as presenting what they regard as ethically difficult situations, and to consider their view of principles, which should govern ethical practice, based on the findings of an empirical venture that I undertook in different parts of China. This chapter comprises three sections. The first section outlines this empirical venture. The second section discusses how nurses in China speak about nursing ethics and the third section attempts to make sense of their conceptualization of ethics in terms of eleven facets of nursing responsibilities.

## 1. The Triangulation Process in Action

The empirical inquiry, which characterizes a triangulation process in action, comprised three phases. As shown in Figure 5.1, it followed a directional flow from one single hospital to different parts of China. The mode of inquiry moved from an unstructured to a more structured one, and the role of the investigator changed from observer to interviewer to surveyor. The first phase was field observation and unstructured interviews in a comprehensive teaching hospital in Beijing. Five vignettes, as shown in Table 5.1, typified the difficult care situations nurses commonly encountered in day-to-day practice regarding information disclosure, withdrawal of treatment, requests for euthanasia, unmet needs of a demanding patient, and unmet needs of a silent patient were derived from the nurses' narratives and observation notes.

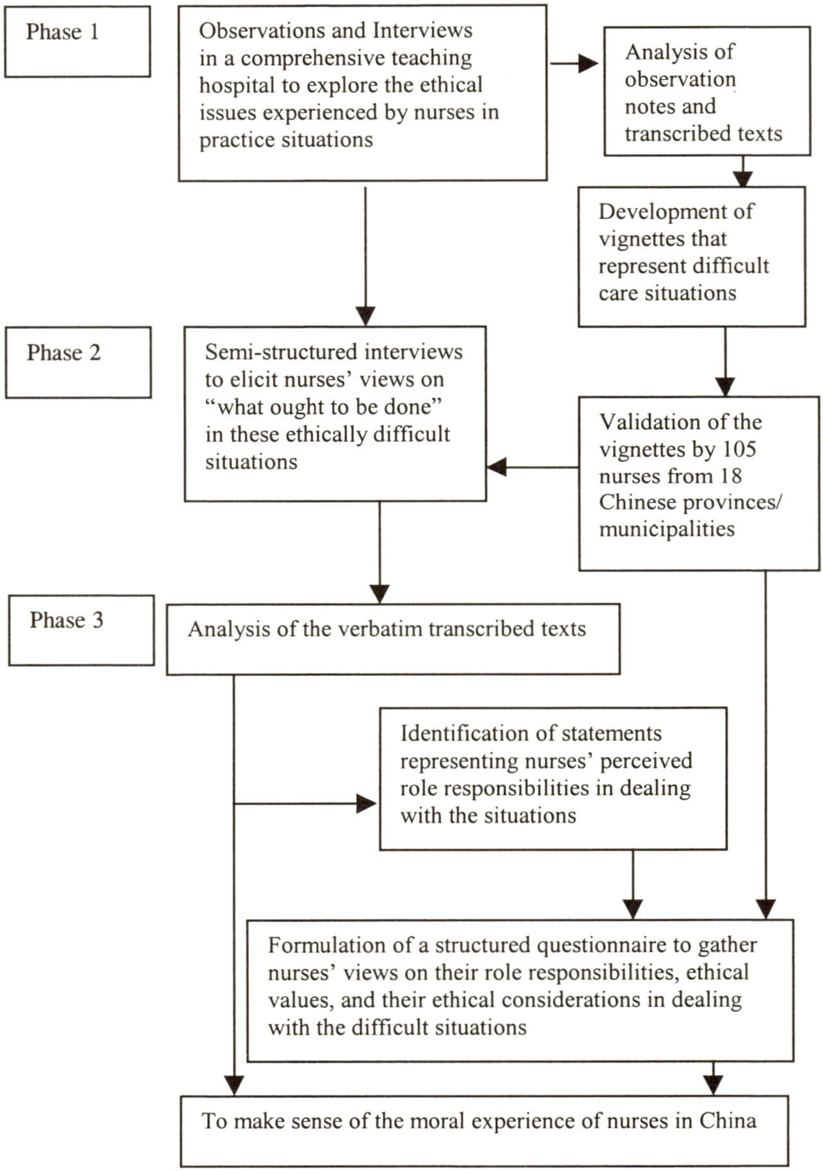


Figure 5.1. Diagrammatic Representation of the Triangulation Process

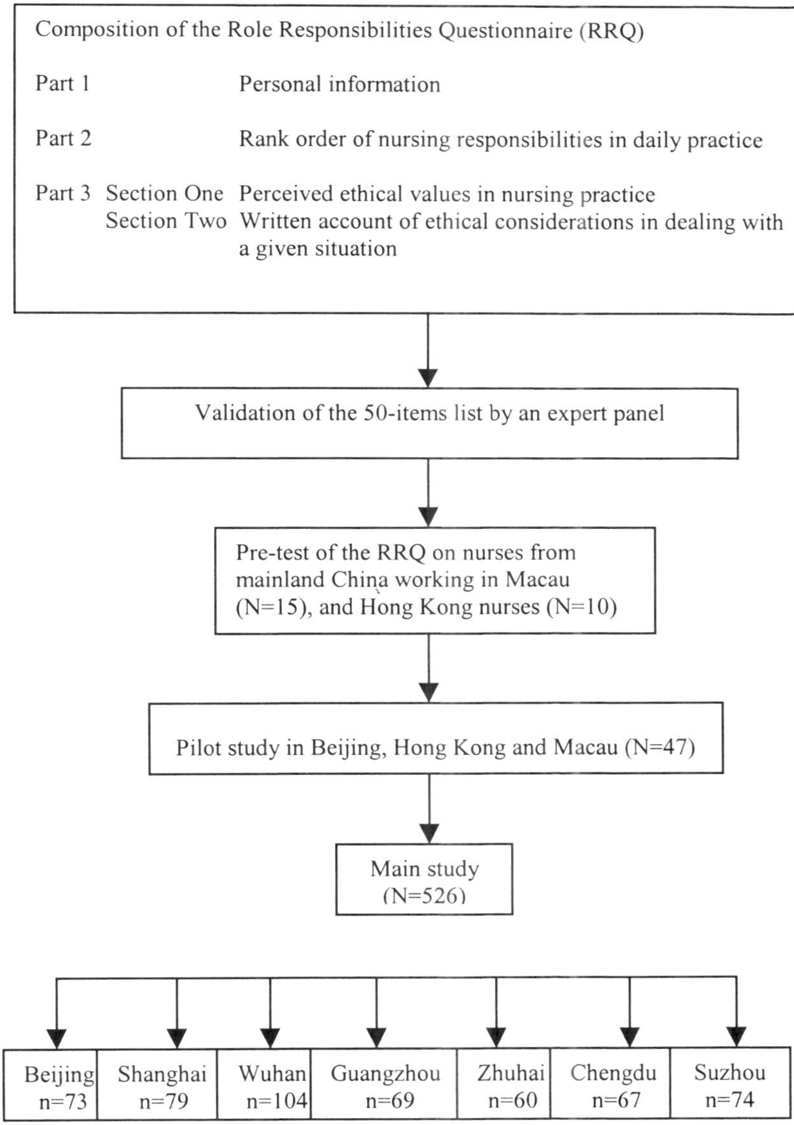


Figure 5.2. Questionnaire Administration

Phase two of the study followed two lines of inquiry. First, I attempted to validate whether the ethically difficult situations identified during the hospital visit also represented nurses' experiences in other parts of China. Second, I continued the dialogue with eighteen of them through semi-structured interviews to learn about their ethical responses to these difficult care situations in particular and their views on nursing ethics in general. Different approaches were then employed to analyze all interview texts that I had collected in two phases of study. (1) the informant's views on nursing ethics and nursing in general were delineated; (2) narratives about similar ethically difficult situations were examined for the range of possible ways these difficult situations could be dealt with in practice. The informants' justifications of their ethical views and their preferred approach in dealing with each issue were analyzed; and (3) statements that the nurses used to express their role requirements while justifying their choices of actions in the interviews were delineated and compiled.

Moving into phase three of the study, the level of inquiry became more focused. As illustrated in Figure 5.2, a structured questionnaire was designed to examine more closely how nurses in seven Chinese cities rank their responsibilities, and the approaches they use to justify their stance in dealing with ethically difficult situations. The questionnaire comprises three parts. Part one gathers respondents' personal information, which includes the place where they work, their age, job title, work unit, work experience, educational level, and any further study related to nursing. Part two includes the list of fifty statements developed in phase two. Respondents were asked to read the fifty items carefully, and then to rank them according to how important they found these statements were in the practice context. The third part consists of two sections. Section one provides space for the respondents to write down six statements that describe ethical values they perceive as more important, and section two includes a vignette that represents one of the five difficult care situations identified in phase one of the study. The respondents were asked to imagine that they were nurses in the situation, and to express in writing what they would consider an ethical way to deal with the situation and a way to deal with it that they consider not to be ethical. Five sets of questionnaires were produced, each set containing only one of the five vignettes. The questionnaires were randomly distributed to the respondents.

526 valid responses were obtained. Descriptive statistics were used to compute the rankings of the statements that represent the nurses' perceived importance of their responsibilities in hospital practice. The statements were subsequently categorized into eleven facets, based on the nurses' conceptions of their role responsibilities in relation to society, healthcare institutions, their practice, the profession, the patient, and the patient's family. Statements that respondents used to represent their ethical responsibilities were listed, and the frequency of similar statements was calculated. The written accounts

in response to the difficult care situations were content-analyzed. These quantified findings, together with transcripts of the interviews from the first two phases of the study were examined to explicate how nurses in China conceptualize ethics in practice situations.[1]

Table 5.1. Vignettes Representing the Five Types of Difficult Care Situations Elicited from Phase One of the Study

5.1.1. Information Disclosure

[Mrs. Chan], aged forty-nine, was an associate professor of art. She suffered from lung cancer with a poor prognosis. Her husband and her sister did not want her to know about her critical condition and requested the doctors and the nurses conceal the truth from her. The family members said that the patient was fragile in character and might not be ready to accept the truth. In order to prevent the patient from discovering the situation, her husband refused to transfer the patient to a cancer ward where she could have had access to more relevant healthcare facilities to treat her condition. The patient remained in the general ward. The nurse found that the patient was sensitive and was keen to know about her condition. She appeared to be optimistic and to have the belief that she would recover one day. She constantly asked the nurses about the kinds of treatment she was receiving. The nurse found that she needed to be extremely careful in responding to her enquires. She avoided talking to her or responding to her directly. For instance, one time the patient asked the nurse to leave the empty medicine bottle behind so that she could read the prescription written on the bottle. The nurse had to make an excuse that the bottle had to be returned to the pharmacy to be checked. The patient eventually died, still ignorant of her disease. The nurse felt uncomfortable and wondered if the patient's ignorance did her more harms than good. She felt that the patient needed psychological support, but she avoided approaching the patient for fear that she would learn about her condition from the conversation. If she had chosen to tell the truth to the patient, she thought that she would not have been able to shoulder the responsibility if the patient collapsed as a consequence. She thought that she might get herself in trouble with the family members if she had told the patient.

5.1.2. Withdrawal of Treatment

[Mrs. Wong], aged forty, suffered from acute endocarditis and had a large thrombus in the heart vessel. She stayed in the hospital for some time but she could not pay the hospital fee. In view of her financial constraint, the physician continued the treatment by using an inexpensive drug, instead of an expensive drug that was known to have a better effect. The hospital administration indicated to her family that they had to take the patient home if the hospital fee could not be settled. Owing to the patient's critical condition, the physician-in-charge and the charge nurse went to the patient's work unit and asked her director to give her more monthly allowance on compassionate grounds. The director agreed to do so. She returned home when her condition was stabilised. Her family paid back the hospital fee in small monthly instalments. After the patient returned home, her condition began to deteriorate gradually. She was never admitted to the hospital again, and died at home six months later.

### 5.1.3. Requests for Euthanasia

[Mr. Huang], aged fifty, suffered from end stage heart failure with severe oedema all over the body. Though the patient required intravenous medication, to do venipuncture for him was difficult because of the oedema. Sometimes, it took more than ten attempts to get to the vein for one injection. The patient suffered a lot since he was in pain but mentally alert. He persistently requested a stop to all treatments and wanted to end his life by taking lethal drugs. His family felt hopeless as well. His department head came to visit him. Since he did not agree with the patient's request, the physician continued the treatment instead of complying with the patient's wish. The patient eventually died in suffering.

### 5.1.4. Unmet Needs of a Demanding Patient

[Mr. Dai], aged forty, a director of a company, was admitted into an intensive care unit because of acute myocardial infarction. Visiting hours were restricted in the unit. Since the patient preferred that his family members take care of him, his family members insisted on staying with the patient and did not comply with the hospital rules restricting visits. The nurses had to spend much time explaining the situation to the patient and relatives. After a detailed explanation by the nurse that the patient's condition was critical and required close monitoring, and that people without professional knowledge could not detect changes in his condition, his daughter at last agreed to co-operate with the nurses. The patient did not feel satisfied with the nurses who took care of his daily living needs. The nurses found the patient quite demanding, such as asking them to serve him for those things that he could do for himself. The nurse felt that the patient still presumed that he was the master of the family and boss of a company. He did not listen to the nurses' words, nor did he show any respect to the nurses. He treated them as if they were his servants. He claimed that he had paid so much for the hospital fee that he deserved good service.

### 5.1.5. Unmet Needs of a Silent Patient

[Mrs. Feng], aged thirty years, was married with one child and lived in the countryside. She had chronic bronchitis since the age of seven. She was admitted to the hospital because of general malaise, fever and cough with profuse purulent sputum. Her younger sister, who was a school teacher, obtained special leave from work, stayed with the patient in the hospital and looked after her. Although the patient's sister had been looking after the patient for some time in the hospital, she had no idea how to dispose of the infected sputum hygienically, and she did not know how to help the patient cough up the sputum. She did not receive any instruction from the nurses how to perform these tasks properly. The patient stayed in the hospital for over three weeks, but her fever persisted despite two courses of antibiotics. The physician at last stopped all antibiotics in order to further investigate the cause of the fever. After a week, the patient's condition remained the same. Apparently the patient's condition did not respond to medical treatment. Since the patient had no insurance coverage, her family had spent almost all their savings to pay the hospital fee. They were thinking of taking the patient home. Her sister felt anxious because she did not know how to take care of the patient properly at home. She was also afraid that her condition was infectious, and might spread to other family members. She did not tell the nurses about her anxiety. She did not think that was a nurse's responsibility to teach her how to take care of the patient, and to handle the sputum hygienically. The patient's sister said that she did not feel comfortable in asking the nurses for help or guidance.

Table 5.2. The Eleven Facets of Nursing Responsibilities

| Facet | Nursing Responsibilities* |
| --- | --- |
| **Nursing Responsibility in Relation to Society** | |
| *The doctrine of socialist humanism* | - Rescue the dying and heal the wounded<br>- Possess a sense of self-sacrifice<br>- Serve the people wholeheartedly<br>- Treat all patients equally, no matter if they are rich or poor, in a high or low position |
| *Healthcare access* | - Prioritize medical resources to treat patients who are curable<br>- The patient has to be given medical care regardless of ability to pay |
| **Nursing Responsibility in Relation to the Patient and the Patient's Family** | |
| *Protectiveness* | - Alleviate the patient's psychological burden<br>- Promote health<br>- Treat the patient as your family member<br>- Avoid doing harm to the patient<br>- Protect the patient from harm<br>- Try hard to preserve the patient's life<br>- Help the patient to comply with medical treatment<br>- Protect the patient from bad news |
| *Quality of care* | - Alleviate the patient's pain<br>- Satisfy the patient's needs<br>- Put the patient's interests first<br>- Promote the patient's comfort<br>- Pay attention to the patient's quality of life<br>- Assure that the patient has a good death |
| *Treating the patient as an individual* | - Respect the patient's rights<br>- Respect the patient's wishes<br>- Be trustworthy in relating to the patient |
| *Holistic inclusion of family members* | - Establish a trusting relationship with the patient and the family<br>- Pay attention to the relationship between the patient and his or her family members<br>- Be trustworthy in relating to the patient's family<br>- Respect the wishes of the patient's family<br>- Alleviate the burden of the patient's family |

Nursing Responsibility in Relation to Practice and the Profession

| | |
|---|---|
| *The nurse's personal qualities* | - Have a sense of responsibility<br>- Be extra cautious when working unsupervised<br>- Possess a heart filled with love to help the patient be restored to health<br>- Have a gentle attitude<br>- Be conscientious in treating the patient<br>- Be a trustworthy person of good character |
| *The nurse's professional qualities* | - Be competent and make effort to improve your nursing skills<br>- Possess professional knowledge in giving health education to the patient |
| *Attitude toward work* | - Don't be afraid of dirty work<br>- Don't be afraid of hard work |
| *Respect for nurses* | - Respect nursing and the nurse's dignity<br>- The nurse's dignity should be respected by the patient and the patient's family |

Nursing Responsibility in Relation to Healthcare Institutions

| | |
|---|---|
| *Institutional rules and regulations* | - Be co-operative in working with other healthcare personnel<br>- Be a good assistant to the physician<br>- Be acquiescent to the law, and be scrupulous in one's conduct<br>- Respect the physician's decision<br>- Comply with hospital rules<br>- Maintain a good relation with patient and family<br>- Follow senior's instructions<br>- Be dutiful about assigned work<br>- Be careful not to make any mistakes that will lead to disciplinary action<br>- The nurse, instead of a patient's family, has to be responsible for care of patient in hospital |

** The statements have been elicited from the verbatim transcription that represented nurses' perception of their responsibilities or attitudes about healthcare in hospital practice*

## 2. Conceptualization of Nursing Ethics

### A. A Nursing Perspective

Reflecting on the Chinese textbooks of medical and nursing ethics, *yide* (醫德) is used to represent professional morality for physicians, nurses and other healthcare workers. Nurses and physicians are seen as different only in their role responsibilities in different practice settings, but their moral responsibilities are grounded in the same set of rules of conduct. The *Regulations on Criteria for Medical Ethics and Their Implementation* (1988 Code) represents the prescribed values for physicians and nurses.[2]

From the interviews, I found that the nurses share a consensual view regarding the meaning of *yide*. Some note that the ethical requirements have evolved over time. An informant, whose life bears witness to the history of China over the past five decades, said,

> In a traditional Chinese society, ethics emphasizes how one should relate to family members and relatives. Previously [in the Mao era] we talked about class relationships. All relationships were basically reduced to two kinds. They were comradeship and class enemies. We were required to serve our comrades selflessly, as we would treat our family members, but to be stern and harsh toward class enemies. Nowadays, we don't emphasize class relationships, and ethics has been extended to different kinds of human relationships. In recent years, we put more emphasis on ethics in professional relationships.

This passage summarizes the informant's experience of the major changes in ethical thinking that China has undergone over the past century. In traditional Chinese society, responsibilities for caring for sick and elderly people are kept mainly within the confines of the family. Since the founding of the People's Republic, the Party leadership mandates that responsibility for the care of the sick be extended beyond the private sphere of the family to the public sphere. People are required to relate to their comrades better than to their relatives, but at the same time to remain wary of those who are identified as class enemies. Ethical thinking in the modern sense puts less emphasis on comradeship. Instead, professional ethics is advocated to regulate the role requirements of different disciplines.[3]

Speaking from their many years of nursing experience, some informants noted that what is required of a nurse in relating to patients has changed. A nurse with forty-five years of nursing experience commented,

> In my early years of nursing [before 1949], I learned how to be humane, that is, to treat others with sincerity, and to take care of patients out of

> love. [My nursing school was run by Christian missionaries] After the liberation of China [after 1949], I learned that everyone has to serve each other.

This emergent notion of "serving others" is mentioned by another informant who has twenty-nine years of nursing experience.

> In the past, healthcare workers viewed patients as asking for a favor of physicians to take care of their medical problems. But nowadays is different; we have to serve the people by putting the patient's interests first.

One informant with fourteen years of nursing experience holds a similar view, but the value that she upholds is different.

> Nursing ethics is having a sense of professional ethics in providing care to patients, respect for patients.

Since the founding of the People's Republic, "serving the people wholeheartedly" has been upheld as the fundamental principle of the doctrine of "socialist humanism." A review of contemporary Chinese nursing literature reveals that one of the predominant themes is the way in which this mandate can be manifested in practice. Obviously these informants have quite different ways of defining how serving others can be realized in practice. Serving others can include taking care of patients out of love, putting the patient's interests first or having respect for the patient. When the nurse informants were asked to describe how they perceive nursing ethics, some had difficulty in finding words to describe it, and some briefly commented that nursing ethics is a complex concept that could not be summarized in a few words.

> We are quite clear from what have learnt, that medical-nursing morality is concerned with how to fulfill the requirements of serving the people by rescuing the dying and healing the wounded. But I prefer not to get to the bottom of the statement. There has been a lot of discussion about what nursing ethics is in theory, but I wonder about its relevance in informing daily practice. I think nursing ethics is more about how I can do my best in taking care of patients using my knowledge and skills and to satisfy patients' needs.

Although nurses in China are required to regularly study the doctrine of socialist humanism at the work place, this informant preferred to talk about nursing ethics out of her experience in taking care of patients. Some nurse informants shared this view, but it does not follow that they are not familiar with the doctrine of socialist humanism, nor that they are unaware of the rules and standards of ethical behavior formulated by the Ministry of Public Health. Most of them were able to recite these rules and standards of ethical behavior. Some found that ethics in a practical sense cannot be reduced to a code of conduct, and a code cannot guarantee ethical practice. Their concern is more to do with whether they can do their best in taking care of patients in practice situations. Articulating nursing ethics in this sense, I would say that their conception of morality is more virtue-based.

In her review of contemporary nursing ethics literature, Joy Penticuff summarizes nursing perspectives.

> Nursing's views of what it means to do good for those who are ill—are derived from the collective narratives of nurses' experiences of caring for patients in countless journeys through illness, recovery, and death. For most nurses, the ethical obligations inherent in each journey must be fulfilled within the boundaries of professional interdependence and complex organizational structures.[4]

Penticuff further points out two aspects of ethical concerns that are special to nursing. First, nurses come to know what is good for patients from a close relationship between nurse and patient. Second, nursing takes place within constraining contexts and multiple obligations. Nurses in China share these concerns.

> Crudely speaking, the primary concern of *lunli* is the qualities of character required of a nurse and patient in relating to each other. The secondary concern is nurses' relationships with patients' relatives, and other healthcare workers. It also concerns nurses' attitudes toward the profession, for instance, whether nurses do their job properly, and the requirements of nurses' role in society.

Nurses in China find that they are taking on multiple roles within practice contexts. With these different roles in mind, the informants give two reasons why they consider patients as their primary responsibility. First, nurses spend most of their time in practice situations with patients. Second, a nurse is required to care for the patient holistically instead of just focusing on the patient's disease. Some nurses say that in relating to patients, a nursing perspective is basically different from a medical perspective.

> While physicians are mainly responsible for treating diseases, the most important aspect of nurses' work is to deal with people.

> Physician's ethics are different from nurse's ethics. The primary concern of a physician is whether to use some therapeutic regime, but nursing ethics emphasizes nurse-patient relationships.

Penticuff has made similar observations when she compared nurses' and physicians' roles in attending patients. Based on the work of C. Baker and N. Diekelmann, Penticuff compares the difference between the nurse-patient relationship and the physician-patient relationship.

> [Nurses] are uniquely situated to attend to the meanings they form around the experience of being ill, of recovering, or of living toward death. In contrast, because physicians' gifts involve attention to the cure of disease instead of to the experience of it, medicine's perspectives are derived from different activities in the employment of medicine's unique talents essential to patients' welfare.[5]

Whether nurses in China share Penticuff's view of nurse-patient relationship has yet to be discussed. What is affirmed here is that nurses in China, as do their Western counterparts, articulate a nursing perspective in making sense of their practice. In one informant's words,

> [Nursing ethics] concerns dealing with people in the public sphere, but not in a kind of formal way. It requires an element of sentiment in taking care of patients, not just to get the job done, but to take note that the person has taken up a sick role, and changes in a patient. Ethical practice is that the patient attains a feeling that he or she is being cared for by the nurse.

This passage is insightful, in the sense that it spells out nurses' role requirements as situated in a place halfway between the private and public sphere of the patient's life. One of the issues that nursing has been facing since its early development in China is how to share the care responsibilities with patients' family members and to draw a qualitative distinction between nursing work and the work of a servant. This issue is still predominant in contemporary nursing. The informant speaks to the reality that between the life in hospital and patients' private sphere of life, nurses are prescribed with a role to take care of patients in such an intimate way that patients can feel it. In sharing the care responsibilities with patients' family members, the goal of nursing is more than getting the task done, as what a servant would. Since taking care of the sick take place in a formal setting, nurses are required to fulfill multiple role requirements encompassing the public and private spheres of patients' life. The question that follows is how nurses in China perceive their care responsibilities within this network of role relationships.[6]

B. Nursing Responsibilities

In examining nurses' views regarding ethical issues in their day-to-day practice, fifty statements that represent nurses' perceived role responsibilities were elicited from the informants, as listed in Table 5.2. These statements were labeled as "nursing responsibilities," based on two observations. First, when the nurses were asked to list six statements that they regarded as more important ethical values, most of them identified "have a sense of responsibility" as a more important value. These findings are similar to those gathered from Anne J. Davis and her associates' survey, in which most nursing students gave the highest ranking to "lack of responsibility/careless" as a characteristic of unprofessional nurse.[7] Second, when the nurses in seven cities (N=526) were asked to rank the fifty statements in terms of their perceived importance in their work place, nurses from five cities ranked "have a sense of responsibility" the highest, and nurses from two cities ranked it the third. This gives it a mean rank of 2.56, which is the highest in comparison with the other forty-nine statements. These observations reveal that nurses in China regard "a sense of responsibility" as the core value. When the informants were asked to describe what they mean by "responsibility," most of them described it as a list of requirements in different role relations.

In relating this statement "have a sense of responsibility" to the other forty-nine statements, all these statements are representations of the kinds of responsibilities that the respondents feel they are obligated to fulfill in hospital practice. When these fifty statements are categorized according to the framework of role relationships, they can be grouped into six major kinds of role responsibilities. They are nurses' responsibilities in relation to society, healthcare institutions, practice, the profession, the patient, and the patient's family. As illustrated in Figure 5.3, these six aspects of role responsibilities can further be categorized into eleven themes. Responsibilities in relation to society comprise two themes: the doctrine of socialist humanism and healthcare access. Responsibilities in relation to practice comprise three themes: (1) the nurse's personal qualities, (2) the nurse's professional qualities, and (3) attitude toward work. Three themes are identified in relation to the patient. They are protectiveness, quality of care and treating the patient as an individual. The theme of the statements in relation to healthcare institutions is institutional rules and regulations; in relation to the profession it is respect for nurses; and in relation to the patient's family it is holistic inclusion of family members. From these fifty statements are derived the six role relationships and eleven facets of nursing responsibilities that characterize nursing ethics in terms of the multiple role responsibilities of hospital nurses in China, as shown in Table 5.2.

In Figure 5.3, doted lines were used to partition the eleven facets in the outer circle to indicate that the items categorized into the eleven facets are not mutually exclusive. Each item is categorized to one facet for two reasons. First, an item is categorized to a facet of responsibility that is seen as most representative of that particular facet. Second, not to place the same item into two or more facets is to avoid possible repetitions in the discussion of nurses' views regarding their responsibilities in the context of multiple role relationships.

Largely the eleven facet of responsibilities are similar to those stated in the 1988 Code, but with three obvious differences. First, the list of responsibilities in relation to the patient is largely expanded in the eleven facets of nursing responsibilities, with the facet of treating the patient as an individual more elaborated, and with the addition of the facet of quality of care. Another obvious expansion is the inclusion of the patient's family in nursing responsibility, which is not explicitly stated in the Code. The third difference is that these eleven facets are conceptualized within a practice context of multiple role relationships, where competing demands and conflicting values posed challenges to nurses in fostering ethical practice.

Comparing the eleven facets with the *International Code of Nursing Ethics* (ICN Code).[8] The contents of the two are in some aspects similar. While six role relationships are identified from the interview texts, the ICN Code groups the crucial aspects of nursing practice into five major headings. They are nurses and people, nurses and practice, nurses and society, nurses and co-workers, and nurses and the profession. They share the similarity of characterizing ethical requirements of nurses in multiple role relationships. In view of these similarities, what follows is to make sense of the eleven facets of nursing responsibilities by comparing them with these two codes.

In the following section, the ways in which nurses in China make sense of these eleven facet of responsibility in their ranking of their responsibilities at the work place and their perceived importance as ethical values will also be discussed. I use primarily three sets of empirical findings. The first set is the results of nurses' rankings of importance of their role responsibilities. The second set is nurses' perceived important ethical values. The third set is content analysis of the nurses' written accounts about their ethical approaches to difficult care situations. The five situations that were used to elicit responses were information disclosure, withdrawal of treatment, requests for euthanasia, unmet needs of a demanding patient, and unmet needs of a silent patient. In this analysis, two statements were added to the list of responsibilities. They are "help the patient to seek financial aid from other sources" and "not to pay no attention to the patient." The first statement is grouped under "healthcare access," and the second under "attitude toward work." Nurse informants refer to those nurses whom I had interviewed with. Nurse respondents were the nurses whose views were elicited via questionnaire. Pseudonyms are given to the patients in the five vignettes described in Table 5.1.

Table 5.3. The First Ten Important Ethical Values as Perceived by Nurses in China

*(N=526)*

| Ethical Value | Facet of Responsibility | No. of nurses choosing this value |
|---|---|---|
| Have a sense of responsibility | The nurse's personal quality | 310 |
| Respect nursing and the nurse's dignity | Respect for nurses | 218 |
| Rescue the dying and heal the wounded | The doctrine of socialist humanism | 199 |
| Be competent and make an effort to improve your nursing skill | The nurse's professional quality | 196 |
| Possess a sense of self-sacrifice | The doctrine of socialist humanism | 181 |
| Serve the people wholeheartedly | The doctrine of socialist humanism | 173 |
| Be extra cautious when working unsupervised | The nurse's personal quality | 155 |
| Treat all people equally, no matter if they are rich or poor, in a high or low position | The doctrine of socialist humanism | 155 |
| Possess professional knowledge in giving health education to the patient | The nurse's professional quality | 135 |
| The nurse's dignity should be respected by the patient and the patient's family | Respect for nurses | 117 |

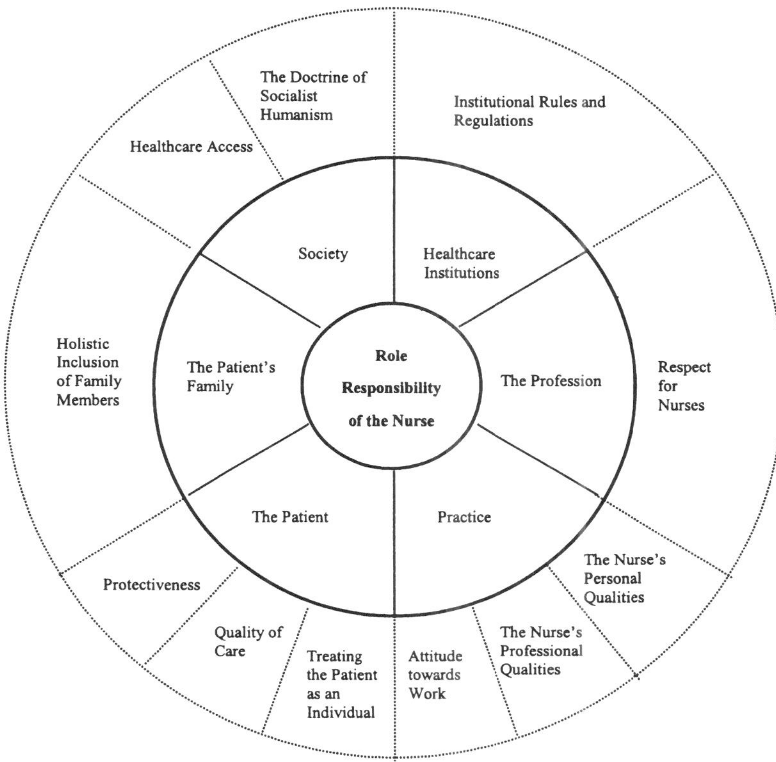


Figure 5.3. Diagrammatic Representation of the Nurse's Multiple Role Responsibilities

Table 5.4. Rankings of Nursing Responsibilities in Seven Chinese Cities*

| Category | Facet of Responsibility | Mean Rankings** | Range of Rankings |
|---|---|---|---|
| In relation to society | The doctrine of socialist humanism | 6.9 | 5.3 – 9.9 |
| | Healthcare access | 45 | 37 – 46.5 |
| In relation to healthcare institutions | Institutional rules and regulations | 35.4 | 31.6 – 38.3 |
| In relation to practice | The nurse's personal qualities | 11.5 | 11 – 14 |
| | The nurse's professional qualities | 7 | 4 – 10.5 |
| | Attitude toward work | 37.5 | 34.5 – 39.5 |
| In relation to the profession | Respect for nurses | 13 | 2.5 – 24 |
| In relation to the patient | Protectiveness | 22.8 | 19.3 – 24.9 |
| | Quality of care | 27.7 | 26 – 29.3 |
| | Treating the patient as an individual | 23.7 | 17.3 – 30 |
| In relation to the patient's family | Holistic inclusion of family members | 41.4 | 39.4 – 43 |

* *The seven Chinese cities were Beijing, Shanghai, Chengdu, Zhuhai, Wuhan, Guangzhou and Suzhou*

** *Rankings ranged from 1 to 50; the smaller the number, the higher the ranking*

## 3. Eleven Facets of Nursing Responsibilities

### A. Nursing Responsibility in Relation to Society

Today's China still avows socialism, and claims that its thorough-going adoption of market mechanisms is essential, and compatible with a basic socialist position. Those holding this view used to be called "capitalist roaders." Their argument must be that Karl Marx was right in saying that the market is an essential stage in human development, but that this can be simulated in less than the form of a full capitalist socio-economic formation of the kind that Marx himself observed, described and analyzed, under a system which remains fundamentally socialist. Some observers, whatever their loyalties or orientations, view this as empty rhetoric.

In this study, nurses' stated adherence to "socialist humanism" and "socialist responsibility" within a medical system that is operated under the mechanism of a market economy presents a remarkable and neat example of a great question in today's China: to what extent and in what way is the adoption of market mechanisms compatible with trying or claiming to maintain a socialist policy? Can we say "these are the correct economic policies for now," but also reconcile them with the communist dictum "from each according to his ability, to each according to his need?"

Marx himself would never have endorsed this distributive principle in today's China. In his *Critique of the Gotha Program*, Friedrich Engels contended that this principle was only suitable for "higher communism," a technologically developed society that can produce a huge material surplus and that is no longer stamped with capitalist ideology. He thought it not suitable for capitalist societies or for "lower communism."[9] These are large and difficult issues, and, possibly, simplistic answers will not do. Some may say that the talk of socialism is just rhetoric, which the Chinese leadership and people no longer believe in. Others may say that no problem exists, since China is in a particular historically transitional stage toward a socialist society. These answers could be too easy. Though this monograph is not concerned with issues of political economy and political science, and although I cannot speak with any authority on these issues, it may be worth saying a little more here, to indicate how the findings of this study raise and may throw light on issues which others would be better placed than I am to pursue. What follows is an attempt to delineate the nurses' views on the two facets of responsibility identified in the present study. They are the doctrine of socialist humanism and healthcare access.

### i. A Sense of Socialist Responsibility

The doctrine of socialist humanism comprises "rescue the dying and heal the wounded," "possess a sense of self-sacrifice," "serve the people wholeheartedly," and "treat all patients equally, no matter if they are rich or poor, in a high or low position." These are familiar propagandistic statements that are found in the first and second statements of the 1988 Code. They also characterize the qualities of virtuous models that the Party leadership promulgates for the people to emulate. As discussed in Chapter One, a sense of socialist responsibility requires a person not to focus on self, family, or in-group interests, but be alert to the thought struggle in all daily life decisions on the basis of whether they contribute to the socialist public good. This virtue of serving the people with a sense of self-sacrifice continues to be upheld in China today. Healthcare workers are required to serve the people through learning from the spirit of Norman Bethune, characterized by a sense of "utter devotion to others without any thought of self." As for nurses, the ideal image would be a socialist humanist Nightingale or an angelic Lei Feng. Activities are regularly held to identify, praise and reward model nurses and physicians whose good deeds reflect the spirit of these models.[10]

Table 5.4 is an overview of the nurses' rankings of the eleven facets of responsibilities according to their perceived importance in practice situations. The nurses gave high rankings to statements representing the doctrine of socialist humanism, with a mean rank varying from 3.43 to 4.18. The nurses ranked "rescue the dying and heal the wounded" second, "possess a sense of self-sacrifice" fourth, "serve the people wholeheartedly" six, and "treat all people equally" ninth among the fifty statements of nursing responsibilities. Of the eleven facets of nursing responsibilities, the nurses ranked the facet of the doctrine of socialist humanism the highest, with a mean rank of 5.3. A majority of nurses also ranked these four statements high on the list when they were asked to write down six statements that most represent their ethical values as shown in Table 5.3.

Apparently, the high rankings nurses in China gave to these statements suggest that the educational and management strategies used by the Ministry of Public Health to indoctrinate healthcare workers with such desirable values are successful. Whether nurses in China strongly believe that the doctrine of socialist humanism is the guiding principle in practice is doubtful, based on two observations of the patterns of the nurses' responses. First, the analysis of the written accounts reveals that nurses seldom used these statements to justify their approach to deal with ethically difficult situations, and not a single nurse used "possess a sense of self-sacrifice" to justify her stance. Second, the responses of the nurses in seven cities to the statement "rescue the dying and heal the wounded" is quite close.

This statement has roots in common with the medical ethics tradition that gives primacy to respect for life. Whereas the rankings of the other three statements that characterize the virtues of socialist responsibility vary more widely, with differences in rankings ranging from two to nineteen. This indicates that significant numbers of nurses have a different view about the importance of these values. These variations are open to interpretation. Nurses who gave high rankings to these virtues might be following a socialist ideal, or they just gave socially desirable responses to show their support of the party line but without a strong belief in it. Those nurses who gave relatively low rankings to the virtues of socialist responsibility might prize this socialist ideal, they do not find these virtues being valued in practice.

### ii. Nurses' Interests

I met a model nurse in the hospital where I conducted my field visit. To identify her was not difficult because she was special. She was a head nurse of a surgical department. She assumed every aspect of her duties with vigilance and compassion, performing routine care of patients, providing direct nursing care to those patients who were in a critical condition, holding case-conferences with the ward staff to better their understanding of patients' conditions. She was knowledgeable and strict in her work, and warm in relating to others. Everyone called her Teacher Yang, and regarded her as the Nightingale of the department.

Virtuous models have been purposely used to foster emulation of socialist values among the people since the Mao era. Donald Munro found that these models are largely selected by the Party leadership to serve three functions. First, national models represent some virtues or attitudes which the government wishes to make widespread. Second, advanced workers demonstrate technical skills and innovative ability contributory to the construction of socialist China. The third function is to spur people on to greater effort. People being selected as model workers can gain peer respect, which is considered to be a greater reward than material gain.[11] In the Mao era people believed that a model worker could set an example and arouse the initiative and enthusiasm of her co-workers by an appeal to morality instead of material reward. As China moves into the era of modernization, methods to motivate workers have changed, but models are still propagated to foster socialist values among the people.

When I asked the ward nurses whether they would like to be Teacher Yang, they expressed the following view,

> What is the point of moving up to the position like Teacher Yang. She works harder than anyone of us. She still has to take night duty like anyone of us. I saw her last night. The prospect of nursing is just like

> this. Everyone regards Teacher Yang as the Nightingale of the hospital. But what for? She works harder than anyone else in the department, but does not enjoy the same promotion prospects as her medical counterparts.

Most nurses appreciate Teacher Yang's noble devotion to nursing, and her commitment to taking care of patients without any thought of self, but not many of them admiring the treatment Yang has received as a model nurse would feel attracted to emulate her. General discontent exists among the nurses on the grounds that their interests are not well looked after in the existing system.

From what I observed in the wards, nurses' work conditions are unattractive. The number of work hours is reasonable, but not the way in which the duty hours are allocated. In the hospital where I stayed, nurses are required to work from 8am to 6pm on a day-shift, with a two-hour break in the middle, from 6pm to 2am on an evening shift, and from 2am to 8am on a night shift. Most nurses are required to stay in the hospital for the evening and night shifts because they find it inconvenient to travel in the middle of the night. Many of them live in suburban areas and have to spend more than an hour in travel. A side room in the ward is allocated to the nurses to rest in-between shifts. Since the crash cart for emergency treatment and some equipment was placed in the room, the person who stayed in the room would be disturbed whenever an emergency happened.

A nurse's salary is no more attractive than that of other professional workers. The standard salary set by the Central Government is relatively low as compared to that of private enterprises. A bitter saying exists among the professional workers that "those who sell eggs are better off than those who build missiles, those who work with razor are better off than those who work with a surgical knife." Most of them say that they would leave nursing given the chance. They contend that requiring nurses to be devoted to others when nurses' interests are not addressed is unrealistic.

The question has been raised in recent years. Does serving the interests of others automatically preclude people seeking benefits for themselves? After making his stance clear that he supports "socialist" instead of "capitalist" market economic system, Han Qingxing contends that such system cannot eliminate the general nature of a market economy, which attributes positive and negative effects on a person's development. On the positive side, it allows individuals to express, realize, and confirm themselves actively and conscientiously through self-advancement, which "essentially liberates individuals engaged in economic activities from personal responsibility for planning and administration," and causes him to "become a self-directed subject of economic operations." He finds that the existing system is in want of reengineering and the most crucial aspect is to introduce a new mode of thinking in the construction of institutions, systems, and organizations that gives due recognition to people who demonstrate "creative and professional and technical abilities." The negative effect of market economy is the expression of human motivation through material gains, such as "worship of money, widespread selfish individualism, and the lopsided development of individuals, etc.." Instead of propagating the virtue of "utter devotion to others without thinking of self" as represented by the model workers, Han supports the notion of seeking material benefit to be tempered through conscientious efforts to "creating conditions for individuals to truly develop creative personalities."[12]

Other arguments are in support of the stance that no contradiction exists between looking after the interests of others and that of oneself. For instance, on the basis of Mo Zi's doctrine of righteousness and benefit, Huang Weihe contends that the notion of "benefit" is in no way synonymous with "selfishness." He did a content analysis of the character *li* (利) that appears in twenty-three of the chapters of *Mo Zi* to argue that Mo Zi gave a more comprehensive interpretation of *li*. He found the character has occurred 246 times, the usage of which represents four meanings. First, reference to the benefit to the community in a sense of approval, for example "the promotion of what is beneficial to the world." Second, derogatory reference to selfish gains at the expense of others, for example "seizing other men's carriages, horses, gowns and furs to benefit oneself." Third, approving reference to individual benefits which do not conflict with those of the community, for example "he who benefits the people will be benefited by them." Fourth, the usage is non-ethical, for example "the *li* (sharpness) of the sword." He further asserts that morality and material well-being can be reconciled, if people uphold the notions of mutual benefit and equitable reciprocity in the pursuit of material goods. "Mutual benefit" constitutes the first and second meanings of *li*, that is, the principle of loving and benefiting others as opposed to behavior that harms others for selfish purposes. Only when this principle is put into effect can there be a state of moral equality, that is, everyone is being treated the same without any element of favoritism. On the other hand, benefit for the majority would be impractical and difficult to realize without looking after individuals' interests.[13]

I would doubt whether Huang's comment on Confucius's notion of *li* is fair, or the representation of Huang's exposition on Mohist views. Nonetheless, Huang's intention to put forward his argument is clear. He does not support the notion of looking after one's self-interests as not virtuous. Chen Congjie supports Huang's viewpoint and proposes that only if the benefits of the tripartite, the country, society, and individual are taken into account can the initiative of an individual be motivated.[14] I find their contention especially relevant to address the nurses' moral tension regarding devotion to serve others and taking care of their self-interests. Equitable reciprocity is what exactly the nurses wish to achieve while fostering a sense of mutual benefit in practice situations.

iii. Healthcare Access

Nurses' response to their responsibilities regarding the doctrine of socialist humanism stood in sharp contrast to the second facet of healthcare access. This facet concerns rationing medical resources to those who are curable and providing the required medical care to those who are in need. The 1988 Code affirms treating patients as equals regardless of the patient's financial situation, it does not state a responsibility for rationing medical resources.

As shown in Table 5.4, contrary to the rankings given to the doctrine of socialist humanism, the nurses ranked this facet the lowest, with a mean rank of forty-five. Ranking of the statement "prioritize medical resources to treat patients who are curable" is also noted to have a comparatively wide variation among the nurses in seven cities, the differences in ranking range from thirty-two to forty-nine. Three reasons may account for this ranking pattern. First, the nurses gave a high ranking to "rescue the dying and heal the wounded" in which the value of respect for life is upheld. For them to give a low ranking to the notion of rationing medical care, where clinical judgment is needed to determine whose life is not worth saving is conceivable. Second, these rankings reflect the realities of China's contemporary medical system in which access to medical services is largely dependent on affordability. Since about 80% of the populace do not have free medical coverage, what concerns people more is how to extend healthcare services to those who do not have access to affordable healthcare. The issues of overspending and rationing medical resources would only concern a minority group which has medical coverage or has the ability to pay.[15] Third, the low rankings can be an expression of the nurses about their lack of control in determining who should have priority in access to medical care.

Contrary to the facet of the doctrine of socialist humanism, the nurses did not choose the nursing responsibilities in the facet of healthcare access as more important ethical values. Many of them justified their approaches in dealing with ethically difficult situations by affirming that patients should be given medical care regardless of ability to pay. As pointed out in Chapter Three, the Chinese government has never intended to provide universal free medical care, nor is affordable healthcare service considered a citizen's right. Many nurses in the present study said that they would help the patient seek medical aid from charity sources instead of asserting that every person should have a right to medical care.

With such a distinct difference in the rankings of these two facets of social responsibilities, nurses in China inevitably face moral tensions in situations where they are required to serve the people wholeheartedly within a system that does not support equal access according to patients' needs. As described in Table 5.1, at least two out of the five difficult care situations identified in Phase One of the study display moral tensions of this kind. The case named "Withdrawal of treatment" that described a woman suffering from acute endocarditis, who ran into financial difficulty regarding the hospital fees and eventually died at home, is a typical moral issue faced by nurses. Regarding the case named "Unmet need of a silent patient" where family members had spent all their savings to pay the hospital fees for a woman with chronic bronchitis who also failed to respond to medical treatment, a moral tension was created when the patient's sister seriously thought of taking her back home. These difficult situations are similar in the sense that they emerge from the competing demands on nurses in fulfilling the requirement of realizing the doctrine of socialist humanism in practice, when they encounter the constraints of the existing system in which medical care is offered as a commodity.

### B. Nurses and Those Who Require Nursing Care

The ICN Code states that the primary responsibility of the nurse is "to those who require nursing care." In the interviews, some nurses in China expressed a similar view that the primary concern of nursing ethics is the way in which nurses should relate to patients and their family members. Of the fifty statements representing the nurses' different ethical stances, seventeen concern a nurse's responsibilities in relation to the patient, and five concern a nurse's responsibilities in relation to the patient's family members. These statements comprise four facets of responsibility: (1) protectiveness, (2) quality of care, (3) treating the patient as an individual, and (4) holistic inclusion of family members.

Three features are noted in the nurses' responses to the facets of responsibilities in relation to the patient and the patient's family. First, nurses in China perceive a large portion of their responsibility as being to patients and their family members. In contrast, only the facets of protectiveness and treating the patient as an individual are explicitly stated in the 1988 Code and the ICN Code.

Second, despite some nurse informants saying that patients are their primary concern in practice, the rankings the nurses gave to these facets are markedly lower than those concerning the doctrine of socialist humanism. As shown in Table 5.4, the mean rank of the facet of the doctrine of socialist humanism is 5.3, while those of the facets of patient responsibilities vary from 22.8 to 27.7. A similar observation is noted in the findings of the nurses' perceived important ethical values. As shown in Table 5.3, none of the first ten values that are most frequently identified by the respondents concerns nursing responsibilities in relation to patients or family members. When the rankings between the facets of responsibility in relation to the patient and those in relation to the patient's family members are compared, another obvious distinction is noted as shown in Table 5.4. The nurses gave significantly lower rankings for their responsibilities of holistic inclusion of family members, with a mean rank of 41.4. We may tentatively say that although nurses in China perceive a large portion of their responsibility as being to patients and their family members, they do not regard these responsibilities as having comparable importance. In particular, these responsibilities are less important as compared to those of the doctrine of socialist humanism in the work place.

Third, contrary to the findings of the nurses' perceived importance of ethical values, the nurses often used the statements of these four facets of nursing responsibilities to justify their approaches in dealing with difficult care situations. Conceivably nurses in China inevitably experience moral tensions if they meet with conflicting interests between the role requirements to fulfill the social responsibility as mandated by the Party leadership and the interests of individual patients and their family members. The stories told by Chi An about her uncomfortable feelings in performing mandatory sterilization for reluctant women in the countryside in the 1970s best characterized this kind of moral tension.[16] What follows is an attempt to make sense of the nurses' rankings given to these four facets of responsibility.

### i. Protectiveness

The 1988 Code and the ICN Code hold that nurses should respect the patient's personality and rights, treat all patients equally and keep the patient's personal information confidential. In the case of the responsibilities listed in the facets of protectiveness and treating the patient as an individual, both codes explicitly do not recognize any right of a patient to information or self-determination. The two Codes, each with its emphasis, indicate the ways in which the patient's confidentiality should be protected. As the ICN Code states

> the nurse holds in confidence personal information and uses judgment in sharing this information.

Making nursing judgments in this regard raises two issues of concern: who owns the personal information, and what should be taken into consideration in making the judgment about who should tell what to whom and how? To clarify the first issue appears straightforward. The ICN Code states that nurses have a primary responsibility to "those people who require nursing care." If the information belongs to "those people," those people should have ownership. Who "those people" are demands further exposition. They may be individuals, family, or a specific group in different situations and in different cultural traditions. As in other parts of the world having a strong familistic tradition, "those people" refer to the patient and the family members in China.[17] Moral tensions inevitably arise if a patient and the family have competing demands on and expectations of the nurse. The nurse has to make a judgment about whom, and for what particular reason, she or he has primary responsibility, in order to resolve the tension.[18] The 1988 Code does not put emphasis on using judgment in sharing the patient's confidential information. Instead, it requires healthcare workers to observe the principle of protectiveness in safeguarding the patient's personal information. The statement reads,

> Keep secrets related to the patient's illness and practice protective healthcare service. In no case is one allowed to reveal the patient's health secret or compromise privacy.

To implement protective medical care carries two meanings. Other than the common understanding that healthcare workers should not disclose patients' information to others, it also means not to disclose medical information to vulnerable patients who may be harmed by knowing their condition. The Chan case described in Table 5.1.1 characterizes the possible ethical dilemma that nurses could encounter if this customary rule of practice is followed without allowing nurses to exercise their professional judgment in situations where letting the patient knows her critical condition can represent the patient's best interests.

The list of responsibilities identified in the present study are congruent with those stated in the 1988 Code instead of the ICN Code. The facet of protectiveness emphasizes the provision of a therapeutic environment for the patient's recovery in two respects. First, it comprises nursing responsibilities that largely reflect the biomedical principles of beneficence and nonmaleficence, in which nurses are required "to protect the patient from harm," "avoid doing harm to the patient," "promote health," and "try your best to preserve the patient's life." The second aspect focuses on the ways in which a nurse should relate to the patient, such as "treat the patient as your family member," "alleviate the patient's psychological burden," "protect the patient from bad news," and "help the patient to comply with medical treatment."

The rankings of the responsibilities "promote health," "avoid doing harm to the patient," "protect the patient from harm," and "try hard to preserve the patient's life" vary from nineteen to twenty-five. These rankings are distinctly lower than the ranking of "alleviate the patient's psychological burden."

These differences can be comprehended in three aspects. First, since medical service is largely provided as a commodity instead of welfare in China, whether a person can get sufficient medical attention depends on his or her status of medical coverage, such as in the cases of Mrs. Wong and Mrs. Feng as described in Table 5.1. Although the nurses ranked "rescue the dying and heal the wounded" high on their list of responsibilities, they are not always possible to implement medical means to "promote health" and "try hard to preserve the patient's life." The nurses can always provide psychological support to the patient because it requires no charge, as was the case with Mrs. Wong.

Second, the new nursing systems of responsible nursing and a systematic approach to holistic nursing care entail individualized and patient-centered care. This approach to nursing explicitly states the requirement of attending to patients' psychological well-being as a nursing responsibility. Third, cultivating the art of communication so as to improve nurses' attitudes and their relations with patients has been high on the agenda in moral education. The therapeutic effect of healthcare workers' words and behavior on patients' psychological well-being is often discussed in medical and nursing ethics literature.[19]

These responsibilities also bear similarities to the ethical requirements listed by Yao Changxu in 1939, which put emphasis on nurses' obligations to try every possible means to provide a psychologically protective environment for the patient. These could include attending to patients' individual needs, using comforting words that could be conducive to healing, gaining patients' trust by treating them with kindness and strictness so that patients would comply with the medical treatment, and relating to patients as one's family members.[20]

Of the eight statements comprising the facet of protectiveness, the nurses gave the highest ranking to "alleviate the patient's psychological burden" (rank order=8). But the nurses gave relatively low ranking to "treat the patient as your family member" (rank order=20), and the lowest ranking to "protect the patient from bad news" (rank order=36). This ranking pattern suggests that the nurses perceive attending to the patient's psychological state as one of their important responsibilities. But the ways in which this responsibility is discharged might not be the same as people would treat their family members. Protecting the patient from bad news is also not a preferred way. The kind of moral tension as described in the Chan case inevitably emerges if the nurse does not find that preventing the patient from knowing her condition, (which is a customary practice under the system of protective medical care), is the best way of alleviating her psychological burden.

## ii. Treating the Patient as an Individual

As for the facet of treating the patient as an individual, which comprises "respect the patient's rights" and "respect the patient's wishes" and "be trustworthy in relating to the patient," the principle of autonomy is apparently upheld. The nurses gave the highest ranking to "respect the patient's rights" (rank order=12) as compared to the other two statements, which ranked twenty-six and thirty-three.

Although patients' right to informed consent is not explicitly stated in the 1988 Code, it does not follow that informed consent is not practiced in China. In my observations at outpatient clinics, patients keep their record of medical consultation. Patients produce their records for the physician in each consultation. The physician writes down the patient's complaints, examination results, diagnosis, and treatment in the record. The arrangement of information sharing among healthcare workers and patients appears to be so spontaneous and casual that we may wonder whether further stipulating patients' right to information is required. What is also interesting to note is that rarely are the doors of the consultation rooms closed. Patients may walk in and out of the rooms freely. Other patients may be present in the room and listen to what the physician says to a particular patient. The concepts of privacy and confidentiality seem not to exist.

As a visiting patient in the outpatient clinic, one unforgettable experience is the embarrassment it caused me to have other patients around while the physician asked me to describe the physical symptoms I was suffering from. I would say that the nurses in China are largely unaware of the need for personal privacy of this kind. The patients' rights to privacy and confidentiality were not noted in the fifty-item list of nursing responsibilities that I elicited from the transcriptions of my interviews with nurses. From an outsider's perspective, I could not agree more with the 1988 Code that healthcare workers should observe patients' rights to privacy and confidentiality in their practice, in the sense of holding in confidence a patient's personal information and not sharing it with others without gaining prior permission from the patient.

A sharp contrast exists in the arrangements for information-sharing in in-patient care. This may be because the principle of protective medical care is more strictly followed in ward situations where patients' conditions are more serious. Informed consent from family members, instead of patient consent, is sought in in-patient care. This practice is also regarded as an edict in recent medical ethics textbooks.[21] In the first legal case involving euthanasia, which received wide public attention in China in 1986, the attending physicians were sued because they administered a lethal dose of painkiller to the patient upon the request of some family members. The case was brought to court by other family members who did not agree with the decision, and was settled after a series of trials that lasted for six years. This case aroused heated public debate about the legalization of euthanasia in China, and has alerted healthcare workers to the possible undesirable legal consequences if consent is not obtained from the whole family.[22]

In the hospital where I undertook my field visit, consent for surgery has to be obtained from a family member, instead of the patient who requires an operation. If a disagreement exists among the family members, or between patient and family members, the family has to resolve it among themselves before consent can be given. If the patient does not have any family member available, the patient's work-unit director will act as a surrogate to sign the consent. In a group interview, the informants expressed these views:

> *Nurse A*: We invite the patient's family member to come before the day of operation. We discuss with them the risks of the operation, anaesthesia, and other possible risks. We also tell them the possible complications. After telling them all these things, we then obtain their consent. If they do not sign the consent form, we cannot do the operation. If we cannot find the patient's family members, we approach the director of his work-unit. We must follow these procedures in obtaining consent for all scheduled operations. Only in case of emergency that the physician will act on the patient's behalf. In case of disagreement among the family members, they have to reach a consensus among themselves first.
>
> *Nurse B*: If disagreement exists between the patient and his wife, his wife will go back home and ask for the opinion of her mother-in-law.
>
> *Nurse C*: If an agreement cannot be reached between the patient and his family member, the physician would not initiate the treatment. An incident occurred, which the patient wanted to have the operation, but his wife was afraid to bear the responsibility. The patient's parents were away. She was hesitant to make the decision. The patient was eventually discharged and went home, since the surgeon would not just take the patient's words for the consent. Likewise, unless the patient is comatose, the physician will not just take the words of patient's family. If the patient insists that he does not want the operation, the surgeon will not proceed.

Since the hospitals are required to earn their running costs, to secure payment from the patients is a matter of administrative convenience. Obtaining consent in treatment decisions from family members or directors of work-units helps ensure that someone will be responsible for the patient's hospital fees. This practice is illustrated in the Wong and the Huang cases as described in Table 5.1.2 and 5.1.3, although the decisions to be made are different. In the Wong case, the family is caught in a dilemma whether to forgo treatment and take the patient back home. The dilemma in the Huang case is whether to comply with the patient's request of withdrawing active treatment and allowing him to die with less pain. The Huang case reveals that practice situations exist where moral tension in nurses inevitably arises if they want to give the best possible care to patients like Mr. Huang and at the same time have to follow the customary rule in dealing with the patient.

In this system of protective medical care, we may argue whose interests are being protected: the patient's, the family's, or the hospital's? It can be held that the interests of the hospital and the family members who legitimately represent the patient's interests cancel each other out. Two nurse informants spoke as follows:

> In China, family members have the largest say in patient care decisions. We would get ourselves into trouble if the family members were not involved. After all, this is a fair system. If an unfortunate event happened to the patient during the procedure, the patient would be unable to bring the case to court. The family would do it instead.

> If the patient suffers from a chronic problem which demands long term care, the family members will have to look after him [or her]. Therefore, to let the family know all the risks related to the procedure and obtain their consent first is more important.

We can see that in this system of protective medical care, family members have primary responsibility for decisions regarding the patient's care. The healthcare workers protect the patient's interests and themselves, by emphasizing the wishes of the family, but at the expense of the patient's right to self-determination in treatment decisions. Moral tension inevitably arises in such situations as the Chan case, if the nurse considers telling the truth to the patient is helping the patient exercise her right to self-determination. The nurse will be caught in a dilemma because the customary belief in protectiveness does not support such a way of dealing with the patient. This is a good example for the difference of rules or virtues are regarded as fundamental in dealing with the situation.

### iii. Quality of Care

The facet of quality of care as identified by the nurses comprises "pay attention to the patient's quality of life" and "ensure that the patient has a good death." With regard to the responsibilities in fostering the patient's quality of life and quality of death, the nurses also see "alleviate the patient's pain," "satisfy the patient's needs," "regard the patient's interests first," and "promote the patient's comfort" as their responsibilities.

This facet of quality of care is not explicitly stated in the two Codes, but it reflects the set of new medical goals developed by the Chinese Medical Association in 1995. These revised medical goals extend the emphasis on the duty to take positive actions to save life, to that of promotion of the quality of life. It also holds that since death and dying is part of life, the provision of a good and comfortable death should be included as parts of medical care.[23]

With the exception of "alleviate the patient's pain," which the nurses ranked relatively high (rank order=15), the rankings of all the other statements comprising the facet of quality of care were between twenty-seven and thirty-nine. The rankings given to "pay attention to the patient's quality of life" and "ensure that the patient has a good death" are thirty-two and thirty-nine respectively, which are specially low as compared to those of other statements. Comparing the rankings of the three facets of patient responsibilities, the facet of protectiveness is ranked slightly higher (mean rank=22.8) than that of treating the patient as an individual (mean rank=23.7). The facet of quality of care is the lowest among the three (mean rank=27.7). This ranking pattern suggests that the traditional role requirement of the nurse is more important than the new role requirement in practice contexts.

The nurses frequently used the statements of the facet of quality of care to justify their ethical stance in dealing with difficult care situations. Since these three facets co-exist in practice situations, which represent customary ethical practice and the newly developed medical goals, moral tension can arise if these responsibilities pose competing demands on the nurse. For instance, the nurse in the Huang case will experience competing demands if the nurse is required to decide whether to conform to the customary practice of protective care or to respecting Mr. Huang's right to choose his way of interpreting quality of life.

### iv. Holistic Inclusion of Family Members

The facet of holistic inclusion of family members is not explicitly mentioned in the 1988 Code or the ICN Code. The ICN Code regards "the individual, the family, and the community" as clients of the nurse, but the orientation is individual-based instead of family-based. The five vignettes elicited from phase one of the study show that nurses often deal with patients' families in patient care situations because they play an active role in providing care for their sick members and making treatment decisions for them. How a nurse should relate to patients' family members is at best superficially dealt with in the textbooks on medical and nursing ethics. Not a single heading concerns the relationship between the nurse and the patient's family in the designated textbook on nursing ethics for Beijing nursing students.[24]

In the present study, the nurse informants include patients' family members in their list of nursing responsibilities. These responsibilities include "establish a trusting relation with the patient's family," "pay attention to the relationship between the patient and his or her family member," "respect the wishes of the patient's family," and "alleviate the burden of the patient's family." The nurses did not give high rankings to these responsibilities as shown in Table 5.4. The mean rank is only 41.4. Apart from the relatively high ranking given to the statement "establish a trusting relationship between the patient and the family" (rank order=17), the other three statements are ranked more than 40.

In comparison with the wide range in ranking the nurses in seven cities gave to the three facets of patient responsibilities, those given to the facet of family responsibility are uniformly low. This suggests that while nurses in China may not share the same sense of importance in relation to the different facets of patient responsibilities, they do share a similar view that their responsibility for holistic inclusion of the patient's family is largely neglected in practice contexts. When we compare the mean ranks between the facets of healthcare access and the patient's family, they are ranked on the low side, 41.4 to 45 respectively. These rankings suggest that holistic inclusion of the patient's family and healthcare access are not responsibilities that nurses find representative of their day-to-day practice.

The reason for this uniformly low ranking may be due to the customary practice in China, as I have discussed in the previous section, of patient's family members participating in providing care to the patient, and bearing the primary responsibility in making treatment decisions for the patient. Therefore nurses in China see the patient's family as a legitimate provider of care instead of as a client who requires the nurse's attention. Since nurses rank their responsibilities to the patient higher than their responsibilities for the holistic inclusion of the patient's family, moral tension can emerge in care situations where family members do not share the nurse's view on matters related to patient care. In such cases, nurses inevitably experience a conflict, as has been described in the cases of Mrs. Wong and Mr. Dai in Table 5.1.1 and 5.1.4. On the other hand, nurses may overlook the needs of the patient and family members if they take it for granted that patients' needs for nursing have already been addressed by their family members, as demonstrated by the Feng case in Table 5.1.5.

### C. Nursing Responsibility in Relation to Practice and the Profession

Three facets of responsibility in relation to practice and one facet in relation to the profession are elicited from the interview transcriptions. They are the nurse's personal qualities, professional qualities, attitudes toward work and respect for nurses. What follows is an attempt to analyze the distinctive features of the nurses' responses to these facets.

### i. Do Not Be Afraid of Hard and Dirty Work

The virtuous nurse models who are given official recognition can best illustrate the attributes comprising the four facets of responsibility in relation to practice and the profession. Of the commendable characteristics these models possess, they all live a plain life, work hard and are willing to do work that most people do not like to do. The nurses in China did not give comparable high rankings to these attributes of "do not be afraid of hard work" and "do not be afraid of dirty work."

While the nurses gave high rankings to the facets of the nurse's qualities and respect for nurses, with mean ranks between seven to thirteen, the mean rank for the facet of attitude toward work is thirty-seven, as shown in Table 5.4. Also, the responses of the nurses in seven cities are quite close, with a difference of less than six in their rankings. This uniform pattern of responses suggests that nurses in China do not consider these desirable attributes propagated by the virtuous models crucial in the work place. They do not find them admirable. An informant commented,

> This is a real problem in nursing, not many people are willing to become a nurse because of the relatively low salary. Apart from this, I think one of the reasons is that the nurse's image is promoted in a negative way. I do not like it. The media always praise nurses for not being afraid of hard and dirty work. Many people know that nurses take care of patients' daily living needs in hospital care. I do not think necessary to promote nursing by just emphasizing this aspect of responsibility. This only gives people an impression that nurses have nothing to do except doing the "hard and dirty work."

The discontent expressed in this passage can be interpreted in two ways. First, these work values, once propagated in the Mao era with the intention of mobilizing the people to construct a socialist China, have given way to another set of work values that emphasizes creativity and industry in the era of modernization. Although the ideal image of a nurse as a socialist humanist Nightingale or an angelic Lei Feng is still promulgated, this image does not attract much admiration. This may explain why the nurse informants did not want to be Teacher Yang although they had a high regard for her.

Second, to present hard and dirty work as the praiseworthy aspect of nursing reinforces the notion that nursing work is the work of a servant. This runs contrary to the efforts that have been made to raise the social recognition of nursing by drawing a qualitative distinction between nursing work and the work of a servant since the early development of nursing in China.

Nurses in China rarely use "do not be afraid of hard work," and "do not be afraid of dirty work" as ethical justifications in dealing with difficult care situations. When they were asked to write down what they would consider as unethical in dealing with the situations, many of them put down a general statement "not to pay any attention to the patient." This statement appears in the written accounts of all five vignettes. Presumably, the nurses in China consider paying attention to the patient is a preferred attitude that nurses should demonstrate in practice contexts. I would say that only if nurses are allowed to exercise their professional judgment can they be responsive to deliver the best possible care in different patient situations.

Moral tensions inevitably emerge if practice context does not provide such a facilitative environment for nurses to pay attention to patients in way which they consider ethical in dealing with the patients' problems in the five vignettes. In short, informants thought that the essential thing was a virtue of being properly attentive to patients. Though this virtue might require some "hard and dirty work," the maxims "do not be afraid of hard work" and "do not be afraid of dirty work" give a misleading picture of what the informants thought the real virtue to be.

### ii. Respect for Nurses

The ICN Code states that nurses are required to promote the profession by maintaining nursing standards, developing nursing knowledge, and improving nurses' status in society. Nurses in China express this sense of professional integrity with an emphasis on respect for nurses. While a consensus exists among nurses that they should respect their profession, they are not so certain whether other people pay due respect to nurses. This is reflected in the nurses' different rankings of these two statements. The mean rank of "respect nursing and the nurse's dignity" is five, and the rankings given by the nurses in seven cities are relatively close, which vary from three to thirteen. This statement is also identified by the nurses as being second in importance in their perceived ethical values. On the other hand, the mean rank of "the nurse's dignity should be respected by the patient and the patient's family" is twenty-one. The ranking for this statement also varies widely among the nurses in seven cities, from two to thirty-five. These contrasted findings suggest that though much lip service is being paid to advocating respect for nurses and nursing, most nurses do not find that they enjoy a respectful status in society. One informant said,

> A common saying exists among nurses that "it doesn't matter how hard we work, if only we can gain people's respect." Respect comes from patients and leaders. Generally speaking, the leaders give more weight to nursing nowadays, but individuals do not. On the surface, physicians are polite to nurses, but I do not find that they really look up to nurses. As for patients, some ask nurses to take care of them as if nurses are servants. They think that they deserve such service because they have paid a high hospital fee. They do not understand that the charge for nursing service is quite minimal, the payment is largely for the pharmaceutical products.

The difficult care situation named "unmet needs of a difficult patient" described in Table 5.1.4 characterizes the kind of moral tension nurses in China inevitably experience in practice contexts where respect for nurses is in question. Only if nurses convince the public of the distinctive nature of nursing work can nurses gain respect from patients.

### iii. The Nurse's Qualities

Much emphasis has undoubtedly been put on strengthening the nurse's qualities in recent years. This is reflected in the high rankings nurses gave to the facets of the nurse's qualities. While the nurses ranked the facet of the doctrine of socialist humanism the highest, the rankings of the facets of professional and personal qualities come second and third among the eleven facets of responsibilities. The mean rank is seven and 11.5 respectively. As shown in Table 5.3, the nurses also identified some of these qualities as more important ethical values. "Have a sense of responsibility" comes first on the list, and "be competent and make an effort to improve one's nursing skills" is fourth. "Be extra cautious when working unsupervised" is seventh, and "possess professional knowledge in giving health education to the patient" is ninth on the list. Also, these statements are frequently found in the nurses' written accounts indicating their ethical stances in dealing with difficult care situations. These rankings suggest that nurses in China see qualities of character as more important in fostering morality in practice.

The statement "have a sense of responsibility" is given the highest ranking. In view of the nurses' rankings of the different facets of nursing responsibilities and their choices of more important ethical values, we may assume that nurses in China gave high priority to socialist responsibility, followed by the nurse's personal responsibilities in relation to the profession and practice. The nurses seldom used the values upheld in the doctrine of socialist humanism to justify their ethical stance. The statements of the nurse's personal and professional qualities are more often used instead. Here, I would suggest that nurses are more concerned about their personal and professional qualities than the doctrine of socialist humanism in practice situations.

The two statements comprising the facet of professional qualities represent two domains of nursing practice. The first domain is a traditional role requirement of possessing technical competence in performing nursing procedures, such as giving injections, or performing oral hygiene. The second domain concerns a new role requirement of extending the focus on care and treatment of the sick to that of health education and health promotion. Of these two domains of nursing responsibilities, nurses in China rank the traditional domain higher. This is reflected in the nurses' uniformly high ranking given to "be competent and make an effort to improve your nursing skills" in seven cities. The mean rank is three, and the difference only varies between two to five. In contrast, the nurses gave a relatively low ranking to "possess professional knowledge in giving health education to the patient." The difference in ranking also varies more widely among the nurses in seven cities, which is between six to twenty. These patterns of response suggest that nurses in China hold a consensual view about their traditional role requirement, but the emergent role requirement of health education and health promotion has yet to be regarded with comparable importance.

The hospital management fosters the traditional nursing role as well. Two observations that I recorded during the field visit can substantiate this suggestion. As a quality assurance measure, the hospital conducts regular assessments of nurses' technical competence on a list of nursing procedures. I was able to attend one demonstration session in a medical ward. In this session, a clinical teacher and a head nurse demonstrated with procedural accuracy and efficiency how to properly make an unoccupied bed, which included damp dusting the bed frame and meticulous folding of sheets. Their faces shone with satisfaction after they completed the task.

I would say that the standard they would like to maintain mirrored nursing in the late nineteenth century, which was characterized by orderliness, cleanliness, and procedural accuracy. As Martin Johnson pointed out, this kind of practice reinforces unthinking compliance with "safe" procedures instead of thoughtful adoption of principles.[25] While this way of practicing nursing has received increasing criticism in the international nursing community, ironically the judgment of nurses' competence remains at the level of procedural correctness in China today.

Second, I noted the "Standard Requirements of Quality Nursing" posted in a medical ward as listed in Appendix 5. The first sentence reads,

> In order to improve the quality of nursing work for its realization in patient care, the following are requirements specified for regular evaluation of the nurse's qualities.

The list comprises six sections: (1) nurse's qualities; (2) therapeutics and nursing procedures; (3) basic nursing care; (4) documentation; (5) emergency trolley; and (6) miscellaneous. They are primarily concerned with etiquette, personal conduct, outward appearance, and rules safeguarding procedural accuracy, cleanliness, orderliness, and efficiency. Some work points will be deducted from those nurses who fail to observe the regulations. This may affect the amount of bonus nurses get at the end of each month. A nurse informant commented that rarely would a head nurse strictly follow these regulations in deducting the work points of the subordinates unless the staff had committed some serious mistakes.

> If a person got a bonus less than the others, he or she should know why. If he or she did not, he or she could ask the head nurse to show him or her the record. The head nurse is responsible for keeping a record of the reasons for deducting our work points.

We may wonder how effective such a penalty system would be for strengthening nursing quality and at the same time motivating nurses to take the initiative in improving the quality of care. The informant commented:

> A common saying exists among us: "A person who never washes the dishes would never break the dishes." Since more chance to do something wrong if one does more, we tend to work according to what is assigned to us, and not more.

In this list of requirements, one item mentions that the nurse should not rely on the patient's relative to perform oral toilet and perineum swabbing if the patient is categorized under grade one nursing, a patient having a severe condition, which requires strict bed-rest. Not a single item concerns providing health education to patients and patients' family members.

Reflecting on these management measures that aim to strengthen nurses' qualities with a primary concern for nurses' procedural accuracy, we may comprehend why nurses in China give such high ranking to competence in some skills. Undoubtedly, these measures foster external compliance to rules and reinforce a sense of external locus of control on the part of nurses in practice contexts. This can inhibit nurses to articulate a moral sense of nursing that is responsive to what constitutes ethical practice in patient care situations where customary rules of practice fail to provide the best possible answer.

I would argue that this view of professional responsibility is restrictive as compared with the ICN Code, which gives a more elaborate description of the nurse's professional responsibilities. It reads,

> The nurse carries personal responsibility for nursing practice and for maintaining competence by continual learning.
>
> The nurse maintains the highest standards of nursing care possible within the reality of a specific situation.
>
> The nurse uses judgment in relation to individual competence when accepting and delegating responsibilities.
>
> The nurse when acting in a professional capacity should at all times maintain standards of personal conduct which reflect credit upon the profession.[26]

The ICN Code emphasizes the nurse's personal responsibility in making professional judgments about how high standards of care can be maintained. Excellence in nursing practice can be achieved by taking account of the realities of practice situations, not by following a list of procedures. Professional judgment of this kind is not noted in the 1988 Code or in the eleven facets of nursing responsibilities.

Of the list of the nurse's professional responsibilities stated in the ICN Code, the nurses in China identify in particular with the requirement to "at all times maintain standards of personal conduct." What the nurses prize is not external compliance to what is stated in the "Standard Requirements for Quality Nursing," but inner virtue. Nurses in China gave relatively high ranking to the statement "be extra cautious when working unsupervised," which is a virtue highly promulgated among nurses in recent years.[27] The intention is to cultivate a strong sense of morality in nurses so that they will do the right thing right even without external regulations. The nurse informants maintained that this virtue is specially crucial for nurses because nurses largely perform duties without supervision. The nurses in seven cities ranked this virtue seventh on the list of important ethical values.

This notion of "be extra cautious when working unsupervised" should be related to the Confucian theory of moral cultivation. As explained in the *Doctrine of the Mean*,

> What Heaven has conferred is called nature; in accordance with his nature is called the path of duty; the regulation of this path is called instruction. The path may not be left for an instant. If it could be left, it would not be the path. On this account the superior man does not wait till he sees things, to be cautious, nor till he hears things, to be apprehensive. There is nothing more visible than what is secret, and nothing more manifest than what is minute. Therefore the superior man is watchful over himself, when he is alone.[28]

According to the Confucians, moral education with a focus on introspective self-evaluation is needed to cultivate desirable qualities so that people act according to principles even when nobody watches over them. The Confucians believe that every person possesses an evaluating mind, and cultivation activates the mind's innate ability to distinguish right from wrong.[29] Introspective self-examination serves three purposes.

First, it causes people to refrain from self-deception, and to be aware of the possible contradiction between their behavior and their real feelings. The second purpose is to help people understand their real nature, which may be obscured by environmental factors. The third purpose is to understand the feelings of others in difficult situations so that people can be sensitized to the principle of reciprocity that "never do to others what you would not like others do to you," and "treat the others as one treats oneself."[30]

This notion of introspective self-examination is found in Sun Simiao's treatise *On the Absolute Sincerity of Great Physicians*. A practitioner is required to constantly engage in self-examination, striving for an improvement in practice (精 *jing*) and remaining compassionate and conscientious in serving their patients (誠 *cheng*). Sun points out that each patient's condition is so unique that physicians to exercise their professional judgment in identifying the best possible treatment for the patient is more important. In his words,

> Nowadays we have diseases which take a similar course with different patients, yet from the outside they appear to be different; and other forms exist, which take a different course with different persons, yet from the outside they appear to be similar.[31]

I would say that Sun's edict bears distinct resemblance to the ICN Code, yet it does not seem to have much effect on the obsession with procedural accuracy and lists of rules.

In recent Chinese publications the Confucian theory of moral cultivation is widely accepted as a method to teach ethics in contemporary China.[32] Two aspects of desirable qualities are specially emphasized in ethics education for nurses.[33] The first aspect is based on the principle of reciprocity. Learning activities are conducted to allow nurses to feel what it is like to be the patient, so that nurses can cultivate good character, a heart filled with love, conscience, and a gentle attitude in relating to patients.[34] The second aspect is to cultivate a sense of being "extra cautious when working unsupervised" in nurses.

"Be extra cautious when working unsupervised" and "be competent and make an effort to improve your nursing skills" are considered to be the two most desirable nurses' qualities. Since the aspect of professional judgment is undermined in nursing ethics education, I would doubt whether nurses are adequately prepared to deal with difficult care situations as described in the five vignettes even though they can well discipline themselves to perform nursing procedures with technical competence. On the other hand, nurses are inevitably required to exercise their professional judgment in dealing with difficult care situations. For instance, as described in Table 5.1, Mr. Huang's nurse could alleviate the patient's pain if the nurse was skilful in putting a needle into Mr. Huang's vein, but the nurse is required to exercise her professional judgment as to what extent to act on Mr. Huang's request to end his suffering. This is like Mrs. Wong's nurse, who is required to exercise professional judgment in finding the best way to deal with Mrs. Wong's request to know more about her disease and treatment regimen.

D. Institutional Rules and Regulations

Ten nursing responsibilities are grouped under the facet of institutional rules and regulations. These statements largely reflect the regulations of hospital ward management, staffs, and patients formulated by the Ministry of Public Health as shown in Appendix 6, which emphasize duty and compliance. The nurses gave a distinctly high ranking to the responsibility to "be co-operative in working with other healthcare personnel." The mean rank is 10, which is the highest when compared with the rankings of the other nine statements. This value of co-operation is stated in the 1988 Code, which reads,

> learn from each other and respect each other, act properly in relating to colleagues and co-workers.

Other responsibilities comprising this facet of institutional rules and regulations include "be a good assistant to the physician," "respect the physician's decision," and "follow senior's instruction." Responsibilities in relating to clients include "maintain a good relationship with the patient and the patient's family," and "the nurse, instead of the patient's family, has to be responsible for care of the patient in hospital." The nurses are also required to "comply with hospital rules," "be dutiful about the assigned work," and "be acquiescent to the law, and be scrupulous in one's conduct." Nurses are more concerned with following the duties assigned to them within the system of hospital care, and maintaining a harmonious relationship with other healthcare workers, patients, and their relatives.

I found that this value of co-operation was highly prized in the hospital where I undertook my field visit. The ward routine was well organized and healthcare workers carried out their assigned tasks dutifully. The allotted tasks of nurses were listed on the work schedule for the day, and the work organization was fundamentally functional in nature. The relationship between physicians and nurses appeared friendly. In the medical department, the nurses and the physicians, together with the students from the two disciplines, gathered together for the morning report before they started the day's work. After the night nurse and the on-call physician gave their respective night reports, the head nurse gave a report about the admissions and discharges of the previous day, which was followed by reports on individual patients from their responsible physicians. The reports mainly concerned clinical progress and therapeutic regimens. The morning report ended with some announcements and reminders for the day given out by the head nurse. The physicians and nurses then worked quite independently of each other in the wards.

The boundary between physicians' and nurses' job responsibilities was quite well defined. A nurse would not assist a physician in therapeutic procedures or during physicians' rounds in routine practice. This may be because the number of physicians was twice that of the number of nurses. The nurses followed the prescribed therapeutic regimens in managing patient care. Quite rarely did a nurse challenge a physician. Not a single nurse informant mentioned to me that they had ever any conflict with their medical counterparts.

This apparent harmony between nurses and physicians may be due to two reasons. First, the two disciplines receive the same doctrine of ethical practice, which requires them to "learn from and respect each other," the fifth statement in the 1988 Code. Second, they enjoy a relatively egalitarian position in the hospital staff establishment. With the introduction of a system of professional titles for clinical nurses, nurses share comparable professional titles of equivalent standing to their physician counterparts.

Paradoxically, nurses in general do not possess high self-esteem. Informants in this study reported similar feelings to nurses studied by Pan Shashan, Fu Aimin and Duan Jiangli.[35] Nursing suffers from low social status, and the notion of "looking up to medicine and looking down on nursing" is still deeply rooted in the Chinese mind. Good relations between nurse and physician may only reflect their distinct job responsibilities within the hospital work organization on the one hand, and nurses' indifferent attitudes toward their professional status on the other. More importantly, the two disciplines have no line authority over each other within the hospital structure. The two disciplines work under the directives of the same hospital management. The source of moral tensions thus is possible not to involve conflicts between physicians and nurses as shown in Table 5.1.

The ICN Code indicates support for co-operation by its statement "The nurse sustains a co-operative relationship with co-workers in nursing and other fields." This notion of co-operation does not advocate loyalty to peers to the extent of condoning morally unacceptable behavior that can jeopardize the fiduciary relationship between the nurse and the patient.[36] The ICN Code states that a nurse has the responsibility to

> take appropriate action to safeguard the individual when his care is endangered by a co-worker or any other person.[37]

Responsibility of this kind is not mentioned in the 1988 Code, nor do the nurses identify it as one of their responsibilities.

In Marsha Fowler's study of the development of codes of ethics for nurses in the United States, it has been pointed out that the requirement of a nurse to be absolutely loyal to physicians and healthcare institutions had been carried forward and prevailed in nursing since the Nightingale era. But this notion of strong loyalty to peers is replaced by fine loyalty in the suggested Code for Nurses formulated in 1926. This implies a loyalty that does not condone morally unacceptable behavior.[38] In the last two decades, the international nursing community has upheld advocacy as a nurse's role. According to Sara Fry, the role of advocacy is to speak on the patient's behalf in the same way that an attorney might plead the case of his client.[39] The notion of being an advocate for the patient on guard against any action that could endanger the patient, which is explicit in the ICN Code, is not included in this list of the responsibilities elicited from the nurses in this study.

When the rankings between the facet of responsibility in relation to practice and healthcare institutions are compared, a clear distinction is noted. The mean rank of the nurse's personal and professional qualities is 11.5 and seven respectively, but the mean rank of the nurse's responsibilities in the facet of institutional rules and regulations is 35.4, as shown in Table 5.4. This can be another source for moral tension in situations where demands from the institutional rules and regulations and what the nurse considered to be desirable approaches in addressing the patient's problem compete with each other. As described in the Chan case in Table 5.1.1, the moral tensions come from the hospital policies of protective medical care in which family members are given the rights and care responsibilities to make treatment decisions for their sick member. Competing demands on nurses also come from hospital regulations of restricted visiting hours and the requirement of nurses not to leave the care of the patient in the hands of the patient's family. The Dai case described in Table 5.1.4 typifies tension of this kind.

### 4. Summary

A common understanding exists among the Chinese that ethics is defined as role requirements enmeshed in a network of relationships. Rule or virtue is considered as fundamental makes a difference in conceptualizing the ethical ways in relating to others. In organizing the fifty statements the nurses use to express their moral stance in this framework, eleven facets of nursing responsibilities have been identified. This list of responsibilities provides a more comprehensive description of nursing responsibilities when compared with the 1988 Code. The list also includes the new values advocated in the newly developed medical goals. This list reflects that nurses in China perceive a large portion of their responsibilities as being related to patients and their family members. Reflecting on the high rankings given to the facets of the doctrine of socialist humanism, the nurse's personal qualities and professional qualities, we can say that nurses give primacy to the virtues that are propagated in recent nursing ethics literature. They are to have a sense of socialist responsibility, skill competence, and qualities of character. These virtues are in congruence with those promulgated in the Chinese medical ethics tradition, the realization of which, is limited by the socio-economic context of practice.

The list is largely comparable to the ICN Code, but with three major differences. First, the ICN Code emphasizes the professional sense of nursing, while nurses in China emphasize personal qualities, with particular concern for skill competence. Second, the ICN Code makes explicit the requirement of a nurse in making professional judgments, such as in situations of sharing information and in taking appropriate actions to safeguard the individual when he or she is endangered by co-workers. Role responsibility of this kind is not identified in the interviews, nor is it included in the 1988 Code. The 1988 Code and the eleven facets of nursing responsibilities emphasize protectiveness in relating to patients and harmonious co-operation in relating to co-workers. Third, nursing responsibilities with regard to the patient and the patient's family is much more elaborate in the list of role responsibilities elicited from the respondents.

Of the eleven facets of nursing responsibilities, three pairs of obvious contrasted rankings exist. The first pair is the difference in rankings between the doctrine of socialist humanism and healthcare access. The second pair is the difference between nursing responsibilities in relation to patients and their family members. The third is between nurses' responsibilities in fostering personal and professional qualities and in complying with institutional rules and regulations. In view of the nurses' high rankings given to the three core virtues, and the variations in their rankings regarding the different facet of responsibility, nurses in China inevitably experience moral dilemmas that emerge from competing role requirements in practice situations as typified in the five vignettes. In the next chapter, I shall continue to explore the nurses' moral experience and to examine the ways in which they deal with difficult care situations with competing demands.

# Six

# DEALING WITH DIFFICULT CARE SITUATIONS

Five types of difficult care situations that hospital nurses often face have been identified from empirical investigation. As described in Table 5.1, they are situations that relate to disclosure of information, withdrawal of treatment, requests for euthanasia, unmet needs of a demanding patient, and unmet needs of a silent patient. Two major concerns are raised in these situations. The first concern revolves around treatment decisions as presented in the first three vignettes. They include treatment decisions for patients who are protected from knowing the nature of their disease, decisions regarding the limit of treatment for patients who are unable to pay their hospital bills, and end-of-life treatment decisions for terminally-ill patients who are suffering from intractable pain. The second concern, as typified in the vignettes of unmet needs of demanding and silent patients, revolves around the competing demands on nurses in dealing with patients and patients' family members. These competing demands reflect challenges posed by the eleven facets of nursing responsibilities.

Three sources of competing demands can be identified. The first source derives from the emergent values that emphasize treating the patient as an individual and quality of care, but encounter the constraints posed by the value of protectiveness, which is predominant in the existing system of medical care. The second source emerges from the role requirement of having a sense of socialist responsibility in practice, but meeting with the constraints of the medical system, which is operated under market economy principles. The third source comes from nurses' emergent sense of professional care, meeting with traditional values that emphasize family responsibility and with institutional policies that require nurses to conform to rules and regulations. In this chapter, the ethical views of the nurses in dealing with these five types of difficult care situations are examined. I will ground my interpretations in the interviews and the 429 written accounts that I collected from nurses in seven Chinese cities.

## 1. Information Disclosure

The problem of how to protect the best interests of vulnerable patients regarding issues of information disclosure has attracted much discussion in recent medical ethics discourse. The most contentious issues are how to identify which patients are vulnerable and need to have decisions made for them, and who can legitimately represent the patient's best interests in making treatment decisions. In defining the vulnerable group who require protection on the part of healthcare workers, the patient's competence to exercise his or her autonomy is the most important consideration.[1] Patients' competence to give informed consent is differently defined. The most generally accepted one is that the patient should demonstrate the capacity to comprehend relevant information, have the ability to weigh the benefits and risks of the proposed procedure, and have the capacity to arrive at a rational decision.[2] These criteria can fall short of including all vulnerable patients who need protection to safeguard their best interests in treatment decisions. People who normally possess the capacity to make rational decisions may be suffering from emotional or physical strain, which renders them unable to bear the burden of making difficult decisions. This could include patients who are in a critical state of illness.[3]

Paul Fulbrook has explored the problems inherent in assessing patients' competence, and argues that the criteria for assessment are ambiguous and value laden.[4] While Fulbrook has illustrated how the values held by healthcare workers have led to biased judgments about patients' mental competence, a recent study conducted by Anne J. Davis and B. A. Koenig suggests that the cultural and societal values embedded in a healthcare system are more subtle and pervasive in influencing the decision of the healthcare workers as to who should be protected and how information should be relayed to patients.[5] The following discussion supports this contention by examining the ways in which nurses in China perceive their ethical responsibilities in safeguarding vulnerable patients.

### A. Ability to Bear the Burden of Knowing One's Condition

In China, healthcare workers disclose medical information to patients and their family members quite liberally except in situations where disclosure is considered to bring harm to vulnerable patients who are suffering from incurable diseases. Under the existing system of protective medical care, the need to tell the truth to the patient is not determined by the person's competence or whether the person demonstrates the ability to comprehend the information, weighs the risks and benefits of different treatment options, and makes rational decisions. In the present study, the informants' viewpoints are consistent in regarding patients' ability to bear the burden of the information as the major consideration. Since family members have a legitimate responsibility in making treatment decisions, it follows that family members also bear the responsibility of deciding whether to conceal potentially upsetting information from the patient. During my stay in the surgical special care unit in a comprehensive hospital in Beijing, I routinely observed charge nurses asking family members if the patient should be informed of the diagnosis. The wishes of the family were usually respected. A patient's wife said,

> The doctor will not discuss in detail with my husband his medical condition. He only tells me how serious his condition is. Of course, the doctor has tried his best to treat the patient. I cannot tell my husband directly, as the doctor told me. I only tell him, "your problem has lasted for so many years, it will take time to treat."

This patient was suffering from hepatic failure due to prolonged bile obstruction. Under common practice, healthcare workers and family members not to allow the patient to make his treatment decisions was regarded as legitimate.

The case of Mrs. Chan typifies the kind of situation nurses face in this system of protective medicine where patients' rights to information and self-determination are largely unacknowledged. Mrs. Chan was fully conscious and well educated. According to the standard of competence, her right to informed consent should have been respected. She was prevented from learning about her terminal prognosis because her husband and her sister did not want her to know about her critical condition. The family members said that the patient was fragile in character and might not be able to bear the burden of knowing the truth. In order to prevent the patient from discovering the situation, her husband refused to authorize her transfer to a cancer ward with better facilities to treat her condition. Mrs. Chan therefore remained in the general ward.

The subterfuge was apparently effective because the patient appeared optimistic, maintaining hope that she would recover one day. In conforming with the family's request to conceal the truth from the patient, the nurse had a difficult time taking care of Mrs. Chan. Because Mrs. Chan was keen to know about her condition, she constantly asked about the kinds of treatment she was receiving. The nurse had to be extremely careful in responding to the enquiries. She avoided talking to Mrs. Chan or responding to her directly. And when she did have to answer questions, she handled them carefully to avoid Mrs. Chan picking up the truth. The patient's hope for recovery was apparently maintained and she was co-operative in receiving the therapeutic regimen. The nurse was able to maintain the deception and, as a result, the patient eventually died ignorant of her true condition.

The family's way of handling Mrs. Chan with her incurable illness was quite similar to the Lee family as described by Jessica Muller and Brian Desmond.[6] The Lee family had emigrated from China to the United States, and both Mr. Lee and Mrs. Lee did not speak English. Mrs. Lee was admitted into the hospital diagnosed with terminal lung cancer. The physicians failed to discuss treatment options with her because of the language barrier, and also because Mrs. Lee's son would not allow them to do so. The Chan and the Lee families asked the physicians not to disclose the disease and prognosis to the patients, and they wanted the physicians to use all possible means to maintain in them hope for a recovery. The major difference between the two cases was the responses that the two families received from the healthcare workers. The wishes of the Chan family were respected, but the Lee family was frustrated and angry with their physician because he hesitated in complying with the family's request for aggressive treatment. Muller and Desmond contended that the conflict might have been resolved if the physician had been more aware of the cultural expectations about the treatment of dying people held by the Lee family. The requests of the two families are considered reasonable, and are accepted practice in the Chinese community.

### B. Nurses' Ethical Dilemma

While the physician in the Lee case was frustrated because he felt he did not treat his patient in accordance with the ethical principles he held, the nurse caring for Mrs. Chan experienced a sense of discomfort, which emerged from her doubt as to whether the patient had received the best possible care. The sources of frustration as experienced by the healthcare workers in the two cases differ. The moral question that worried Mrs. Lee's physician is understandable in the Western ethical tradition, which gives primacy to the individual and his or her rights to self-determination and privacy. The physician found himself unable to observe the principle of respect for the patient's autonomy because the Lee family insisted on dictating the plan for Mrs. Lee's therapeutic regimen. The physician continued with the treatment in accordance with the wishes of the family, but he perceived that the treatment was futile in the sense that it only delayed the patient's death and inflicted suffering on her. This is inconsistent with the principles of beneficence and nonmaleficence. The physician's sense of justice was violated because he felt the medical resources expended on Lee could have been better utilized on patients with a better prognosis. The cardinal ethical principles, namely the principles of autonomy, beneficence, nonmaleficence and justice, were all compromised because the physician had to accept the family's dominance in treatment decisions.

The nurse caring for Mrs. Chan experienced a different kind of frustration as Mrs. Lee's physician. The nurse was uneasy in relating to the patient. She felt that the patient needed psychological support, but she avoided approaching the patient for fear that she might accidentally let slip Mrs. Chan's condition in conversation. She was afraid that she could not shoulder the responsibility if Mrs. Chan collapsed as a consequence of learning the truth. She also thought that she might be in trouble with the family members if she told the patient of her condition. The nurse wondered whether this policy did more harm than good. Hence, moral tension emerged in Mrs. Chan's nurse because what was customarily regarded as ethical nursing practice did not produce the desired benefit for the patient.

The experience of the moral tension experienced by nurses in Hong Kong is quite different than that experienced by nurses in mainland China. In a study of Hong Kong nurses' moral experience regarding information disclosure, Pang Meiche and Chow Laiwan found that the nurses encountered most difficulty in handling situations in which physicians and nurses held different views on disclosure of the patient's illness to the patient and to the patient's family. The nurses in the Hong Kong study quite often found themselves caught in the dilemma of whether to comply with the physician's decision not to inform the patient, or to protect the patient's right to be informed.[7] Disagreement among healthcare workers has been reckoned as a source of ethical dilemmas for nurses in other parts of the world where patients' right to informed consent has been formally enacted.[8] While the dominance of physicians over nurses often constrains nurses from acting as advocates for their patients, I would argue that the tension can also be due to different approaches to ethical justifications on the part of physicians and nurses. A collaborative model for ethical decisions among healthcare workers has been suggested as an alternative to resolve the tension.[9] Yet, the same moral tension has not emerged in mainland China. The difficult situations nurses there often face do not revolve around the relationship between nurses and physicians, but between patients' family members and nurses.

### C. Protective Truthfulness as an Alternative to Safeguarding the Patient's Best Interests

While healthcare workers manage to work cooperatively in the protective medical system, tension is inevitable if they and family members do not share the same opinions over what they regard as the best interests of the patient. Healthcare workers can find themselves in a moral dilemma of whether to respect the family's wishes or to safeguard what is considered to be good for the patient. When the nurses, who came from eighteen Chinese provinces (N=105), were asked whether they had faced such a situation, 93% of them said they had. Some provided examples where patients gave up their fight against disease or emotionally collapsed after they learned of their terminal diagnoses, but they also told of experiences where patients peacefully prepared for their impending death when they learned of their condition. The nurses considered the issue of how patients and family members should be cared for the most delicate aspect in fostering ethical practice.

It would have been a difficult decision for the caregivers, the family members and the nurses, to disclose the terminal prognosis to Mrs. Chan. In a community that cherishes family relationships, family responsibility to bear the burden of their sick members is a deeply seated belief. This includes protecting the patient from emotional stress or loss of hope. Hence, by excluding the patient from discussions of his or her disease and the cost of medical treatments, the healthcare workers and the family members are shifting the burden of illness from the patient to the family. The following written account reflects the socially approved way of a family to take care of their sick relative.

> If I were the family member, I would not tell the patient the truth. I would encourage the patient and give her psychological support. As for treatment, I would try my best to provide her with the best treatment possible.

Disclosing a terminal diagnosis to the patient might denote a lack of compassion and love on the part of the caregiver. A Chinese saying goes, "a sentence of blessing makes a person feel warm for three years, but bad words cause a person to feel cold even in the month of June." Words represent a voice from the heart, and "what the heart thinks, the tongue speaks." Since the concept of ill health is associated with misfortune, suffering, burden, despair, and sorrow, a person with compassion for others would find it difficult to utter these words. Telling someone he or she has a poor prognosis would appear insensitive and cruel, and therefore should especially not be done to a family member. Since nurses are expected to possess a parent's heart in taking care of patients, they may share the same difficulty encountered by families in disclosing bad news to patients. In the words of one informant,

> Being a nurse, one has to conform to one's professional conduct of practice. One has to try to satisfy the family's request, that is, not to tell the patient the truth. If the patient has any suspicion, one has to handle it carefully and at the same time to support her psychologically. Withholding the fact is a good measure to help the patient live in hope as life comes to a close.

The informant's account summarizes precisely the doctrine of protective truthfulness found in the major medical and nursing ethics textbooks. Whether textbook knowledge of this kind can address the moral tension embedded in the Chan case is doubtful.

Ninety-one written accounts of nurses' descriptions of what they would consider as ethical and unethical practice in handling the Chan case were gathered in Phase Three of the study. Content analysis revealed that the common ethical justifications used by the nurses could be expressed as "tell the truth to the patient," "help the patient to comply with medical treatment," and "alleviate the patient's psychological burden." The concept expressed as "respect the wishes of the patient's family" was used relatively less often by the nurses to justify their stance. Although most nurses expressed the concern that patients might lose hope once they learned of their terminal prognoses, they found that the patients could be better handled if they were informed of their clinical progress and therapeutic regimens. Some argued that concealment was futile because the patients would inevitably learn of their conditions as their diseases progressed, and avoiding direct communication with the patient only increases the patient's burden.

> The patient [Mrs. Chan] may have already sensed the severity of her illness since she was a well-educated individual. Nurses in such circumstances should talk to the patient, give her support, help her through the critical psychological state and help her comply with treatment; eventually, to help her die in peace.

Some nurses found that the case was not handled ethically. They argued that "the patient was deprived of her right to know her condition," "this is not fair to the patient," "lying to a patient is unethical," "fear of taking responsibility and staying away from the patient will only increase her psychological burden." Some respondents saw the issue from the point of view of the patient when they explained their thoughts on the matter.

> If I were the patient, I would like to know about my condition. I would prepare to face my work and my family reasonably. I would plan to settle all unfinished business. I would face my life more positively.

> If I were the patient, I would like to know more about my condition. I would actively comply with hospital's arrangement for treatment. ... I hope to know my condition when I die.

Most nurses valued telling the truth regardless of the possibly undesirable consequences for the patient. Some said telling the truth should be valued for its sake, as we value honesty in a person. Furthermore, truth telling is considered crucial in sustaining relationship. An informant said,

> Everyone has to face death one day. I cannot see the point why we need to lie. I knew a charge nurse—her husband died of liver cancer. She said that she previously had never lied to her husband. They were

> honest to each other. She regretted that she did not tell the truth to her husband about his terminal prognosis.

The concept of the patients' right to information emerges in the nurses' accounts of ethical justification of open disclosure, but not a single nurse suggested that the patient should be given the right to self-determination in treatment decisions. So, though telling the truth to the patient was ethically justifiable in comparison with respect for family's wishes in the Chan case, it did not follow that the nurses preferred to override the family's decisions. The findings only indicate that truth telling was considered by most nurses as beneficial to the patient in this particular situation. The slogan "rescue the dying and heal the wounded" which underpins the concern for the patient's compliance with therapeutic regimens was considered by the nurses at large as their primary responsibility. Apparently, the ethical concept of protectiveness is overriding, in the sense that in some cases at least to withhold the truth for protective reasons is considered as right or acceptable, with the goal of helping the patient to comply with therapeutic regimens.

The nurses tended to offer rational arguments to balance out the competing values at stake in the Chan case, and were able to propose alternatives to resolve the moral tension between the nurse, the patient, and the family members. A preferred way to handle the situation was to tell the patient the truth together with the family members, or to counsel the family members so that they could tell the patient and provide psychological support to the patient.

> We may discuss with the family the patient's character, and choose the right time and right method to disclose the condition to her. One may not require detailed explanation. One can also introduce some successful examples to the patient so as to build up her confidence in her fight against the disease.

The primary concern is not to assert the patient's right to self-determination, but how to maintain hope and confidence in the patient so that he or she could comply with the therapeutic regimen. This, I would say, is a more important aspect to note in relaying medical information to vulnerable patients even when the person believes that patients have the right to know. The empirical study reported by Merja Kuuppelomaki and Sirkka Lauri revealed that patients suffered negative experiences because they learned about their incurable illness, and the knowledge came from insensitive healthcare workers whose presentation was blunt and straightforward.[10]

Table 6.1. Content Analysis of the Written Accounts: Information Disclosure

Total number of responses=91

| Facet of Responsibility | Statement | Frequency Count* |
|---|---|---|
| Treating the patient as an individual | Tell the truth to the patient | 68 |
| Protectiveness | Help the patient to comply with medical treatment | 68 |
| | Alleviate the patient's psychological burden | 35 |
| | Respect the wishes of the patient's family | 19 |
| | Protect the patient from bad news | 19 |
| Quality of care | Ensure that the patient has a good death | 13 |
| Treating the patient as an individual | Respect the patient's rights | 11 |
| Quality of care | Alleviate the patient's pain | 9 |
| Holistic inclusion of family members | Be trustworthy in relating to the patient's family | 8 |
| Attitude toward work | Not to "pay no attention" to the patient | 8 |
| Holistic inclusion of family members | Establish a trusting relationship with the patient and the family | 5 |
| Quality of care | Pay attention to the patient's quality of life | 5 |

** Most respondents gave more than one ethical justification for their preferred ways in dealing with the given situation. Those statements with a frequency count less than 5 are not listed.*

## D. Summary

In the existing system of protective medical care, healthcare workers are expected to alleviate patients' psychological burden so as to enable healing to occur. But most nurses are ambivalent about telling the truth to patients, which comes with a strong paternalistic consideration. Truth telling would become a vicious act if the patient were to lose hope and confidence in life after learning of his or her disease. It does not follow that nurses in China prefer to be untruthful to patients, but the truth must come in the form of protective truthfulness. Being truthful to the patient is regarded as a prima facie duty among the nurses. Some expressed the view that they value truth telling in such a situation regardless of the possible undesirable consequences. A majority of them would prefer telling the truth to Mrs. Chan, but their primary ethical justification was not that of respect for the patient's autonomy, nor safeguarding patient's right to self-determination. Instead, the practice was basically beneficent in nature, since they based their decision to reveal the truth on whether the patient would receive more relevant treatment and better nursing care. To this end, a family's right to informed consent has been observed instead. In clinical practice, nurses shared their experience in caring for patients who collapsed soon after they learned of their disease, and patients who refused further treatment for fear of imposing too much financial burden on the family after learning of the cost of treatment. Hence, nurses found that their consideration of information disclosure is not whether the patient is competent to make rational decisions, but whether patients can bear the burden of knowing their condition. The definition of vulnerability based primarily on patients' competence, which is found in other parts of the world, does not appear to be held by the nurses whose views were investigated in this study. Given such a social and ethical context, the moral tension typified in the Chan case cannot be resolved without changes in the social and ethical values, which underpin the protective system of medical care.[11]

## 2. Withdrawal of Treatment

The ethical debates on withdrawal of treatment found in the Western literature primarily concern the ways in which the defining criteria in making decisions to limit treatment for a vulnerable patient group can be justified. Examples of these decisions are withdrawal and withholding of artificial nutrition and hydration, or do-not-resuscitate orders. The vulnerable group usually refers to patients who have incurable diseases or are in a persistent vegetative state. The judgments based on the notions of quality of life, medical futility, ordinary and extraordinary medical means, patients' right to self-determination, and legitimacy of surrogate decision involving vulnerable patient groups are most often debated.[12] Arguments based on healthcare cost and burden of care are also used as reasons to justify decisions of limiting treatment. The extent of concern is not so overwhelming in the case of mainland China.

As pointed out in Chapter Four, forgoing treatment for the terminally ill was practiced in ancient China. It prevailed for two reasons. One reason is that people commonly believed that if they die away from home, their souls cannot return home. Hence, patients and families wish to take the sick home during the terminal stage of their illness. The second reason is financial. It has been a common practice that people are not willing to spend money on medical treatments without an assurance of complete cure. Since medical care is now offered as a commodity and the majority of people do not have medical insurance coverage, withdrawal of treatment is often related to the ability to pay. Decisions to forgo or continue treatment are usually made by the patients' families, with or without the patients' participation. Physicians provide information about the patients' disease condition, treatment options, and prognosis, but they often avoid making the final decisions. When family members have decided that treatment should be withdrawn, they are required to sign a statement to the effect that they had made the decision to discontinue treatment voluntarily, and that they will bear responsibility for the decision.

This phenomenon is observed in this empirical study as illustrated in the Wong case. Mrs. Wong was a middle-aged woman who suffered from acute endocarditis. She did not belong to the privileged group entitled to free medical coverage, and her family ran into financial difficulties in paying her medical fees. The healthcare workers were caught in a dilemma because the patient's condition was manageable, provided relevant medical care was given. They were forced to limit treatment because of the patient's financial position. I will now examine the moral experience of nurses in China in dealing with this type of difficult care situation.

### A. Patient's Ability to Bear the Burden of Medical Expenses

Mrs. Wong's condition was apparently not incurable because the physician continued treatment regardless of the financial constraints. The nurse informants held a similar view. When they were asked to comment on Mrs. Wong's medical condition, they indicated that patients with a similar condition should have a high chance of recovery. In analyzing the issue at stake in the Wong case, this is not a case concerning patients' rights to information and self-determination because no argument existed between Mrs. Wong, her family members or the healthcare workers whether the patient should continue or forgo treatment. The case would be a straightforward one that if the hospital bill could be settled, Mrs. Wong would continue receiving the best possible medical treatment with a good prognosis. Hence, the primary issue is obviously who should bear the responsibility for the medical expenses.

### B. Nurses' Responsibility in Making a Profit

Market forces often put nurses in China in difficult ethical circumstances. In some of the clinical departments in the hospital where I undertook field research, workers have to take responsibility for the department's income. If the department manages to gain a profit, every worker will enjoy a larger salary bonus. Likewise, the bonus will be reduced if the account cannot be balanced. If a patient fails to pay a hospital bill after receiving treatment, the department has to incur the cost, which reduces the amount of money available for staff bonuses. This bonus system was introduced in the 1980s primarily to strengthen the motivation of workers, which is meant to be performance-related to bolster individual responsibility in improving work quality. The extent to which individual staff motivation can be enhanced in a system where all staff will be given a penalty of a bonus reduction if one fails to comply with the institutional regulations is doubtful. As shown in Appendix 5, not a single item in the list of nursing regulations concerns rewarding a nurse who has done something positive. Furthermore, bonuses are divided equally among the staff instead of rewarding individuals who have performed better. Lu Feng pointed out that this arrangement avoids upsetting an egalitarian group dynamic, which is intended to maintain harmonious co-worker relationships. The most important value this system upholds is safeguarding smooth institutional operations.[13]

In relation to the issue of overcharging, some informants admitted that the current bonus system tends to encourage workers to find ways to increase income at the expense of patients' interests by using unnecessarily expensive medication and including more medical expenses on patients' hospital bills. The informants also reported incidents of arguments between nurse and patient for to two main reasons. In the first kind of case, patients suspected nurses of inaccurately recording their medical expenses. In the second, patients refused prescribed treatments in order to save money, but thereby caused the condition to get worse. An informant stated,

> This patient has dyspnoea and requires continuous oxygen therapy. Since the charge for oxygen depends on the length of time of use, the patient finds it too expensive and avoids using it unless he feels bad. To convince him of the possible adverse effects is difficult.

What preoccupied the nurse informants most were situations where patients could not afford to pay their medical fees. In phase two of the study as illustrated in Figure 5.1, 90.5% of the nurse respondents (N=105) indicated that they had encountered similar situations in practice contexts, and only 18.1% indicated that this kind of situation rarely happened in their work place. In other words, nurses in China quite often face situations where treatment-limiting decisions must be made on the basis of patients' financial circumstances. An informant expressed her feelings of powerlessness regarding this system of contract responsibility.

> We often come across situations of this kind [patients who need medical care but cannot afford to pay the fee]. This problem … may be … you can see that our salary is quite low, we can only manage a basic standard of living with the money we can get. If we want to help

> those who are in financial difficulty ... those who cannot pay the hospital fee, I feel quite helpless, I think I can't offer any help.

This apologetic comment was probably provoked by the comparison of herself with the good deeds done by Lei Feng, who lived a frugal life so he could spend every penny possible to help those in need.[14] Although most informants shared this feeling of being unable to help their neediest patients, they also shared in the spirit of Lei in the sense that not a single nurse whom I interviewed showed any ill feelings to those people who left the hospital quietly without paying their medical bills. The nurses most often felt that these patients are to be pitied. They commented that such patients usually had genuine reasons to leave the hospital without paying their bills. An informant commented,

> The hospital cannot find a solution for over 90% of those patients who cannot pay the medical fee. The hospital will give special consideration in exempting the medical fee of some patients, such as excellent students who come from the countryside. The quota is small, only a few each year.

Concerning how they felt when patients ran away without paying the hospital fee, an informant replied,

> I [pause] … I do not have any [ill] feeling. They are already quite pity. They have left their village and come to work here, and then they became sick. They have no relatives around, and are so lonely. I don't think they would run away if they could afford to pay.

Nurses often face the dilemma of how to meet the healthcare needs of those patients who are unable to pay. An informant aired her concern in a group interview,

> A socialist society should be superior to other forms of society because every person is supposed to have equal access to healthcare, but this system is not working now. I am a people's representative and so I have heard a lot of grievances about this issue. I doubt whether we can achieve the goal of "health for all by the year 2000." Heated debates often result whenever we discuss issues related to medical coverage, but we cannot sort out any solution. The fact is that people cannot stay in hospital if they don't have any money. The hospital is not a charity organization. It has to rely on income in order to run the service. This is a big issue, but the problem does not lie in hospital. This is a nationwide issue.

The nurses find that they are unable to fulfill their socialist responsibility to serve the people wholeheartedly under this perverted medical system that does not foster access to medical care for every citizen.

> Every person should have a right to life, but not everyone is eligible to seek medical care nowadays. It depends on a person's financial status. The poor should be treated the same. This is not fair. Medical care should serve all people, and should be equally accessible to every person. Those with no money and cannot receive medical care is a pity.

Medical care in mainland China is supposedly based on the principle of socialist humanism, while in Hong Kong the tenets of capitalism prevail. Ironically the system of medical care is closer to the socialist ideal in Hong Kong than it is in the mainland. The Hong Kong government funds over 90% of hospital facilities, which offer reasonably good medical services affordable to the people at large.[15] Patients who have financial difficulties can always request an exemption of the medical fees. The voice from the public in affirming that the government should shoulder this responsibility is also clear and loud. In 1991, the front page of a local newspaper reported the miserable case of a family whose fifty-eight year old mother was denied peritoneal dialysis. The woman was suffering from chronic renal failure. She was conscious, but partially dependent because of an earlier cerebral vascular accident. But her physician decided to withdraw dialysis. The patient's husband said the act of withdrawing dialysis was the equivalent of homicide. The physician-in-charge defended himself by saying that he made the decision reluctantly, in view of the hospital's limited resources for this type of treatment. According to the rationing criteria, a person over fifty-five was not eligible to receive the treatment. The issue raised a public concern about the ways in which medical funds should be allocated. An estimation of the cost of waiving the age limit for peritoneal dialysis of this patient group was found to be affordable. The public's voice was heard, and the age limit for providing long term treatment for chronic renal patients has now been lifted in Hong Kong.[16]

The provision of medical services in Hong Kong stands in sharp contrast to that in the mainland. The public expectations also differ. The nurse informants in China expressed no strong feelings that the government should fully subsidize the hospitals and provide free medical care. Some nurses complacently accept that the problem of healthcare access is not easy to solve. Content analysis of the eighty-four written accounts of the nurses' ethical viewpoints toward the Wong case, shown in Table 6.2, reveals that the most common ethical justification used by the nurses is that "the patient has to be given medical care regardless of ability to pay."

Table 6.2. Content Analysis of the Written Accounts: Withdrawal of Treatment

Total number of Responses=84

| Facet of Responsibility | Statement | Frequent Count* |
|---|---|---|
| Healthcare access | The patient has to be given medical care | 74 |
| | Help the patient to seek for financial aid from other sources | 55 |
| Protectiveness | Help the patient to comply with medical treatment | 19 |
| Attitude toward work | Not to "pay not attention" to the patient | 14 |
| Protectiveness | Alleviate the patient's psychological burden | 13 |
| | Try hard to preserve the patient's life | 11 |
| The doctrine of socialist humanism | Rescue the dying and heal the wounded | 9 |
| The nurse's personal quality | Possess a heart filled with love to help the patient be restored to health | 7 |
| Treating the patient as an individual | Respect the patient's wishes | 5 |
| Institutional rules and regulations | Comply with hospital rules | 5 |

** Most respondents gave more than one ethical justification for their preferred ways in dealing with the given situation. Those statements with a frequency count less than 5 are not listed.*

Instead of stating that the government should shoulder the responsibility in providing minimal care to patients who are not able to pay, many nurses suggested seeking help for patients from charitable sources in the community or by an appeal for public donations. Apparently, China's public does not expect universal access to free medical care, nor apparently is it the intention of the Chinese government to provide such access. The nurses' written accounts reveal that obtaining donations through public appeal are most frequently suggested as a means to help the poor in different parts of China. The nurses supported setting up charitable foundations for the poor and a medical insurance system for the public, but they did not want to turn hospitals into charity organizations. In their view,

> Hospitals are not charity organizations. The community should share the burden by mobilizing various resources. Hospitals should contribute their part, but not all.

C. Responsibilities of Medical Care Facilities

The nurses suggested two obligations that hospitals should fulfill. The first obligation is to provide medical care for any patient in a life-threatening situation. An informant stated,

> Once, we admitted a patient suffering from acute pneumonia. He had come from the countryside, and had no medical coverage. His elder brother was preparing to take him back home. We knew that he would die if he left the hospital. Our medical consultant asked him to stay. He recovered after treatment, but his brother was unable to borrow money to pay the bill. We therefore raised some funds for them to buy the tickets back to their village. The patient promised to come back when he had raised the money. But he did not return.

Although the hospital may suffer financial losses in providing emergency care to patients in life-threatening conditions without prior determination of their ability to pay, the nurses expressed the view that the hospital should at least bear this basic responsibility as its service to the public.

The healthcare workers' handling of the Wong case illustrates the second obligation the nurses said hospitals should fulfill. The physician used a cheaper drug with similar effect, instead of an expensive drug that was known to have a better effect, in order to save some medical expenses for Mrs. Wong. Some nurse informants reported that they had done similar things to cut medical expenses for their patients, such as recording fewer billable items for those patients who had no medical coverage, and using the medication left over by previous patients. The physician and the patient would receive pressure from the medical affairs office, which indicated to Mrs. Wong's family that they had to take the patient home if the hospital fee could not be settled. The nurse in the Wong case would inevitably experience moral tension if she or he strongly believed that the patient has to be given medical care regardless of the ability to pay.

Most respondents considered that Mrs. Wong's nurse had tried her or his best to deal with the situation, but they did not agree that Mrs. Wong should die at home with no further medical attention. They expressed the view that the patient was relatively young, and that she had a high chance of recovery if relevant treatment were available. One respondent expressed the view that financial support should be provided for the patient by whatever means in view of her curable condition.

> I think this patient should stay in the hospital to continue treatment. The financial problem can be resolved by the hospital and her work unit, or by asking for donations. The patient's life needs to be saved.

As listed in Table 6.2, only a few nurses indicated that complying with the hospital rules is the ethical way of dealing with the situation. More respondents thought that the ethical way to deal with the situation could be expressed as "help the patient comply with medical treatment," and "try hard to preserve the patient's life." Some further suggested that to help the patient build confidence in fighting against the disease was more important, not to let her worry about the hospital fee and to relieve her of psychological burden. Some suggested that the patient should not be discharged. Even though she was discharged from the hospital, regular follow-up was required to assess her condition. The nurses justified active treatment with statements such as, "the patient has a right to life," "to practice socialist humanism, that is, to save life first." Some nurses shared the view that the ethical way in dealing with Mrs. Wong is to "possess a heart filled with love to help the patient be restored to health."

Some respondents assumed the perspective of Mrs. Wong's family, and supported the stance of active treatment.

> If I were in the patient's family, I would try hard to help her continue treatment, by borrowing money, selling my property, or asking for donations from society. I should feel sad if the patient died because I could not pay the medical bills.

Fan Ruiping has made similar observations in his study of the autonomy principle that governs treatment decisions in East Asian culture, which is primarily oriented toward family-centered decision making.[17] As he noted

> Family sovereignty works in accepting treatment for the patient is one thing. For the family to withhold or withdraw treatment on behalf of the patient is another thing.

Some respondents preferred to respect the patient's wishes. When the nurses commented from Mrs. Wong's point of view, they responded quite differently as compared to a family member's view.

> If I were the patient, and the work unit did not agree to cover my medical expenses, I would forgo treatment and end my life so as not to be a burden on my family.

Wanting to help a member of the family, and not wanting to cause difficulties to other members are two sides of the same coin. People regard taking care of their sick family members at all cost as a moral duty, but when the roles are reversed they will also feel obligated not to be a burden to their family members. People who are in favor of legalizing euthanasia note that a considerable number of people commit suicide during the terminal stage of their illness because they do not want to be a burden to others and prefer to have a dignified death. They conclude that euthanasia can offer these people a better way of ending their lives.[18] I would question using this view to argue for legalizing euthanasia in China, on the ground that individual patients' best interests may not be best safeguarded by advocating individuals' voluntary consent. Patients in similar situations to Mrs. Wong would most likely be forced into a situation where the only moral option for them is to choose death in order to avoid having the family members run into debt. Perhaps the suggestion made by Guo Qingxiu, Jing Fengling, and Gen Honggang of letting the patient's family and the physician make the euthanasia decision would better prevent abuse.[19] But this would open to another kind of abuse, if the patient has no voice.

### D. Treating the Patient with the Same Standard of *Ren*

Although most respondents indicated that to impose a treatment-limiting decision in the case of Mrs. Wong is not ethical, they considered Mrs. Wong's nurse to have dealt with the situation ethically. In response to the dilemma, the physician-in-charge and the charge nurse went to the patient's work unit and asked her director to give her a larger monthly allowance on compassionate grounds. The director agreed to do so. She was discharged after her condition stabilized. The patient and her family members showed their gratitude to the ward staff, and paid back the hospital fee in small monthly instalments. After the patient returned home, her condition began to deteriorate gradually. She was never admitted to the hospital again, and died at home six months later.

Regardless of the sad situation, Mrs. Wong and her family left the hospital thankful to the hospital staff. Their gratitude may be due to four reasons. First, the physician had fulfilled his fundamental responsibility by continuing the treatment although he was notified by the hospital administration that the patient's bill had not yet been settled. This could have reduced the amount of bonus the ward staff could get at the end of the month. Second, the healthcare workers had fulfilled their caring responsibilities regardless of the patient's ability to pay. Although a cheaper drug had been used in order to reduce the medical expenses, the patient's condition was kept under control. Third, the nurse and the physician showed their consideration for the patient and her family member by persuading her work unit to give her more allowance to cover the bill, so that they did not need to go into debt. Above all, the patient and her family might feel that their dignity was protected by the healthcare workers, who had acted as their advocate, and had provided the best possible care to the patient within the constraints of the medical system.

Despite the fact that discriminatory treatment is unavoidable in this market-driven medical care system, the nurse who told of this incident said that she just tried her best to treat the patient equally.

> For patients who cannot afford to pay for expensive drugs, we use cheaper ones. As a nurse, I cannot make the treatment decision. But as far as nursing is concerned, we have to treat every patient equally. I ask my juniors not to discriminate against those who cannot afford to pay. This is not their problem. This is a social problem. Society should bear the responsibility. Therefore, as long as they are admitted to the hospital, we have to treat them the same.

Likewise, Marsha Fowler contends that even though to limit treating the patient on medical grounds is justifiable, nursing should go beyond limiting treatment by providing worthy surroundings of care for those whom we know we are not going to be able to treat.[20] The sense of care equality can be represented in a Chinese idiom "treating every person with the same *standard of ren*" (一視同仁). An informant, who is a patient's wife, described this sense of equality while expressing her perception of ethical nursing practice. In her words,

> Medical morality is treating every person with no discrimination, treating all equally well. Be good to people of special status, and be equally good to common people.

The patient's wife elaborated what she meant by good nursing.

> Nurses stay with the patients most of the time. Nurses should … show concern for their patients, and also show concern for the patient's family. … Physicians only come once or twice a day. It depends on the nurses to contact physicians if anything happens to patients. Nurses should take more initiative, not to wait for the patient or the patient's relative to ask for their attention. They should regularly attend patients, and monitor the patient's condition.

Sun Simiao's notion of absolute sincerity can best characterize this informant's expectation of good nursing. As discussed in Chapter Four, a person who possesses the virtue of *cheng* understands the nature of things, the self, and other people. This enables him or her to see into others, to foresee the good and the evil in things, and to acquire right ways of relating to others. In this regard, nurses who possess absolute sincerity demonstrate understanding of the patients under their care, and can master the necessary skills in treating the patients so as to help them recover from illness. Although nurses may feel helpless in situations of imposed limitation of treatment, they can always treat their patients with benevolence. According to Sun, a physician with *cheng* will treat patients as they would treat their family members, as represented in the popular Chinese saying, "a person who professes medicine should have a father's and a mother's heart." According to this notion of the good, Mrs. Wong's nurse had treated the patient and her family equally. She tried her best to take care of the patient. She also showed concern for the patient and her family members, and took initiative to help them resolve the payment issue so that the dignity of the Wong family could be safeguarded.

## E. Summary

Nurses in China perceive that two facets of nursing responsibilities in meeting societal healthcare needs exist. On the one hand, they uphold the doctrine of socialist humanism, and on the other hand, they find that the existing system of medical care greatly compromises the principle of equality in terms of accessibility to medical care. Nurses in China did articulate a sense of equality in fostering ethical practice. This sense of equality, which emphasizes treating every person with the standard of *ren*, has its roots in Sun's notion of absolute sincerity.

Decisions regarding limitation of treatment characterized in the Wong case inevitably pose moral dilemmas for nurses who strongly believe that every patient has to be given medical care regardless of their ability to pay. In recent years, debates on whether to save life at all costs is always justifiable have emerged in China. On the one hand, some people argued that not life itself is, but the value of life matters. On the other hand, some argued that medical resources have to be used more discerningly to improve the health of those with better prognosis instead of lengthening the dying process.

The new medical goals formulated by the Association of Chinese Medical Ethics in 1995 can be seen as representing the official view in the debates. One of the renewed medical goals is to broaden the medical goal of prolonging life to include promotion of quality of life and quality of dying.[21] Guan Guanying further argues that this expanded medical objective supports of the practice of euthanasia.[22] The association has not stated its position regarding the issue of limited access and the constraints posed in realizing the medical goals. The revised medical goals may offer Mrs. Wong's nurse a wider perspective. Concern should be extended to include the patient's quality of life, and basing treatment decisions on other criteria such as prognosis, treatment efficacy, and resource implications.

The moral tension central to the Wong case is still not resolved without further reforms. At least two major aspects demand reform. One is to improve the working conditions of the nurses so as to improve their morale and motivation, and the other is to establish a social security system so that every person has medical coverage enabling them to gain access to decent medical care. I share the nurses' view that these are nationwide problems that need to be addressed at the central level. The least that the government can do is to substantially increase its budget for health care, not for advancing medical technology, but for ensuring that all citizens have access to essential healthcare regardless of their ability to pay, and improving availability of healthcare services to those without medical coverage.

### 3. Requests for Euthanasia

In the Chan and Wong cases, the patients were prevented from actively participating in making treatment decisions although they were competent and able to make informed decisions. Mrs. Chan's exclusion from her treatment decisions, was justified (within the existing practice of protective medical care) by maintaining that the patient might not be able to bear the burden of knowing her condition. In the Wong case, the treatment decision was influenced by whether her family could afford the treatment. It would be logical to suggest that patients who are permitted to be actively involved in making treatment decisions are required to be competent, able to appreciate their disease condition, and belong to the privileged group who has medical insurance. As illustrated in the Huang case, this may not be the case even though the patient can meet the above criteria. The reason was Mr. Huang made his request for a lethal drug to end his hopeless suffering, a procedure not allowed to be performed by physicians in the medical ethics tradition.

The story would have been different if Mr. Huang had made his request in Holland. A Dutch court specified that active euthanasia can be justified if the following conditions are met.

The request must come only from the patient and must be entirely free and voluntary.
The patient's request must be well considered, durable, and persistent.
The patient must be experiencing intolerable suffering, with no prospect of improvement.
Euthanasia must be a last resort; other alternatives to alleviate the patient's situation must have been considered and found wanting.
Euthanasia must be performed by a physician.

> The physician must consult with an independent physician colleague who has experience in this field.[23]

While healthcare workers in Holland would have honored Mr. Huang's request, their counterparts in China responded differently. First, instead of further exploring the opinion of Mr. Huang, the opinion of his family members and the head of his work unit were sought. Second, treatment was continued in spite of the patient's request for a painless death. Even though Mr. Huang's request would not be fulfilled in other parts of the world that do not permit euthanasia, the way in which the Huang case was dealt with was obviously not in accordance with the biomedical principles of autonomy and beneficence that are well accepted in Western societies.[24] Mr. Huang was fully alert and showed acceptance of his terminal condition. He was prevented from exercising his autonomy when he was excluded from participation in decisions over his treatment. The principle of beneficence was not honored in the sense that the patient continued to suffer from intractable pain till he died. We may suggest that the principle of justice is also called into question because Mr. Huang continued to receive medical treatment when he had no chance of recovery, whereas medical resources would be better utilized by being diverted to treat similar patients as in the Wong case. In the following paragraphs, I will make sense of nurses' ethical viewpoints about the ways in which requests for euthanasia are dealt with in China. First, their general attitude toward euthanasia will be examined. Second, their views of ethical ways of dealing with Mr. Huang's request will be discussed.

### A. Nurses' General Attitude Toward Voluntary Active Euthanasia

The original meaning of euthanasia is "happy" or "noble" death, and is in no way confined to the medical context. There have been many different answers from different cultures over the question of whether suicide can be a noble or happy death. Furthermore, some who might object to medical personnel assisting a patient's suicide, or killing a patient on the basis of a living will, might nevertheless find "ordinary" suicide acceptable, or even good. The concerns raised by Chan Homan and Ko Wingman in their article "Misconception, medical goal, and patient's right to self-determination" (written in Chinese) represented this view. Although there has been little public debate on legislating euthanasia in Hong Kong, Chan and Ko saw that with an increasing emphasis on patient participation in treatment decisions, healthcare professionals in Hong Kong will inevitably face euthanasia issues just as their counterparts do elsewhere. They argue that active euthanasia cannot be accepted as a medical practice on the grounds that it goes contrary to the code of professional practice that requires respect for life and equal treatment for all. They consider the practice of euthanasia a breach of the public's trust and counter to the expectations for healthcare professionals.[25] Requests for euthanasia in clinical contexts bring to the forefront the possible conflict between the virtues of healthcare professional as such and the "humanitarian" use of medical skills to end life. Plato and Aristotle thought that some skills were neutral and they could be used for good or ill. Medical skills could be used to cure a patient or to kill a patient. Their good use depends on the virtues befitting doctors. Since the days of Hippocrates, doctors have been clear that an euthanasia act is "contrary to the doctor's role deliberately to kill patients, even at their request."[26] This raises the question whether the concessions or compromises made in advocating euthanasia are compatible with the virtues of healthcare personnel.

Recent opinion surveys on euthanasia reflect that increasing numbers of healthcare workers in China support the idea. In their review of euthanasia-related cases in China in the past decade, Yu Lin and Shi Dapu argued that euthanasia should be legalized in China so that physicians who are suspected of assisting in euthanasia would not be prosecuted for murder.[27] These findings suggest that a majority of healthcare workers would comply with requests for euthanasia once the act is permitted by law. An international study conducted by Anne J. Davis and her associates supports this conclusion. The survey reveals that 26 out of 30 nurses in Beijing would honor voluntary requests for euthanasia if it were legalized.[28]

Similar findings are obtained in the present empirical study. Among the thirty-four nurses that I interviewed in Phases One and Two of the study, only two indicated that they could not accept the idea of euthanasia. One nurse gave the following reason:

> China is basically an ancient society in which children are expected to pay filial devotion to parents. For me, I will try my best to make my parents happy. I should feel guilty all my life if I used euthanasia to end my parents' lives.

The other informant opposed to euthanasia also indicated that she should know how to take good care of her family members when death is approaching. Although she did not accept euthanasia, she commented

> Euthanasia can be seen as a kind of social consciousness, a culture: I think if this idea is continually promulgated in society as is now being done, people will gradually accept it.

Most informants accepted using euthanasia as a medical measure to relieve the suffering of dying patients. This gives an impression that the traditional attitude of healthcare workers in regarding themselves as a healer whose role is to "rescue the dying and heal the wounded" is compromised. First, the nurses concede that some lives are not worth further medical attention. Second, justifying euthanasia on the grounds of unbearable suffering is to concede that medical care is not always able to control patients' pain and suffering. These are, I think, the views of the key persons who advocate legalizing euthanasia in China.

This attitude of the nurses in China is disturbing, in the sense that their attention can be diverted from dealing with the immediate and real issues in the care of the dying, such as improved pain, symptom control, and provision of comfort care. Taking into account that access to healthcare is not yet a citizen's right, and that development of hospice care is a recent and limited phenomenon in China, much room still exists for improving other alternatives to alleviate the patient's situation in particular and the healthcare system in general. In view of this national condition, to justify active voluntary euthanasia without raising the danger of abuse is difficult, even though supporters claim that such act would only be used as a last resort to relieve the patients' unbearable suffering. More importantly, the concessions made in advocating euthanasia are incompatible with a proper view of the virtues of healthcare workers, which is rooted in the tradition of medical ethics. In recent years, this view challenged in arguments for euthanasia on the grounds that using medical measure to prolong life does not necessarily uphold the value of respect for life. Requests for euthanasia come from people who do not want to continue living a suffering and undignified life. By paying due respect to patients' dignity and their life as they will it, some argue that euthanasia is a beneficent act of a compassionate practitioner to help those who have expressed their will to end their suffering.[29]

### B. The Unit Head as a Decision-Maker?

One major concern in euthanasia-related treatment decisions is how to safeguard patients' best interests in the decision making process. Mr. Huang and Mrs. Wong's situations are similar in the sense that the two cases involve making treatment decisions that can influence the patients' length of life and quality of dying. The pattern of decision making is similar in the two cases as well. The two families were indecisive in response to the patients' situations. The decision-making process involved the patients' family members and healthcare workers, and the heads of the patients' work units. Furthermore, the medical treatments that Mr. Huang and Mrs. Wong finally received depended on the approval of the heads of their work units, albeit in different ways. Mrs. Wong's unit leader did not actively participate in the treatment decision, but was persuaded to pay the patient's deficit medical expenses. Mr.

Huang's unit head acted as an authority figure who explicitly stated his view that treatment should be continued.

Heads of work units have played a significant role in people's private and public lives in urban areas since the 1950s. Urban workers were assigned to work units, which were originally established as part of a national plan to restrict migration of rural residents into cities, and to develop a rational system of job allocation and distribution of goods and services. They then evolved to serve political, social, and economic functions. Work units allowed for distribution of jobs, housing, goods, and services to the people. They also served as the locus of political activity.[30] Lu maintains that one of the basic features of a work unit is that "every unit performs simultaneously its political and social functions, and the functions of its professional division of labor."[31] More importantly, work units as the representative of the State take care of the day-to-day needs of their members. Lu compared work units to traditional clans, and found that they

> exercised patriarchal authority over members, and the individual's obligation to the group outweighed his personal rights, and the group assumed overall responsibility for its members.[32]

Work units replaced traditional clans in providing welfare and protection to their workers, and unit heads represented a patriarchal authority in controlling more important decisions for their subordinates, such as granting approval of marriage, allocation of housing, or granting permission for transfer.[33] Against this backdrop, Mr. Huang's unit head only did what was expected of him in his leadership role. The appearance on the scene of Mr. Huang's unit head is significant in two respects. First, he showed his good will in not wanting Mr. Huang abandoned in his suffering. Second, his presence indicated that the work unit continued to cover the patient's medical expenses. This may explain why the physician conformed to the unit head's opinion by continuing the treatment until the patient died. As pointed out by Lu, the role of work units in providing social security for its workers has been diminishing since the beginning of market reforms in China in the 1980s. This in turn shifts the responsibilities and authority of the unit heads back to individual families. The Wong case is an example of this shift.

From the respondents' comments on the role of the unit heads in the Wong and the Huang cases, we can note that their expectations were quite different. The nurses expected Mrs. Wong's unit leader to shoulder the responsibility of insuring adequate medical coverage. Only a few respondents mentioned the role of the unit head in the Huang case. One respondent commented that the unit head should not have acted so as to lengthen the patient's suffering. Presumably then, most nurses hold the view that treatment decisions should be made among family members only, but the work unit should continue its social security function.

C. Alleviating Unbearable Suffering

In contrast to the Wong case, most nurses agreed that Mr. Huang was terminally ill and was in a state of suffering. The nurse who told of the incident doubted whether not to comply with Mr. Huang's wish was ethical. She noted that Mr. Huang's request was not acceptable in current practice. In Phase Two of the study, 66 out of the 105 nurses indicated they had never encountered a similar situation. In contrast, only nine indicated that they had never met a case related to withdrawal of treatment. As one nurse informant commented

> We need a clear definition of euthanasia, to let death naturally come or to allow a patient to end his life. No legislation exists yet. We find it difficult to differentiate. I have come across similar cases before, but I cannot tell whether they constitute a kind of euthanasia. Anyway, if a patient says that he does not want to continue treatment, we will consult his family members. If they agree to sign the form indicating their consent to withdrawal of treatment, they must take the patient back home. … As long as the patient stays in the hospital, he has to undertake active treatment.

Since the hospital I observed in the field visit is a comprehensive teaching hospital, patients who do not require active treatment are not supposed to stay. If the notion of euthanasia includes using passive means to hasten a person's death, most informants would say that they had had experience with euthanasia. Likewise, if the customary practice of forgoing treatment is followed, one possible alternative in addressing Mr. Huang's request would have been to let his family take him back home. Since in this case the family was unable to manage taking care of the patient in such a critical condition at home, the patient's family felt hopeless and brought the unit head in to try and influence the patient.

The content analysis of ninety-six written accounts of nurses' descriptions of what they would consider as ethical and unethical practice in handling Mr. Huang's request is shown in Table 6.3. Obviously more respondents gave higher priority to the nursing responsibilities in relation to quality of care and treating the patient as an individual than to that of protectiveness. Most respondents considered to "ensure that the patient has a good death," "alleviate the patient's pain" and "respect the patient's wish" as their primary concerns. Over 40% of the respondents indicated that the patient's wishes should be respected, ten respondents would accept Mr.

Huang's request based on the value of respect for the patient's rights. It does not follow that all of them agreed to override the wish of his family members. Sixteen respondents noted that the inclusion of the family members by respecting the wishes of the family would be an ethical way in dealing with Mr. Huang's request. Less than 25% of nurses indicated that the ethical ways in dealing with Mr. Huang's request were to "try hard to preserve the patient's life" and "help the patient to comply with medical treatment." These findings suggest that nurses in China are able to see their role requirements beyond the traditional role that emphasizes helping the patient to comply with medical treatment. They understand that there may be patient care situations that priority is given to caring for the patient's quality of life and assuring that the patient has a good death.

Although most respondents accepted euthanasia as an ethical means to alleviate Mr. Huang's suffering, assuring a peaceful and painless death, many respondents did not equate the idea of a good death with active euthanasia. Fewer than 10% of the respondents justified their stance in support of Mr. Huang's request using the publicized view such as "alleviate the burden of the patient's family" and "prioritize medical resources to treat patients who are curable." Instead, most respondents suggested terminating active treatment while trying all possible palliative measures that could help alleviate the suffering. To this end, nurses should possess competent skills in nursing the patient physically and psychologically, such as "alleviate the patient's psychological burden," "pay attention to the patient's quality of life," "promote the patient's comfort," and "satisfy the patient's needs." In addressing the difficulties that the nurse encountered in giving intravenous medication to Mr. Huang, sixteen respondents felt that the nurse did not act ethically. They suggested that the nurse should find other means to minimize the number of unsuccessful needle insertions. In other words, the respondents found that an array of nursing measures exists that Mr. Huang's nurse could have used to ensure that the patient had a good death.

As shown in Tables 6.1, 6.2, and 6.3, a similar response "pay no attention to the patient" was elicited from the respondents' written accounts when they were asked to describe the unethical way in dealing with the situations. In comparison with the number of similar responses collected in the situations of information disclosure (n=8) and withdrawal of treatment (n=14), more nurses (n=19) used this statement in the Huang case. This gives the impression that nurses value open communication with patients and patients' families in order to understand the best possible ways for providing comfort and care to alleviate the suffering of patients.

Table 6.3. Content Analysis of the Written Accounts: Requests for Euthanasia

Total number of Responses=96

| Facet of Responsibility | Statement | Frequency Count* |
|---|---|---|
| Quality of care | Ensure that the patient has a good death | 67 |
| | Alleviate the patient's pain | 63 |
| Treating the patient as an individual | Respect the patient's wishes | 41 |
| Protectiveness | Try hard to preserve the patient's life | 23 |
| | Help the patient to comply with medical treatment | 21 |
| Attitude toward work | Not to "pay no attention" to the patient | 19 |
| Holistic inclusion of family members | Respect the wishes of the patient's family | 16 |
| The nurse's professional quality | Be competent and make an effort to improve your nursing skill | 16 |
| Protectiveness | Alleviate the patient's psychological burden | 12 |
| Treating the patient as an individual | Respect the patient's rights | 11 |
| Quality of care | Pay attention to the patient's quality of life | 8 |
| | Promote the patient's comfort | 6 |
| Holistic inclusion of family members | Alleviate the burden of the patient's family | 6 |
| Quality of care | Satisfy the patient's needs | 5 |
| Healthcare access | Prioritize medical resources to treat patients who are curable | 5 |

** Most respondents gave more than one ethical justification for their preferred ways in dealing with the given situation. Those statements with a frequency count less than 5 are not listed.*

Comparing the reactions of nurses to the three situations, most informants expressed their admiration for Mr. Wong's nurse for two reasons. First, Mrs. Wong's nurse was able to facilitate an open communication between all parties concerned and work out a solution that could safeguard the patient's dignity and at the same time maintain the fiduciary relationship between healthcare workers and the patient's family. Second, Mrs. Wong's nurse presented a positive example of treating the patient in accordance with the standard of *ren*. On the other hand, the informants expressed ambivalent feelings toward the protective medical care system that posed constraints on Mrs. Chan's nurse in having open communication with the patient. The nurse could only resort to avoiding or pretending to relate with the patient. The informants considered this approach to be unethical since the nurse could not provide psychological care to the patient in a responsive way. Mr. Huang's nurse did not encounter the same constraint Mrs. Chan's nurse experienced since Mr. Huang and his family accepted that the patient was dying. She could encounter difficulties in finding the best possible ways to address the needs of a dying patient who wanted to die instead of lingering in unbearable suffering. Additionally, a euthanasia request may indicate a plea for help instead of a genuine intention to end one's life. Hence, to communicate with the patient is more important in order to understand what is most beneficial to him or her.

## D. Summary

The findings of this empirical study are apparently congruent with similar studies of nurses' attitude toward euthanasia in China. Most nurses accept euthanasia as a medical measure to relieve the suffering of dying patients along as protection under the law exists. This gives the impression that a shift in emphasis on the role responsibilities of healthcare workers is happening in China today. As suggested by the findings of this study, most nurses in China support the practice of euthanasia in clinical contexts, on the grounds that it can uphold the patient's autonomy and assure a good death for the terminally ill. Their notion of euthanasia does not imply using active measures to end a patient's life. They see it as positive measures to alleviate the patient's suffering. The findings of the nurses' responses to the Huang case suggest that nurses in China are able to comprehend their role requirements beyond the traditional one that emphasizes positive measures to save life. They can see that patient care situations require them to put priority on caring for the patient's quality of dying. Although most respondents accepted euthanasia as an ethical means to alleviate Mr. Huang's suffering, many did not equate good death with active euthanasia. The difficulties in dealing with such situations do not emerge from the conflict between the virtues of the healthcare professional as such and the "humanitarian" use of medical skills to end life. Most respondents suggested terminating active treatment and at the same time trying all possible palliative measures that could help alleviate the suffering to a state bearable to Mr. Huang. This view is in congruence with the ICN Code, which states that the four fundamental responsibilities for nurses, one of which is alleviation of the patient's suffering. The existing system of protective medical care does not foster this practice, and thus accounts for the moral dilemmas faced by Mr. Huang's nurse.

### 4. Inclusion of Family Members in Meeting the Patient's Needs

How to deal with family members and at the same time provide care to patients without reducing nursing work to that of a servant has remained a dominant issue in nursing in China since its early development. Nursing practice in the Nightingale tradition regarded the family's presence as a hindrance to maintaining a clean and orderly environment favorable for healing. Restricted visiting privileges and the preparation of professionally trained nurses were seen as ways of resolving the issue. Once a belief among nursing pioneers existed that the participation of patients' relatives and friends would not be necessary to bedside care if an adequate number of properly trained nurses existed. The servant image of a nurse would be changed if nurses came from good families and were professionally trained. Obviously though, these good intentions overlooked the logic of care within Chinese family tradition.

Findings of the empirical study show that traditional care practices continue to exert a pervasive influence on the ways in which nurses assume care responsibilities in hospitals. Nurses are ambivalent about the extent they should include family members in taking care of the sick. The Dai and the Feng cases as described in Table 5.1 typify issues of this kind. While the Dai case came from the interviews, I developed the Feng case from my field observations and informal interview with Mrs. Feng's sister. Although the situations of Mr. Dai and Mrs. Feng have many differences, their primary concern is similar. It revolves around the long-standing issue of how nurses should relate to patients and family members. The manifested caring issues vary in two extreme ways. In the case of Mr. Dai, the patient's family members were totally restricted from participating in the care for Mr. Dai, to the extent that the patient's demand for more tangible care from his family members was not attended to. Whereas in the Feng case, care of the patient was left totally in the hands of her sister. The following discussion attempts to make sense of nurses' experience regarding these caring issues and their ethical viewpoints in dealing with situations as experienced in the Dai and Feng cases.

#### A. The Dai and Feng Cases

The primary source of conflict in the Dai case was the hospital's policy of restricting visitors and the refusal of the patient and his family members to comply with it. The hospital has strict rules on visiting, and nurses are responsible for their enforcement. In the hospital's "Standard Requirements for Quality Nursing" states

> Relatives are allowed to stay from 8am to 9pm. Two relatives are allowed in a room with one patient. One relative is allowed in a room with more than one patient. No visiting is allowed in the intensive care unit. A nurse, who fails to keep the rules accordingly, will have one work point deducted for each exceeded head count.[34]

In the Dai case, the patient stayed in an intensive care unit where visiting was virtually prohibited. Visitors were allowed to enter the unit three days a week for one hour each day. Mr. Dai came from a wealthy family and worked in a high position. He suffered from acute myocardial infarction and required special nursing care. Mr. Dai's nurse assumed full responsibility for taking care of the patient, but had to deal with his anxious family members who wanted to stay by the patient's bedside, and a demanding patient who did not feel satisfied with how the nurse took care of his daily living needs. He treated the nurse as if she were his servant. The nurse spent much effort to gain the co-operation of the patient and the family members. While the patient's family eventually accepted the arrangement, the nurse continued to find Mr. Dai a difficult patient. Presumably, the issue would not be so acute if Mr. Dai had been in Mrs. Feng's situation.

In contrast to the Dai case, the Feng case took place in a general ward where patients' relatives were allowed to stay at the patients' bedside during the daytime and were expected to provide personal care to their sick relatives. Nurses were almost invisible except while tidying the ward and dispensing medicine. Although the patient's sister had been looking after the patient for some time in the hospital, but she did not know how properly to help the patient cough up sputum, and she had no idea how to dispose of the infected sputum hygienically. She had not received any instructions from nurses on how to perform these tasks properly, and she did not tell nurses about her anxiety. The patient's sister said that she did not feel comfortable in asking nurses for help or guidance.

B. Representation of the Dai and Feng Cases in Day-to-Day Practice

When the nurses (N=105) were asked whether they had met similar situations before, 88.6% of the group said yes to the Dai case, and 76.2% to the Feng case. When they were asked how often did they meet similar situations as in the Dai case, 17.2% of the group indicated "rarely" or "never." This percentage is much higher in their responses to the Feng case. Sixty one percent of the group indicated "rarely" or "never." Presumably, the Feng's sisters of this world are so self-effacing as to be invisible, while the Dais make their presence obvious.

There might be three reasons for these contrasting responses to the two cases. First, the Feng case did not pose any difficulty for nurses. Only the patient's sister experienced difficulties in taking care of the patient. As I have pointed out in the previous chapter, nursing practice is still centered on the domain of technical competence that emphasizes procedural accuracy and efficiency. Nurses ranked the domain of nursing responsibilities regarding health education and health promotion as comparatively less important. This suggests that nurses would more likely overlook the difficulty encountered by Mrs. Feng's sister. Alternatively, it means that most relatives are capable of taking care of the sick, and the case of Mrs. Feng's sister is exceptional. When I asked the informants whether they often encountered family members who did not know how to take care of the patients properly, many said they had. One informant told of the following incident.

> The patient came from the countryside. He had gastro-intestinal bleeding. His daughter came and gave the patient a piece of cake to eat on the morning that he was scheduled for operation. Poor girl, she was not aware that her father was not allowed to drink or eat anything prior to an operation. The patient's internal bleeding became worse. As a result, the family had to spend even more money on medical fees.

If this case were reported in Hong Kong, the public would blame the nurse for not giving clear instructions to the patient and his family about the risks of eating anything before the operation. I found this noteworthy that the informant did not indicate a sense of failure on her part in not instructing the patient and his family on the proper pre-operation procedures. Nor do hospital rules foster the practice of giving health information in clinical wards. According to one informant,

> Regulations regarding nurses' job responsibilities comprise "soft" and "hard" guidelines. Providing health education to patients belongs to the category of soft guidelines. No penalty will be imposed on the nurse who fails to follow a soft guideline. Also, no one will take note of the issue because the patient and her relatives would most likely not make a complaint to the hospital. Nursing procedures such as the administration of medicine and the preparation of intravenous infusions belong to the category of hard guidelines. A nurse who commits this kind of mistake will bear disciplinary consequences.

The "Standard Requirements for Quality Nursing" is a good piece of evidence of this. Since the role requirements of a nurse in providing health education to patients and their primary care providers are less obvious in practice situations, this may explain why nurses are possibly not aware of the issue demanding nursing's concern.

The third reason is that the institutional ethos emphasizes maintenance of co-operative relationship and prevention of conflicts. When the informants were asked to give their general impressions about the relationship between the nurse and the patient and the patient's relatives, most of them said that they would maintain a certain distance with patients and at the same time try to maintain a harmonious atmosphere by avoiding any direct confrontation. As one informant commented

> Basically we try to maintain a kind of peaceful atmosphere in the ward, in which we are not particularly close with patients but we avoid getting into trouble with them. This is not worthwhile anyway. On the one hand, it will give me stress. On the other hand, my senior will criticize me. Even though I have strong reasons, I would be considered in the wrong simply because I quarrel with others.

The common strategy nurses used to resolve possible conflicts with patients and the patients' families is not to deal with the patient directly, but to refer the case up the chain of authority to head nurses and physicians-in-charge. If they cannot settle the issue at ward level, the director will be informed. According to one informant,

> We often encounter difficulties in dealing with patients and their family members. For instance, this morning we admitted a critically ill patient who required special care. Since the beds were already full, we needed to transfer a patient to another ward in order to admit this patient. The patient refused. I could not solve the problem and so I referred the patient to the physician. ... If the physician cannot convince the patient, he will seek help from the medical affairs office.

In such cases, front-line nurses can avoid direct confrontations with patients. Nurses are impeded in open communication with patients and family members, which also reinforces that maintaining a safe distance from patients is more preferred. In addition, these practices foster a work-to-rule attitude, which may explain why nurses were cautious in dealing with the Dai family, but had a relatively low awareness of the needs of Mrs. Feng and her sister.

The content analysis of seventy-seven and eighty-one written accounts of nurses' descriptions of what they would consider as ethical and unethical practices in dealing with the Dai and Feng cases is shown in Tables 6.4 and 6.5 respectively. Similar to the findings of the previous three vignettes, the concept expressed as "paying no attention to the patient" was elicited from the written accounts when the respondents were asked to describe the unethical way of dealing with the Dai and Feng cases. This response to the two cases was seen nineteen times for the Dai case, and thirty-two times for the Feng case. In other words, more nurses indicated that the attitude of "paying no attention to the patient" is more unethical in the Feng case than in the other four cases. The respondents elaborated in the written accounts what they meant by "paying no attention to the patient." These are situations where the nurse "attends to the patient with an indifferent attitude," "carries out his or her work without any communication with the patient," "does not respond to the patient's request," "does not communicate with the patient so as to understand her condition," "does not attend the patient even though you know the patient has a problem," and "does not take initiative to help the patient's sister." In contrast to the institutional ethos that discourages nurses from taking initiative toward having open communication with patients, the respondents consider a non-responsive attitude unethical.

Table 6.4. Content Analysis of the Written Accounts: Unmet Needs of a Demanding Patient

Total number of Responses = 77

| Facet of Responsibility | Statement | Frequency Count* |
|---|---|---|
| Respect for nurses | The nurse's dignity should be respected by the patient and the patient's family | 31 |
| Institutional rules and regulations | Help the patient to comply with medical treatment | 25 |
| | Comply with hospital rules | 22 |
| | The nurse, instead of a patient's family, has to be responsible for care of the patient in hospital | 20 |
| Attitude toward work | Not to "pay no attention" to the patient | 19 |
| Institutional rules and regulations | Maintain a good relationship with patient and family | 17 |
| | Be co-operative in working with other health care personnel | 16 |
| Respect for nurses | Respect nursing and the nurse's dignity | 13 |
| Holistic inclusion of family member | Establish a trusting relationship with the patient and the family | 12 |
| The nurse's professional quality | Possess professional knowledge in giving health education to the patient | 11 |
| Holistic inclusion of family members | Pay attention to the relationship between the patient and his or her family members | 10 |
| Protectiveness | Treat the patient as you would treat your family member | 9 |
| Treating the patient as an individual | Respect the patient's wishes | 8 |
| Quality of care | Satisfy the patient's needs | 8 |
| The doctrine of socialist humanism | Treat all patients equally, regardless if they are rich or poor, in a high or low position | 6 |
| Protectiveness | Alleviate the patient's psychological burden | 5 |
| The nurse's professional quality | Be competent and make an effort to improve your nursing skill | 5 |
| Quality of care | Put the patient's interest first | 5 |

** Most respondents gave more than one ethical justification for their preferred ways in dealing with the given situation. Those statements with a frequency count less than 5 are not listed.*

Table 6.5. Content Analysis of the Written Accounts: Unmet Needs of a Silent Patient

Total number of Responses=81

| Facet of Responsibility | Statement | Frequency Count* |
|---|---|---|
| The nurse's professional quality | Possess professional knowledge in giving health education to the patient | 64 |
| Attitude toward work | Not to "pay no attention" to the patient | 35 |
| Institutional rules and regulations | The nurse, instead of a patient's family, has to be responsible for care of the patient in hospital | 32 |
| Protectiveness | Help the patient to comply with medical treatment | 28 |
| Healthcare access | The patient has a right to health care regardless of ability to pay | 26 |
| The nurse's personal quality | Possess a heart filled with love to help the patient be restored to health | 12 |
| Healthcare access | Help the patient to seek for financial aid from other sources | 12 |
| Institutional rules and regulations | Be co-operative in working with other health care personnel | 10 |
| The nurse's personal quality | Have a sense of responsibility | 8 |
| Protectiveness | Alleviate the patient's psychological burden | 7 |
| The doctrine of socialist humanism | Rescue the dying and heal the wounded | 7 |

** Most respondents gave more than one ethical justification for their preferred ways in dealing with the given situation. Those statements with a frequency count less than 5 are not listed.*

## C. Respect for Nurses

Mr. Dai's nurse found the patient quite demanding since he asked her to serve him for things that he could have done for himself. As described in the vignette,

> The nurses felt that the patient still presumed that he was the master of the family and boss of a company. He did not listen to the nurses, nor did he show any respect for them. He treated them as if they were his servants. He claimed that he was paying so much for his hospital stay that he was entitled to good service.

Mr. Dai's attitude toward nurses typifies the ancient Chinese attitude that nursing is the work of servants. In response to Mr. Dai's apparently arrogant behavior, thirty-one respondents indicated that "the nurse's dignity should be respected by the patient and the patient's family." Thirteen of them said nurses should "respect nursing and the nurse's dignity" as an ethical response in dealing with Mr. Dai's antagonistic attitude.

They felt that respect is due to a person in correspondence to the dynamic of social role relationships, which is in line with the Confucian notion of respect.[35] They were concerned that respectful relationships should be grounded in equality. This notion of equality is different from the sense of equality prized by Mrs. Wong's nurse. Mrs. Wong's nurse is concerned with treating patients with the same standard of good nursing care. The responses to the Dai case are concerned with respect due to each other in their role relationships. One informant suggested,

> The Patient, his or her relatives and nurses should treat each other on an equal basis. First, we should respect patients. Patients should respect us as well. Hospital rules and regulations have specified everyone's role requirements. If we do not act as required of us in our roles, we cannot build a respectful relationship with each other.

This passage highlights two aspects in building a respectful relationship. First, people should fulfill the requirements of their roles in correspondence to situational changes, patient and nurse should fulfill their role requirements appropriately. According to the respondents' expectations, when a person is hospitalized, he should act within the normal role requirement of a patient. Hence, Mr. Dai should cooperate with healthcare workers and comply with the therapeutic regimen and the hospital rules and regulations. He should be aware that he is under the nurses' professional care instead of treating the nurse as if she was his subordinate. An informant shared her expectations of a patient's role.

> I would tell the patient in an affirmative but soft voice so that he could pick up the message that I have reasons to support what I say. I will tell him that "When you are at home, you are the master, and you expect your children to listen to your words. You are also the boss and your subordinates are required to listen to your orders. This is right. You get ill and are admitted into this ward. I am responsible for managing this ward, and what I do for you is for your well-being. Isn't that right? Therefore I think you have to listen to my words."

Hospital rules and regulations are functional in two respects. First, the role requirements of healthcare workers, patients, and regulations for ward management are defined.[36] Hence, each party should know what is proper behaviour in each role relationship. Second, most informants found hospital rules functional to back them up in declining the patient's demanding requests.

In this dynamic role relationship, accordingly Mr. Dai's nurse should have fulfilled her role requirements to the hospital and the patient's expectations. According to the hospital, nurses must help the patient comply with medical treatment, be responsible for care of the patient and not to rely on the patient's family, maintain a good relationship with patient and family, and be co-operative in working with other healthcare workers. Some respondents also considered that Mr. Dai's nurse should have taken into account meeting the patient's wishes, satisfying the patient's needs and alleviating the patient's psychological burden. In sum, the informants emphasized that respect is built on equality, in the sense that each person should act "equal" to what is required of his or her role. Hence, this notion of equality has a strong paternalistic basis, in which a patient is expected to be compliant and follow the instructions of healthcare workers, and a nurse is expected to do what is best for the patient just as a mother would treat her child.

The second aspect of building a respectful relationship is that respect does not come spontaneously. The two parties should make an effort in order to gain respect from others. An informant quoted a Chinese idiom to illustrate this sense of respect.

> If a person gives me allowance that measures one foot long, I will give the person allowance ten times in return. In such dealings, we can gain respect from others.

The process of gaining respect demands a person to act according to his or her role requirements even though the other party does not honor theirs. In a nurse's words,

> Nurses have to give detailed explanation patiently so as to gain the patient's trust. Being a nurse, one has to meet the patient's needs and think from his or her point of view. Nurses have to respect the nursing profession, themselves, and others. If patients and relatives do not understand the responsibility of a special care nurse, the nurse has to make them understand so that they can appreciate the positive aspects of nursing.

The first concern of the respondents in gaining respect is to let the patient and his family members in the Dai case understand the qualitative distinction of nursing work from that of the work of servants. To this end, they need to demonstrate their professional competence and knowledge while taking care of the patient. The second concern is to let the patient know that the care he receives from the nurse is better than his family can give. The respondents interpreted the statement "treat the patient as your family member" quite differently in this context. It comprises the common understanding that nurses should treat patients as if they were their family members. The respondents would like Mr. Dai's nurse to show that the care his family members can provide him is qualitatively distinctive from that which the nurse provides him. Her care requires medical knowledge and technical skills and can contribute to hastening his recovery in ways his family's care cannot. Two respondents noted at least two aspects of care that a patient's relative cannot provide. The first aspect is close monitoring of the patient's medical condition, and the second is provision of a therapeutic environment that can hasten the patient's recovery. In sum, the old concern for gaining respect for nurses is still a predominant issue in contemporary China. Nurses commonly believe that only if they can replace family members in providing qualitatively distinctive professional care to the patient will the servant image of nursing work diminish.

### D. Inclusion of Family Members

Many nurses indicated that the most difficult issue in ward management is management of visitors. In the Dai and Feng cases, respondents shared the view that "the nurse, instead of a patient's family, has to be responsible for care of the patient in hospital." An informant disclosed that hospitals used the number of visitors staying in the ward as an indicator of care quality. If nurses can provide better care to patients, an assumption that family members do not need to be there is made. This practice is in confrontation with the cultural preferences for being cared for by the family when sick.

The respondents held different views regarding hospitals' visiting policies. Some found strict visiting rules reasonable on the grounds that the rules are necessary to prevent cross infection and to maintain a clean and quiet environment for patients. Others noted that patients would become more emotional when their relatives were present, which could do patients more harms than good. The nurses used the same justifications for restricted family involvement as they were practiced in the Nightingale tradition. When no visitors are allowed, the respondents noted that they have the responsibility to treat the patient as their family members so that the patient might feel at home and be co-operative with the nurse. Some respondents doubted whether they could perform the role of a family surrogate. As an informant commented

> One should allow visitors to come. Visits are good for the patient because it brings affection and reassurance. Also, nurses can learn from the patient's family members about the patient's habits. Nurses cannot understand the patient's habits in such a short time. The patient is now sick and has to adapt to a new hospital routine. Misinterpretation of the patient's need creates conflicts easily.

Some nurses considered restricted visiting as not ethical, mainly because the kind of support and affection that family members can give to the patient is irreplaceable. A preferred approach is to allow more flexibility in the visiting regulations, and to get patient's family members involved in planning nursing care. Furthermore, the current practice that requires nurses to be a surrogate for the patient's family discourages nurses from identifying the problems family care providers encounter, as illustrated in the Feng case.

Concerning the ethical way of dealing with the situation, the predominant response is that nurses should give health education to the patient and the family member. This preferred practice is undermined in practice situations where the hospital rules and regulations do not allow room for nurses to develop this dimension of care. I would like to see at least two changes in this respect. First, instead of minimizing patients' families as the least important aspect of the role responsibilities of nurses, hospital management should advocate patient-focused and family-centered care by emphasizing the nurses' roles in empowering family members to participate in taking care of the sick. Second, the penalty system that monitors nursing quality in terms of procedural accuracy and technical competence should be transformed into a responsive system that awards good practices that positively promote the quality of patient care.

## E. Summary

How to draw the boundary between nurses' legitimate claim they provide qualitatively distinctive care from that of family members in caring for the sick is undoubtedly a major source of tension in practice situations in China. The Dai and the Feng cases typify issues of this kind, but expose them in two extreme ways. In the case of Mr. Dai, the patient's family members were totally restricted from participating in taking care of Mr. Dai, to the extent that the patient's demand for more tangible care by his family members was not attended to. Whereas in the Feng case, care of the patient was left totally in the hands of her sister so that the demand for nurses' professional input was neglected. The primary source of tension does not originate from nurses' attempt to expand their legitimate sphere of professional practice by excluding family members in taking care of the sick. It lies in the institutional rules and regulations that emphasize clear lines of authority, well-defined roles, procedural accuracy, technical competence, and maintenance of an harmonious atmosphere. This institutional ethos fosters a strong work-to-rule attitude that restricts healthcare workers responsiveness in addressing individual patients' needs. In the Dai case, the tension emerges from the hospital rules restricting visitors and the refusal of the patient and his family members to comply with them. The neglect of Mrs. Feng and her sister's health educational needs is understandable since health education is regarded as a "soft" nursing responsibility. In contrast to committing an error in, say, giving medication, which could result in disciplinary action, no penalty is imposed on nurses who fail to follow a "soft" guideline. In order to maintain a peaceful and co-operative atmosphere, most nurses prefer to maintain a safe distance from patients while trying to avoid any direct confrontation with patients and their relatives. This practice impedes nurses in openly communicating with patients and family members, and prevents nurses from providing care based on a good understanding of the patient's individual needs.

Analysis of the written accounts of nurses' descriptions of their views of ethical and unethical practices in dealing with the Dai and Feng cases reveals that many nurses reckoned an attitude of unresponsiveness is unethical. In sum, ethical practice demands nurses to overcome three hurdles in current practice. First, they need to expand nursing's concerns beyond those responsibilities stipulated by hospital rules and regulations, so as to create personal space for open communication between nurses and patients. Second, nurses have to see their job descriptions beyond the scope of technical competence, so that they can refocus nursing from a task orientation to a patient orientation. Third, they have to go beyond the commonly held belief that the only way nurses can dispel the traditional view of nurses as servants is to replace family members in providing qualitatively distinctive care. Inclusion of family members in caring for patients and extending the scope of nursing responsibility in health education would be a more positive approach to demonstrate nurses' professionalism. This could also ease tensions between nurses and patients' families over the distribution of care responsibilities.

# Seven

# FROM VIRTUE TO VALUE: A DIALOGUE TO BE CONTINUED

## 1. Summary

I have shown that, in the modern development of Chinese nursing, three essential virtues have been identified in academic writing, official documents, and in the opinions of nurses themselves. They are a sense of socialist responsibility, a desire for excellence in practice and sincerity in relating to patients. These virtues have their roots in traditional Chinese medical ethics, but are expressed within the ideological framework of "socialist humanism." The criteria for medical ethics formulated in 1988, in which Mao's mandate for healthcare workers is promoted as the fundamental principle, upholds the importance of these virtues. Embedded in this mandate is an advocacy of respect for life that demands both a negative duty not to do harm, and a positive duty on the part of healthcare workers to protect life and treat patients with altruistic motives.

Over the past ten years, education and management measures have been instituted to foster these virtues in nurses. Only if nurses possessed these virtues and at the same time follow the rules of conduct set forth by the Ministry of Public Health, they believe that undesirable practices brought about by the introduction of market factors to healthcare could be counteracted. To this end, nurses are required to be angelic Lei Fengs or socialist humanist Florence Nightingales. I question how realistic these ethics-inducing measures are, in the sense that nurses are able to put the mandate into practice. In reviewing the competing values emerging from the contemporary issues that healthcare workers are required to deal with, I remain doubtful.

Three issues have been examined. They are healthcare access on a fee-to-service basis, population control policies, and changing views of society about legalizing active euthanasia. I argue that another set of values based on the notion of "quality of life" promulgated by the Party leadership poses direct challenges to the adequacy of the mandate in informing practice. Nurses in China were apparently silent about their ethical viewpoints. In this context, where old and new values meet, I started a dialogue with nurses in China, with the objective of letting their voices be heard, in a context of their place and time and culture, and of broader and perhaps universal ethical issues.

I adopted triangulation as a method of study for two purposes. The first purpose was to ground my interpretations of nurses' moral experience with "demonstrable sophisticated rigor," and second was to sustain a dialogue between nurses in China and their counterparts in other parts of the world. This process of inquiry comprised three phases. It followed a directional flow from one single hospital to different parts of China. The mode of inquiry moved from an unstructured field study to a more structured questionnaire survey, and the role of the investigator changed from observer to interviewer to surveyor. The empirical findings reveal that nurses in China comprehend nursing ethics in the context of multiple role relationships expressed in eleven facets of nursing responsibilities. Nurses gave high rankings to the doctrine of socialist humanism and the nurses' personal and professional qualities in importance to nursing responsibilities, which are congruent with the three core virtues that are propagated in recent nursing ethics literature. Apparently, the educational and management strategies used by the Ministry of Public Health to indoctrinate healthcare workers with such desirable qualities have been successful. Three pairs of contrasted rankings emerged from the pattern of nurses' rankings given to the eleven facets of responsibilities. This suggests that nurses in China inevitably experience moral dilemmas that emerge from competing role requirements as typified in the five vignettes. They are situations in relation to disclosure of information, withdrawal of treatment, requests for euthanasia, unmet needs of a demanding patient, and unmet needs of a silent patient. The following section is an attempt to base my arguments on interpretations of the nurses' ethical responses to see how they conceptualize ethical practice. I hope this can provide better alternatives for resolving the ethical dilemmas embodied in contemporary healthcare practices.

## 2. Conceptualization of Ethical Practice

In her thesis on the ideal of service and the historical reality of nursing and ethics, Marsha Fowler observed that the list of virtues held in the 1980s closely resembles those drawn from the nursing literature over the past century. As she argues

> the major shift in the virtues and excellencies relevant to nursing has not been in the identification of which virtues and excellencies are necessary. Rather, the shift is an interpretive one.[1]

She further suggests that in ranking these virtues, what concerns nurses changes over time, and interpretation of these virtues and their implication for practice also varies.[2] This observation is noted in the history of Chinese nursing. In the Republican period, the list of ethical requirements compiled by Yao Changxu puts less emphasis on the requirements of excellence in practice, but more on the ways in which a nurse ought to relate to patients so as to foster healing. Nurses were required to treat a patient as they would treat their family member. In the Maoist era, the notion of "serving the people" was promoted encompassing the virtues of "utter devotion to others without thinking of yourself," "boundless warm-heartedness in serving others," "willingness to endure hardship," and "loyalty to the Party's leadership." Excellence in practice was largely devalued. To demonstrate that they did possess a high sense of socialist responsibility, people were required to put the interests of the common good first. During this period, the traditional fiduciary relationship between healthcare worker and patient was weakened. Ironically though, the notion of "treating the patient better than your family member" continued to be upheld. As nursing entered into the era of China's reforms, primacy was given to excellence in practice, with the objective of improving the quality of nursing and reconstructing the professional identity of nurses. Along with the introduction of market factors in healthcare provision and material incentives to motivate workers' initiative, the virtue of "socialist responsibility" was questioned. How the nurse should relate to patients in a professional sense also became problematic.

In view of the empirical findings, this "interpretive shift" occurs over the three periods of nursing development in China, and was also articulated by nurses when they were asked to give their ethical viewpoints on the five difficult care situations. When the nurses were asked to rank the importance of the fifty statements that represent aspects of qualities of character or rules of conduct, their responses fell into a pattern. They gave uniformly high rankings to statements representing the doctrine of socialist humanism and the nurse's personal and professional qualities, but they gave uniformly low rankings to statements representing the holistic inclusion of family members and healthcare access. When they were asked to express their views on ethical ways of dealing with the five difficult ethical situations, their responses did not suggest a similar pattern. Most nurses justify their stances using statements that represent treating the patient as an individual and protectiveness as in the Chan case, access to healthcare as in the Wong case, and quality of care and treating the patient as an individual in the Huang case. As for the Dai case, they valued institutional rules and regulations and the holistic inclusion of family members, and in the Feng case, the nurses' professional qualities.

Some respondents commented that ranking the fifty statements was difficult because they found them all relevant to nursing, and thus how these statements should be ranked depends on the situation. I agree, and would further suggest that this is the reason why nurses are required to be responsive to different patient care situations and to be able to exercise ethical judgment for discerning the best possible care in practice. The ICN

Code makes explicit the requirement of a nurse to make professional judgments, such as in situations of sharing information and in taking appropriate action to safeguard the individual when he or she is endangered by co-workers. Nonetheless, in China today, institutional rules that reinforce a system of protective medical care and external regulations for standard practice pose a restricted view of the interpretation of nursing virtues.

According to Sun Simiao, excellence in practice (精 *jing*) and sincerity (誠 *cheng*) in relating to patients require continuous efforts on the part of medical practitioners to expand their knowledge, and to give "undivided mental attention to the last details" in diagnosing patients' problems. I argue that the first aspect is highly commended in current practice, but not the second aspect. For instance, the criteria for medical ethics states that healthcare workers are required to "be rigorous in learning and practicing medicine," and they should "work hard to improve [their] knowledge, ability, skills and service." But no mention of the importance of clinical judgments as stated in Sun's thesis exists. The notions of responsible nursing and a systematic approach to holistic nursing care have been introduced as measures to promote professionalism in nursing. I have strong reservations about the possibility of this professional sense germinating in a system where strong emphasis is placed on rules and regulations.

Empirical findings suggest that nursing is primarily seen as a set of technical tasks. Knowledge that arrives from a dialogical understanding of individual patients is not valued, and inhibited in practice. With the exception of Mrs. Wong's nurse, all nurses in the other four vignettes experienced tensions in relating to the patients and family members due to customary practices or restrictive institutional rules and regulations, and their scope of responsibility was limited to performing nursing procedures. Their responses analyzed in this study demonstrate that they do possess these qualities of character. They are able to articulate a moral sense of nursing that demands a move away from a rule-based ethic to one which is more flexible, pluralist, contextualised, individualized, and subjectively informed, in short, to one which is virtue-based. These findings support Mencius's view that virtues should precede rules of conduct.

On the basis of my analysis of the nurses' ethical responses to the five difficult care situations, three major aspects of the multiple role responsibilities have undergone an "interpretive shift" in their attempt to conceptualize how ethical practice could be fostered. Figure 6.1 summarizes the ways nurses in China articulate ethical practice in the context of multiple role responsibilities. In contrast to Figure 5.3, three major changes of the diagrammatic representation of the eleven facets of nursing responsibilities are made. First, the boundary between the patient and the patient's family has been lifted. Second, the boundary between the profession and practice is removed; and third, virtue-based practice is identified as the core value.

On the assumption that family members are playing a significant role in taking care of the sick in hospital care, requiring nurses to treat patients better than their family members is unrealistic. Yet, to leave total care responsibilities to patients' family members is equally unethical. As shown in the Chan, Huang, Dai, and Feng cases, none of these situations foster the best possible care for patients. Furthermore, conflicts in practice contexts are largely due to a lack of direct communication between nurses, patients, and patients' families. Nurses in China should be more proactive in starting a dialogue with society so as to gain agreement on nursing as a legitimate sphere of practice.

The existing issues embodied in the tripartite relation between nurse, patient, and patient's family could be critically appraised and reconstructed in a way that fosters responsive care to patients and society on the one hand and the professional integrity of nursing on the other. To draw a qualitative distinction between nursing work and the work of a servant has been a major concern for nurses who want to protect their professional integrity and to gain respect from society. This conception of nursing tends to place high value on technical tasks instead of patient care, which in turn prevents nurses from seeing their profession as a practice that supports the well-being of patients through responsive care. Therefore I suggest that an interpretive shift is needed to conceptualize virtue-based practice as the core value. Traditional virtues would be reinterpreted in the context of contemporary practice. Furthermore, the central task of making a qualitative distinction in nursing work has to focus on inquiring into practical ways to make a difference in improving care for individual patients.

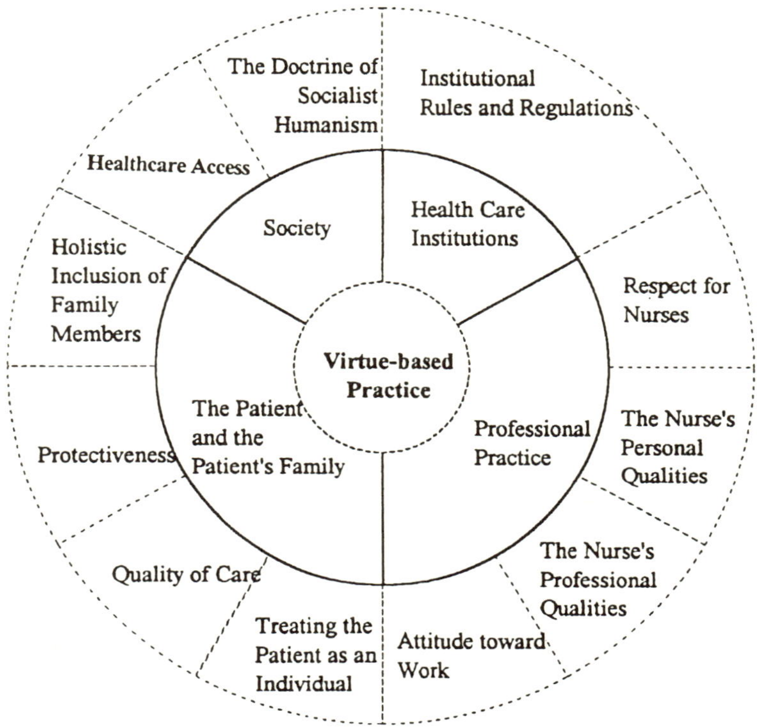


Figure 7.1. Conceptualization of Ethical Nursing Practice

## 3. Cultivating a Moral Sense of Nursing: A Dialogue to be Continued

I cannot recommend how mainland nurses can foster virtue-based nursing practice, I believe that recent discussion in the international community of nursing as a caring practice may provide insights for Chinese nurses. As defined by Anne Bishop and John Scudder, "[nursing] is a practice, in that it is made up of practical ways of fostering the good, that is the well-being of persons."[3] They further argue that the search for an understanding of nursing as a caring practice has to begin with the recognition of the moral sense of nursing within the clinical context. Though much has been said about the eminence of caring pertinent to nursing practice, no consensus exists regarding the definitions of caring, the components of care, or the process of caring.[4]

After many years of work in transcultural nursing, Madeleine Leininger constructs a theory of transcultural care diversity and universality. She contends that though some of the care patterns, processes, and acts may be universal, the diverse expressions, meanings, patterns, and modalities of caring are culturally devised. In order to reduce the ambiguities inherent in providing culturally congruent care, a cross-cultural knowledge of ethical and moral values is essential to help nurses make meaningful care judgments, decisions, and actions.[5] In what respect caring is an aspect of the moral nature of nursing has invited many debates in recent years. Stanley Hauerwas explains the ambiguity inherent in the concept of care. He finds that care is not meant to provide a basis for judgment on specific actions in the medical context. Instead, care is the source of all particular obligations and one's court of final appeal for deciding the features of actions and practices that make what we do right or wrong in any context.[6] Arguing from a relational ethics tradition, Nel Noddings suggests that care means to be charged with the protection, welfare, or maintenance of something or someone. Therefore, to care is to engage in some behaviors that have moral dimensions. This view is affirmed by Jean Watson and further delineated by Sara Fry.[7] Human caring is a moral concept when caring is directed toward human needs and is perceived as a duty to respond to need. Patricia Benner suggests that caring as a foundation of ethical responses is rooted in relational values of openness and responsiveness that are required for a respectful meeting of other people.[8] In sum, consensus exists among the theorists that nursing should be articulated as a caring practice, but there are competing views as to whether caring should be considered as a moral concept as such.

Over the past decade, much scholarly effort has been invested in explicating what caring practice is within the clinical context, with an intention of articulating the moral sense of nursing. Among other nursing scholars, Benner, and Bishop and Scudder find the pheno-menological approach especially appropriate for inquiring into the new possibilities inherent in practice which in turn give insight into what is in nursing that makes a difference in caring for the sick, and how to improve practice. While Benner used expert models to uncover the domains and competencies of nursing practice, Bishop and Scudder argued that a sense of morality is what is crucial to excellence in nursing practice. They used exemplary practices in nursing to illustrate how the moral sense is realized and how better practice can be encouraged.[9]

Using exemplary practices as a strategy to cultivate desirable attributes has been widely used in China. Virtuous models are used as examples to illustrate the desirable attributes which healthcare workers should possess. The life and work of these models reflect the prescribed moral virtues, but are raised to the level of sainthood. Since these examples are presented abstractly, outside the context of practice, whether most healthcare workers can identify with these models in a way that motivates emulation is debatable. The notion of model emulation deviates from a crucial notion of the importance of cultivating a person's evaluating mind. It creates a situation in which mere imitation is fostered, impeding a person from actively discerning right from wrong, and conceiving new possibilities that could improve practice.

On the assumption that model emulation is not learning by mere imitation, but an interplay of presenting virtuous models and cultivating an evaluating mind, I experimented on using a dialogical process in order to see how it could facilitate behavioral and attitudinal changes in my students. I deliberately structured their learning experiences to foster learning from the exemplary nursing practice. In classroom teaching, I put emphasis on cultivating the students' power of evaluation through readings of symbolic models of a sincere inquirer. The students were encouraged to express and discuss in class their viewpoints on abstract concepts, such as love, freedom, equity, the meaning of life, illness, suffering, and death. The dialogical process exemplified by Plato's Socratic dialogues was encouraged in classroom discussion, with an intention to help students recognize the tentativeness and finitude of the inquiring process, but at the same time surrender themselves to the "truth" uncovered, with a willingness to be tested and to be challenged. Although a dialogue of this kind may end in uncertainty about which view is more justifiable, it helps the students to explore among themselves their underlying assumptions and unreflected views on issues. This in turn helps them develop a more tolerant attitude toward ambiguity on the one hand and a desire to search for the best possible answer through rational arguments on the other.

When the students underwent clinical training, they were asked to capture their experiences of positive and negative examples of nursing practice by keeping journals of their clinical practice. The journals include the aspects of nursing they have learned, their experience of positive and negative examples of nursing practice, and what they have learned from these examples. These written accounts were not graded, but served two more important purposes. First, the students were given an opportunity to express their experience of good and bad nursing in words. By expressing their experience verbally, the students were forced to interpret their experiences, and at the same time enter into introspective self-examination of the moral sense of nursing. Second, the written accounts helped to maintain the dialogical process between students and teachers for examining the possible ways of fostering the good in different practice situations. The findings of this experimental teaching are encouraging in the sense that the students were able to recognize positive and negative examples of nursing practice in a variety of patient-care situations, and they were able to give suggestions about the possible ways to improve practice.[10]

I would suggest nurses in China engage in this dialogical process, which I believe can open their minds to all possibilities of how virtue-based practice can be realized within the clinical context. At least three levels of change in current practices are required to make this dialogical process possible. They are healthcare policy, management and education. As I have shown in the empirical research, a gap between public rhetoric of nursing ethics in China and the moral experience of nurses exists. That gap is partly because the state does not provide free or subsidized healthcare to many Chinese. The message is clear that the state should guarantee decent healthcare to all its citizens if we want to "take virtue seriously." Over the past ten years, educational and management measures have been instituted to foster a sense of morality. These are believed to be crucial in counteracting the undesirable practices resulting from the introduction of market factors to healthcare. The empirical findings in the present study reveal that these ethics-inducing measures impose a restricted interpretation of nursing virtues, instead of allowing nurses to actively engage in finding positive ways to improve practice. Advocating a genuinely virtue-based ethics for nursing may be controversial, given the problems on the ground, in particular for the Chinese nurses whose voices I have tried to make heard in this study. But if my interpretation is right, they are saying, or almost saying, something of universal interest and importance: do not concentrate on a set of procedural or ethical rules. Concentrate instead upon not just delineating but cultivating the virtues of a good nurse.

# NOTES

## Chapter One

1. Merja Kuuppelomaki and Sirkka Lauri, "The Ethical Decision-making of Nurses Associated with the Feeding of Demented Patients and Terminally Ill Elderly Cancer Patients in Seven Countries," *Hoitoece*, 3:4 (1991), pp. 146–153. Anne J. Davis, B. Davidson, M. Hirschfield, S. Lauri, J. Y. Lin, A. Norberg, L. Phillips, E. Pitman, C. H Shen, R. V. Laan, H. L. Zhang, and L. Ziv, "An International Perspective of Active Euthanasia: Attitudes of Nurses in Seven Countries," *International Journal of Nursing Studies*, 30:4 (1993), pp. 301–310. Surname comes first in Chinese names, and this rule is followed in the main text. For consistency in presenting English references in the notes, the rule of having surname as last name is followed. However, for publications in Chinese surname remains as first name.

2. Alasdair MacIntyre, *After Virtue: A Study in Moral Theory* (London: Duckworth, 2nd ed., 1985), p. 191.

3. *Ibid.*, p. 185.

4. 徐少錦、溫克勤編，《中國倫理文化寶庫》。北京：中國廣播電視出版社，頁 3，1995。

5. James Legge (trans.), *Confucian Analects, the Great Learning and the Doctrine of the Mean* (New York: Dover, 1971).

6. Dimcheuk Lau (trans.), *Mencius* (Hong Kong: Chinese University Press, 1984), Vol. 1, Bk. 2, Pt. A., p. 67.

7. *Ibid.*, Bk. 4, Pt. A, pp. 155–157.

8. Weiming Tu, "Selfhood and Otherness in Confucian Thought," *Culture and Self: Asian and Western Perspectives*, eds. Anthony J. Marsella, George A. DeVos, and Francis L. K. Hsu (New York: Tavistock Publications, 1985), pp. 231–251.

9. Peng Lei, "The Practical Significance of Confucian Moral Cultivation," *Social Sciences in China*, 18:2 (1997), pp. 45–43.

10. Donald J. Munro, *The Concept of Man in Early China* (Stanford: Stanford University Press, 1969), pp. 3–4.

## Chapter Two

1. Donald J. Munro, *The Concept of Man in Contemporary China* (Ann Arbor: University of Michigan Press, 1977), p. 5. Christina B. Whitman, "Privacy in Early Confucian and Taoist Thought," *Individualism and Holism: Studies in Confucian and Taoist Values*, ed. Donald J. Munro (Ann Arbor: Center for Chinese Studies, University of Michigan, 1985), pp. 85–99.

2. Paul U. Unschuld, *Medical Ethics in Imperial China: A Study in Historical Anthropology* (Berkeley: University of California Press, 1979), pp. 238–239.

3. 王琇瑛，《護理發展簡史》。上海：上海科學技術出版社，1987。

4. *Ibid.*, 頁 78~79。

5. Thomas K. S. Wong and Samantha M. C. Pang, "Holism and Caring: Nursing in the Chinese Health Care Context," *Holistic Nursing Practice*, 15:1 (2000), pp. 12–21.

6. Ann Brashaw, "The Historical Tradition of Care," *Caring: The Compassion and Wisdom of Nursing*, ed. Gosia Bryjznska (London: Arnold, 1997),

pp. 10–31. Marsha D. M. Fowler, *Ethics and Nursing, 1893–1984: The Ideal of Service, the Reality of History*, Ph. D. Thesis (Los Angeles: University of Southern California, 1984).

7. Lin Nan, "Chinese Family Structure and Chinese Society," *Bulletin of the Institute of Ethnology Academia Sinica*, 65 (Spring 1988), pp. 59–129. Thad J. Barnowe, "Chinese Attempts to Reform Organizational Cultures," *Advances in Chinese Industrial Studies*, I, Pt. A. (1990), pp. 332–333. 孫隆基，《中國文化的深層結構（修訂版）》。香港：集賢社，1992。Yong Zhu and Yaping Cheng, "Kinship and Legal Duties in Ancient China," *Social Sciences in China*, 18:3 (1997), pp. 99–105.

8. Chunghsing Sun, "The Five Interpersonal Relationships in the Four Books: A Study in Confucian Ethics," *National Taiwan University Journal of Sociology*, (1993), p. 3.

9. 朱熹，《四書章句集注》。上海：上海書局，1987。

10. Sun, "The Five Interpersonal Relationships in the Four Books," pp. 3–4.

11. James Legge (trans.), *Confucian Analects, the Great Learning and the Doctrine of the Mean* (New York: Dover, 1971), p. 409.

12. Sandra A. Wawrytko, "Confucius and Kant: The Ethics of Respect," *Philosophy East and West*, 32:3 (1982), p. 237.

13. 孫隆基，《中國文化的深層結構》，頁 175~204。Dimcheuk Lau (trans.), *Mencius* (Hong Kong: Chinese University Press, 1984), Vol. 1, Bk. 4, Pt. A, p. 152.

14. *Ibid*., Vol. 2, Bk. 7, Pt. A, p. 281.

15. Legge, *Confucian Analects*, p. 270.

16. Plato "Euthyphro," trans. Hugh Tredennick and Harold Tarrant, in *The Last Days of Socrates* (New York: Penguin Classic, 1993), pp. 1–28.

17. Jingyu Wu (trans.), *Twenty-four Stories of Filial Devotion* (Singapore: Asiapac Publication, 1997).

18. *Ibid*., pp. 127–130.

19. Unschuld, *Medical Ethics in Imperial China*, p. 2.

20. 孫隆基，《中國文化的深層結構》，頁 131~204。 Nelson W. S. Chow, "Western and Chinese Ideas of Social Welfare," *International Social Work*, 30 (1987), pp. 31–41. Veronica Pearson, "Community and Culture: A Chinese Model of Community Care for the Mentally Ill," *International Journal of Social Psychiatry*, 38:3 (1992), pp. 163–178. Annie Lau, "Family Therapy and Ethnic Minorities," *Family Therapy in Britain*, eds. Eddy Street and Windy Dryden (Milton Keynes: Open University Press, 1988), pp. 270–290. Veronica Pearson, "Families in China: An Undervalued Resource for Mental Health?" *Journal of Family Therapy*, 15 (1993), pp. 163–185.

21. Tsungyi Lin and Meichen Lin, "Love, Denial and Rejection: Responses of Chinese Families to Mental Illness," *Normal and Abnormal Behavior in Chinese Culture*, eds. Arthur Kleinman and Tsungyi Lin (Dordrecht, Mass.: D. Reidel and Hingham, 1981), pp. 387–401.

22. Veronica Pearson, *Mental Health Care in China: State Policies, Professional Services and Family Responsibilities* (London: Gaskell, 1995).

23. Unschuld, *Medical Ethics in Imperial China*, p. 57.

24. *Ibid*., p. 27.

25. Ilza Veith, "Changing Concepts of Health Care: An Historian's View," *Western Journal of Medicine*, 133:6 (1980), pp. 532–538.

26. Unschuld, *Medical Ethics in Imperial China*, pp. 72–73.

27. 王琇瑛，《護理發展簡史》，頁 4。

28. China Medical Commission of the Rockefeller Foundation, *Medicine in China* (Chicago: The University of Chicago Press, 1914), p. 58.

29. Lystra E. Gretter, *The Nightingale Pledge* (Detroit: Harper Hospital, 1893). Sara T. Fry, "The Code for Nurses, International Council of Nurses (ICN Code)," *Ethics in Nursing Practice: A Guide to Ethical Decision Marking* (Geneva, Switzerland: International Council of Nurses, 1994).

30. China Medical Commission of the Rockefeller Foundation, *Medicine in China*, p. 58.

31. *Ibid*., pp. 70–71.

32. *Ibid*., pp. 96–97.

33. Chungtung Liu, "From *San Gu Liu Po* to 'Caring Scholar': The Chinese Nurse in Perspective," *International Journal of Nursing Studies*, 28:4 (1991), p. 317.

34. 《辭海》(*Word Encyclopaedia*).

35. Unschuld, *Medical Ethics in Imperial China*, pp. 40–42. Renzong Qiu, "Philosophy of Medicine in China (1930–1980)," *Metamedicine*, 3 (1982), p. 64.

36. Tao Lee, "Medical Ethics in Ancient China," *Cross Cultural Perspectives in Medical Ethics: Readings*, ed. Robert M. Veatch (Boston, Mass.: Jones and Bartlett Publishers, 1989), p. 133.

37. 徐少錦、溫克勤編，"女誡"，《中國倫理文化寶庫》。北京：中國廣播電視出版社，頁 476，1995。

38. William Theodore de Bary, *Asian Values and Human Rights* (Cambridge, Mass.: Harvard University Press, 1998), pp. 126–127.

39. 劉詠聰，《女性與歷史：中國傳統觀念新探》。香港：香港教育，頁 89~108，1993。呂美頤、鄭永福，《中國婦女運動：1840–1921》。鄭州：河南人民出版社，頁 38~41，1990。

40. Chiang Jung, *Wild Swans, the Three Daughters of China* (London: Flamingo, 1992), p. 31. Delia Davin, *Woman Work: Women and the Party in Revolutionary China* (Oxford: Clarendon Press, 1976), p. 12.

41. 王琇瑛，《護理發展簡史》，頁 88~89。

42. Zedong Mao, *Quotations from Chairman Mao Tse-tung* (Peking: Foreign Language Press, 1972), p. 294.

43. *Ibid*., pp. 294–298.

44. Liu, "From *San Gu Liu Po* to 'Caring Scholar,'" p. 321.

45. Lau, *Mencius*, Vol. 1., Bk. 7, Pt. A, p. 151.

46. Qiu, "Philosophy of Medicine in China," p. 65. Lee, "Medical Ethics in Ancient China," p. 133.

47. Barbara Spencer, *Desert Hospital in China* (London: Jarrolds Publishers, 1954), pp. 128–138.

48. 王琇瑛，《護理發展簡史》，頁 77~82。 China Medical Commission of the Rockefeller Foundation, *Medicine in China*, pp. 68–73.

49. 姚昶緒，《病人看護法》。上海：商務印書館，頁 1~3，1939。Charles E. Rosenberg, *The Care of Strangers: The Rise of America's Hospital System* (New York: Basic Books, Inc., 1987), p. 212.

50. 王琇瑛，《護理發展簡史》，頁 79~80。

51. Chimin Wong and Lienteh Wu, *The History of Chinese Medicine: Being a Chronicle of Medical Happenings in China from Ancient Times to the Present Period* (Shanghai: National Quarantine Service, 1936), pp. 805–806.

52. Wong and Wu, *The History of Chinese Medicine*, p. 61.

53. Myron E. Wegman, Tsungyi Lin, and Elizabeth F. Purcell (eds.), *Public Health in the People's Republic of China: The Macy Foundation Series on Medicine and Public Health in China* (New York: The Josiah Macy, JR. Foundation, 1973), p. 33.

54. 王琇瑛，《護理發展簡史》，頁 79~86。

55. Rosenberg, *The Care of Strangers*, pp. 234–235.

56. Liu, "From *San Gu Liu Po* to 'Caring Scholar,'" p. 322.

57. Rosenberg, *The Care of Strangers*, p. 219.

58. Fowler, *Ethics and Nursing*, pp. 121–122.

59. P. Esterhuizen, "Is the Professional Code Still the Cornerstone of Clinical Nursing Practice?" *Journal of Advanced Nursing*, 23:1 (1996), pp. 25–31. Trevor Hussey, "Nursing Ethics and Codes of Professional Conduct," *Nursing Ethics*, 3:3 (1996), pp. 250–258. 佘雲楚、彭美慈，"專業守則：實務或霸權？評「香港護士專業守則」"，《專業交叉點：專業倫理的理念與實行》。香港：青文書局，頁 66~101，2000。彭美慈、曾熙媛、王春生、張志君、劉書琴、汪國成、賴錦玉，"採用特爾非法撰寫新世紀中國護士倫理準則"，《中華護理雜誌》，35 卷，9 期，頁 517~518，2000。

60. 姚昶緒，《病人看護法》，頁 1。

61. Li Feng, "I am a Nurse," *Women of China Special Series: Half the Sky (1)* (Beijing: Women of China, 1985), pp. 185–186.

62. *Ibid*., p. 186.

63. Liu, "From *San Gu Liu Po* to 'Caring Scholar,'" p. 324.

64. 姚昶緒，《病人看護法》，頁 2~3。

65. Lee, "Medical Ethics in Ancient China," pp. 132–139.

66. Unschuld, *Medical Ethics in Imperial China*, pp. 72–73.

67. Sara E. Parsons, *Nursing Problems and Obligations* (Boston: Whitcomb and Barrows, 1916), pp. 26–55.

68. Steven W. Mosher, *A Mother's Ordeal: The Story of Chi An* (London: Warner Books, 1995), p. 54.

69. 司務道，《陝西羚蹤：司務道教士自傳之一》。香港：靈實醫院靈實福音佈道團，1985。Spencer, *Desert Hospital in China*.

70. Victor Sidel and Ruth Sidel, *The Health of China: Current Conflicts in Medical and Human Services for One Billion People* (London: Zed Press, 1982), p. 3.

71. Zedong Mao, "In Memory of Norman Bethune," *Selected Works of Mao Tsetung* (Peking: Foreign Languages Press, 1965), Vol. 2, p. 337.

72. *Ibid*., pp. 337–338.

73. Eileen P. Bluenthal, *Models in Chinese Moral Education: Perspectives from Children's Books*, Ph. D. Thesis (Ann Arbor: University of Michigan, 1976), pp. 84–87.

74. B. B. Burch, "Models as Agents of Change in China," *Value Change in Chinese Society*, eds. Richard W. Wilson, Amy A. Wilson, and Sidney L. Greenblatt (New York: Prager, 1979), pp. 122–137. Gay G. Reed, "Moral/Political Education in the People's Republic of China: Learning Through Role Models," *Journal of Moral Education*, 24:2 (1995), pp. 99–111.

75. *Ibid*., p. 105.

76. Mao, *Quotations from Chairman Mao Tse-tung*, p. 40.

77. Mao, "On Contradiction (August 1937)," *Selected Works of Mao Tsetung*, Vol. 1, p. 314. "On the Correct Handling of Contradictions among the People (27 February 1957)," *Quotations from Chairman Mao Tsetung*, p. 18.

78. Bluenthal, *Models in Chinese Moral Education*, pp. 9–10. Mosher, *A Mother's Ordeal*, pp. 44–85.

79. Kunyen Huang, "Infectious and Parasitic Diseases," *Medicine and Public Health in the People's Republic of China*, ed. Joseph R. Quinn (Bethesda, Md.: National Institutes of Health, 1973), pp. 241–264. Judith Banister, *China's Changing Population* (Stanford: Stanford University Press, 1987), p. 51. Davis M. Lampton, *The Politics of Medicine in China: The Policy Process 1949–1977* (Folkestone, Kent: Western Press, 1977), pp. 13–16.

80. Mao, *Quotations from Chairman Mao Tse-tung*, p. 118 and p. 124. Raymond L. Whitehead, *Love and Struggle in Mao's Thought* (Maryknoll, N.Y.: Orbis Books, 1977).

81. Lampton, *The Politics of Medicine in China*, pp. 56–61.

82. Sidel and Sidel, *The Health of China*, p. 4.

83. Lampton, *The Politics of Medicine in China*, pp. 242–244.

84. Banister, *China's Changing Population*, pp. 61–62.

85. Lampton, *The Politics of Medicine in China*, pp. 242–244.

86. Tienhis Cheng, "Disease Control and Prevention," *Public Health in the People's Republic of China*, p. 191.

87. Banister, *China's Changing Population*, p. 62.

88. Renzong Qiu, "The Fiduciary Relationship between Professionals and Clients: A Chinese Perspective," *Ethics, Trust, and The Professions, Philosophical and Cultural Aspects*, eds. Edmund D. Pellegrino, Robert M. Veatch, and John P. Langan (Washington, D. C.: Georgetown University Press, 1991), pp. 255–256.

89. David M. Lampton, "Economics, Politics and the Determinants of Policy Outcomes in China: Post-cultural Revolution Health Policy," *Australian and New Zealand Journal of Sociology*, 12:1 (1976), pp. 43–49. Veronica Pearson, "Health and Responsibility, But Whose?" *Social Change and Social Policy in Contemporary China*, eds. Linda Wong and Stewart MacPherson (Hong Kong: City University of Hong Kong, 1995), p. 91.

90. Guangde Sun, "Health Care Administration in China," *Public Policy in China*, eds. Stuart, S. Nagel and Miriam K. Mills (Westport, Conn.: Greenwood Press, 1993), p. 55. Xiaoming Chen, Weihu The, and Zihua Lin, "The Rise and Decline of the Co-operative Medical System in Rural China," *International Journal of Health Services*, 23:4 (1993), pp. 731–742.

91. World Bank, *Health: Sector Policy Paper* (Washington, D. C.: World Bank, March 1975), p. 39.

92. Yangpei Lin, Vivian Lin and James Lawson, "Health Policy Reform in the People's Republic of China," *International Journal of Health Services*, 21:3 (1991), pp. 481–491. Jane M. Orient, "A Critique of Western Medical Commentary on the People's Republic of China," *Archives of Internal Medicine*, 144 (1984), pp. 106–109.

93. AnElissa Lucas, *Chinese Medical Modernization: Comparative Policy Continuities, 1930s–1980s* (New York: Praeger Publications, 1982), pp. 78–79.

94. 鄭韓生，“爲護理事業奮鬥一生”，《中華護理雜誌》，30 卷，6 期，頁 383~384，1996。楊曄，“論護理教育的價值取向”，《中華護理雜誌》，30 卷，8 期，頁 476~477，1995。

95. D. M. Baltzan and W. S. Maddin, “Medicine in China,” *Canadian Medical Association Journal*, 93:21 (1965), pp. 1118–1122. Richard Garfield, “China's Nurses: Redefining Roles to Improve Health,” *International Journal of Nursing Studies*, 15 (1978), pp. 129–134.

96. Victor Sidel and Ruth Sidel, “The Healthcare Delivery System of the People's Republic of China,” *Health by the People*, ed. Kenneth W. Newell (Geneva: World Health Organization, 1975), pp. 1–12. Susan B. Rifkin, “Health Care for Rural Areas,” *Medicine and Public Health in the People's Republic of China*, ed. Joseph. R. Quinn (Bethesda, Md.: National Institutes of Health, 1973), p. 147.

97. Lampton, *The Politics of Medicine in China*, p. 243.

98. Qiu, “The Fiduciary Relationship between Professionals and Clients,” pp. 247–259.

99. Lampton, *The Politics of Medicine in China*, p. 243.

100. 王琇瑛，《護理發展簡史》，頁 107~108。

101. Garfield, “China's Nurses: Redefining Roles to Improve Health, ” pp. 129–134. Gail E. Henderson and Myron S. Cohen, *The Chinese Hospital: A Socialist Work Unit* (New Haven: Yale University Press, 1984), pp. 80–85. Renee C. Fox and Judith P. Swazey, “Medical Morality is Not Bioethics: Medical Ethics in China and The United States,” *Perspectives in Biology and Medicine*, 27:3 (1984), pp. 336–360.

102. “On Question of Party History: Resolution on Certain Questions in the History of Our Party since the Founding of the People's Republic of China,” *Beijing Review*, 24:7 (6 July 1981), pp. 20–21.

103. 天津市護士學校，“認真總結經驗，努力辦好護士學校”，《中華護理雜誌》，15 卷，5 期，頁 229~231，1980。曾竹平，“關于護理教育的討論”，《中華護理雜誌》，16 卷，3 期，頁 98~102，1981。鄭韓生，“爲護理事業奮鬥一生”，頁 383~384。

104. Kathleen M. Dirschel, “Teaching Nursing in China: An Exchange Programme,” *Nursing Outlook*, 29:12 (1981), pp. 722–726.

105. Henderson and Cohen, *The Chinese Hospital: A Socialist Work Unit*, pp. 80–85.

106. 宋珍英，“如何做好在職護士的思想教育工作”，《中華護理雜誌》，16 卷，3 期，頁 118~119，1981。

107. 吳行正，“護理責任制的探討”，《中華護理雜誌》，17 卷，5 期，頁 228~266，1982。

108. Marie Manthey, *The Practice of Primary Nursing* (London, England: King's Fund Centre, 1992). R. K. Shukla, “Primary or Team Nursing? Two Conditions Determine the Choice,” *Journal of Nursing Administration*, (November 1982), pp. 12–15. Sue T. Hegyvary, *The Change to Primary Nursing: A Cross Cultural View of Professional Nursing Practice* (St Louis: Mosby, 1982). Samantha M. C. Pang and Eva Y. H. Tang, “An Evaluative Study on Individualizing Patient Care in a Hospital Ward in Hong Kong,” *Hong Kong Nursing Journal*, 63 (September 1993), pp. 13–20.

109. Florence Nightingale, "Commentaries by Contemporary Nursing Leaders," *Notes on Nursing: Commemorative Edition* (Philadelphia: Lippincott, 1992), pp. 1–85.

110. Virginia Henderson, *Basic Principles of Nursing Care* (Geneva: International Council of Nurses, rev. ed., 1997), p. 22.

111. Ann Bradshaw, "What are Nurses Doing to Patients? A Review of Theories of Nursing Past and Present," *Journal of Clinical Nursing*, 4 (1995), pp. 81–92.

## Chapter Three

1. Colin Mackerras, Pradeep Taneja, and Graham Young, *China Since 1978: Reform, Modernisation, and Socialism with Chinese Characteristics* (Melbourne: Longman Cheshire, 1994), p. 1.

2. Zedong Mao, *Selected Works of Mao Tse-tung* (Beijing: Foreign Languages Press, 1965), Vol. 2, p. 633.

3. Jie Wu, "The People's Daily, 17 November 1987," *On Deng Xiaoping Thought* (Beijing: Foreign Languages Press, 1996), p. 110.

4. Wu, *On Deng Xiaoping Thought*, p. 117. Kuilang Zhan, "Marx's Vision in His Late Years and Deng Xiaoping's Theory of Building Socialism with Chinese Characteristics," *Social Sciences in China*, 16:4 (1995), pp. 143–152.

5. Wu, *On Deng Xiaoping Thought*, pp. 121–122.

6. Xiaoping Deng, *Selected Works of Deng Xiaoping (1975–1982)* (Beijing: People's Publishing House, 1983), pp. 148–149.

7. *Ibid*., p. 172.

8. 羅國傑編，《人道主義思想論庫》。北京：華夏出版社，頁 199~229，1993。

9. Wu, *On Deng Xiaoping Thought*, p. 131.

10. Zhuo Zhang, "An Analysis of Some of the Objectives of China's Modernization," *Social Sciences in China*, 14:3 (1993), pp. 5–16. Xueyi Lu, "China's Social Structure in the 21st Century: On the Transformation of the Social Structure," *Social Sciences in China*, 18:2 (1997), pp. 73–76.

11. Wu, *On Deng Xiaoping Thought*, pp. 124–125.

12. *Ibid*., p. 125.

13. Godwin Chu, "The Changing Concept of Self in Contemporary China," *Cultural and Self: Asian and Western Perspectives*, eds. Anthony Marsella, George Devos, and Francis Hsu (New York: Tavistock Publications, 1985), p. 277.

14. 王琇瑛，《護理發展簡史》。上海：上海科學技術出版社，頁 108~111，1987。

15. *Ibid*., 頁 153~154。

16. 《中國衛生年鑒》。北京：人民衛生出版社，頁 393，1996。

17. Anne J. Davis, Lanjun Gan, Juyin Lin, and Virginia L. Olsen, "The Young Pioneers: First Baccalaureate Nursing Students in the People's Republic of China," *Journal of Advanced Nursing*, 17 (1992), pp. 1166–1170.

18. 馮運華，"中國護理近年之發展"，《香港護理雜誌》，33 卷，4 期，頁 41~43，1997。

19. 衛生部，"中華人民共和國護士管理辦法"，《全國醫院分級與疾病分類標準及醫院工作制度，職責配備規範》，柴瑞震、程廷安、姜任華編。成都：成都科技大學出版社，頁 186，1995。See Appendix 1.

20. 裴顯俊，“醫學模式轉變與護理人員知識結構的優化”，《中華護理雜誌》，25 卷，2 期，頁 110~111，1990。李鈺霖，“關于中等護士職業教育的改革”，《中華護理雜誌》，25 卷，3 期，頁 144~145，1990。

21. 楊以成、王偉智，“如何在護理大專教育中貫穿‘護理程序’教學”，《中華護理雜誌》，26 卷，11 期，頁 523~524，1991。張芳，“改進‘病人生活護理’課的教學法”，《中華護理雜誌》，26 卷，11 期，頁 524，1991。陳命家、李和林，“護士專業設公共關係課可行性探討”，《中華護理雜誌》，29 卷，1 期，頁 51~52，1994。黃劍琴，“爲中專護生講授現代護理新概念的做法和體會”，《中華護理雜誌》，29 卷，5 期，頁 293~296，1994。周曼穎、楊以成，“關于中等護士專業增設護理程序課程的探討”，《中華護理雜誌》，29 卷，1 期，頁 40~42，1994。余夢萍、張黎明，“ 應用護理診優化，護理人員再教育”，《中華護理雜誌》，30 卷，1 期，頁 33~35，1995。嵇芸、吳布生、常桂琴，“論護理學的研究對象”，《中華護理雜誌》，31 卷，3 期，頁 185~187，1996。

22. 陳靈艷，“談談「醫教護」和「醫學護」”，《中華護理雜誌》，25 卷，3 期，頁 145~146，1990。

23. 衛生部，“醫院工作人員職責 1982”，《全國醫院分級與疾病分類標準及醫院工作制度，職責配備規範》，頁 115~131。See Appendix 3.

24. Guangde Sun, “Healthcare Administration in China,” *Public Policy in China*, eds. Stuart S. Nagel and Miriam K. Mills (Westport, Connecticut: Greenwood Press, 1993), pp. 53–62. Liping Sun, Hansheng Wang, Sibin Wang, Bin Lin, and Shanhua Yang, “Changes in China’s Social Structure Following the Reforms,” *Social Sciences in China*, 16:3 (1995), pp. 70–80.

25. Sun, “Healthcare Administration in China,” p. 57.

26. *Ibid.*, pp. 59–60. Veronica Pearson, “Health and Responsibility; But Whose?” *Social Change and Social Policy in Contemporary China*, eds. Linda Wong and Stewart MacPherson (Hong Kong: City University of Hong Kong, 1995), pp. 99–100.

27. Zhikuan Zhang, “A Major Reform in Hospital Management System in China: Grading and Assessment,” *Chinese Medical Journal*, 107:4 (1994), p. 244.

28. 衛生部，“醫院工作人員職責 1982”，《全國醫院分級與疾病分類標準及醫院工作制度，職責配備規範》，頁 115~131。

29. 衛生部，“衛生技術人員職稱及晉升條例（試行）1979”，《全國醫院分級與疾病分類標準及醫院工作制度，職責配備規範》，頁 199。

30. 馮運華，“中國護理近年之發展”，頁 41~43。

31. 郜敏芳、劉蘇君、謝貞，“關於護理科研成果社會效益和經濟效益的調查分析”，《中華護理雜誌》，31 卷，3 期，頁 163~164，1996。

32. 張立紅、李素平、朱月珍，“對 6 所三級甲等醫院護理科研現狀的調查分析”，《中華護理雜誌》，31 卷，8 期，頁 468~469，1996。

33. Gail E. Henderson and Myron S. Cohen, *The Chinese Hospital: A Socialist Work Unit* (New Haven: Yale University Press, 1984), pp. 54–55.

34. Marie Manthey, *The Practice of Primary Nursing* (London: King’s Fund Centre, 1992). S. T. Hegyvary, *The Change to Primary Nursing: A Cross-Cultural View of Primary Nursing Practice* (St. Louis: C. V. Mosby, 1982). Alan Pearson, ed. *Primary Nursing: Nursing in the Burford and Oxford Development Units* (London:

Chapman and Hall, 1989). Steven Ersser and Elizabeth Tutton (eds.), *Primary Nursing in Perspective* (Kent: Scutari Press, 1991). Samantha M. C. Pang and Eva Y. H. Tang, "An Evaluative Study on Individualising Patient Care in a Hospital Ward in Hong Kong," *Hong Kong Nursing Journal*, 63 (1993), pp. 13–20.

35. Manthey, *The Practice of Primary Nursing*, pp. 26–39.

36. 林菊英，"中國護理訪問團赴美參觀訪問情況介紹"，《中華護理雜誌》，1 期，頁 46~48，1981。張惠蘭，"接待美國護理考察團情況介紹"，《中華護理雜誌》，2 期，頁 62~64，1982。朱雅琪，"日本醫院護理工作的概況"，《中華護理雜誌》，6 期，頁 374~376，1982。

37. 宋珍英，"如何做好在職護士的思想教育工作"，《中華護理雜誌》，3 期，頁 118~119，1981。吳行正，"護理責任制的探討"，《中華護理雜誌》，5 期，頁 266~268，1982。

38. 陳坤惕，"中華護理學會第十八屆理事會工作報告"，《中華護理雜誌》，18 卷，5 期，頁 261~265，1983。

39. 黃穎，"我擔任責任護士的體會"，《中華護理雜誌》，19 卷，4 期，頁 235~236，1984。党桂芝，"當好責任護士的體會"，《中華護理雜誌》，21 卷，9 期，頁 407~408，1986。

40. 編輯部，"全國責任制護理研討會討論情況簡介"，《中華護理雜誌》，22 卷，3 期，頁 102~103，1987。

41. 陶乃煌，"系統工程及其在護理管理中的應用(四) '臨床護理是一個系統' 護理過程"，《中華護理雜誌》，20 卷，4 期，頁 237~240，1985。李維光，"正確判斷護理問題(護理診斷)"，《中華護理雜誌》，22 卷，3 期，頁 100~101，1987。毛乾雯，"怎樣掌握書寫護理計劃的方法"，《中華護理雜誌》，22 卷，3 期，頁 97~99，1987。

42 王偉智、翁素貞，"從兩次病人調查看責任制護理的深化"，《中華護理雜誌》，24 卷，4 期，頁 193~195，1989。

43. 鄺秦桂，"全深化責任制護理按職稱上崗學校流與研討會議紀要"，《中華護理雜誌》，27 卷，12 期，頁 2，1992。

44. *Ibid*., 頁 2。

45. 王隴德，"在全國整體護理研討會上的講話"，《中華護理雜誌》，31 卷，11 期，頁 621~624，1996。楊惠芳，"全國整體護理研討會會議紀要"，《中華護理雜誌》，31 卷，11 期，頁 678~679，1996。

46. 袁劍雲、金橋、杜新柱、王鴻飛，"論系統化整體護理與 '模式病房' 建設"，《中華護理雜誌》，31 卷，2 期，頁 118~120，1996。蘇蘭若、于豔秋，"以病人爲中心建設模式病房"，《中華護理雜誌》，32 卷，5 期，頁 274~275，1997。

47. Anne J. Davis, Marcia Petrini, Juying Lin, and Virginia Olsen, "Values and Visions: Academic Nursing Students in the People's Republic of China," *Asian Journal of Nursing Studies*, 4:2 (1998), pp. 33–38.

48. 鄧穎超，"爲「護士之歌」、「家庭護理」題詞"，《中華護理雜誌》，18 卷，5 期，頁 255，1983。

49. 王琇瑛，《護理發展簡史》，頁 113~115。

50. 李華，“向護士前輩學習”，《中華護理雜誌》，1 期，頁 2，1981。李向明、陳光曼、王瑞廷、辛翠蘭編，《中國現代醫學家傳略》。北京：科學技術文獻出版社，頁 309~312，319~322，1984。

51. "'I am a Nurse' Wang Xiuying, Winner of the Nightingale Prize," *Women of China Special Series: Half the Sky(1)*, ed. Feng Li (Beijing: Women of China, 1985), pp. 183–190.

52. Renee C. Fox and Judith P. Swazey, "Medical Morality is Not Bioethics: Medical Ethics in China and the United States," *Perspectives in Biology and Medicine*, 27:3 (Spring 1984), pp. 340–341.

53. 蘇州醫學院附屬第一醫院，《建院 110 周年紀念刊》。蘇州：蘇州醫學院，頁 32，1994。

54. 劉旭東，“讓理想之花開得絢麗多彩記上海市第一人民醫院護士卜凡”，《中華護理雜誌》，6 期，頁 321~322，1982。

55. 劉瑩，“護士姐姐萬歲”，《中華護理雜誌》，24 卷，8 期，頁 489，1989。

56. 黃雪華、歐清，“醫德教育應注意發揮典型人物的作用”，《中華護理雜誌》，26 卷，8 期，頁 382~383，1991。

57. 黃黨發，“天使聖潔芙蓉爭輝”，《中國醫學倫理學》，總 34 期，2 期，頁 54~56，1994。

58. 姚昶緒，《病人看護法》。上海：商務印書館，頁 22，1939。

59. 王桐，“熱愛護理專業做好本職工作”，《中華護理雜誌》，4 期，頁 193~197，1982。張靜茹，“護士，其實就是一個沒有翅膀的天使”，《中華護理雜誌》，20 卷，3 期，頁 183，1985。

60. 魏桂芳，“獻給我最敬愛的人：護士”，《中華護理雜誌》，26 卷，5 期，頁 215，1991。

61. 王三虎，“護士形象簡史”，《中華護理雜誌》，27 卷，11 期，頁 518~519，1992。

62. 潘紹山，“試談醫院護士的職業道德”，《中華護理雜誌》，22 卷，9 期，頁 428~429，1987。

63. 傅愛民，“醫院改革開放後護理工作見開及反思”，《中華護理雜誌》，23 卷，10 期，頁 620，1988。

64. 段江麗，“從尊嚴的需要談護士行爲”，《中華護理雜誌》，25 卷，1 期，頁 49~50，1990。

65. 黃雪華、歐清，“醫德教育應注意發揮典型人物的作用”，《中華護理雜誌》，26 卷，8 期，頁 382~383，1991。

66. 衛生部，“醫院工作人員守則，1981”，《全國醫院分級與疾病分類標準及醫院工作制度，職責配備規範》，頁 131。

67. Eileen P. Bluenthal, *Models in Chinese Moral Education: Perspectives from Children's Books*, Ph. D. Thesis (Ann Arbor: University of Michigan, 1976), p. 5.

68. 張維慶，“和護士同志們談幾句話”，《中華護理雜誌》，19 卷，6 期，頁 362~363，1984。沈宗雲、楊以成，“淺談護理人才培養中的倫理教育”，《中華護理雜誌》，26 卷，4 期，頁 182~183，1991。侯琳、朱友明，“注重人才培養提高護士素質”，《中華護理雜誌》，28 卷，11 期，頁

652~653，1993。林翠芬，“培養護士優良心理品質淺見”，《中華護理雜誌》，30 卷，6 期，頁 355~356，1995。

69. 王桐，“熱愛護理專業做好本職工作”，《中華護理雜誌》，4 期，頁 193~197，1982。陳坤惕，“中華護理學會第十八屆理事會工作報告”，頁 261~265。顧美儀，“國際護士社節寄語”，《中華護理雜誌》，27 卷，5 期，頁 194，1992。楊惠芳，“全國整體護理研討會會議紀要”，《中華護理雜誌》，31 卷，11 期，頁 678~679，1996。

70. Mao, “On Coalition Government (24 April 1945),” *Quotations from Chairman Mao Tse-tung*, p. 171.

71. *Ibid*., p. 255.

72. 衛生部，“醫務人員醫德規範及實施辦法 1988”，《全國醫院分級與疾病分類標準及醫院工作制度，職責配備規範》，頁 131~132。“Regulations on Criteria for Medical Ethics and Their Implementation 1988,” trans. “Section II: Ethical Directives for the Practice of Medicine.” *Encyclopedia of Bioethics*, ed. Reich Warren Thomas (New York: Simon and Schuster Macmillan, rev. ed., 1995), p. 2691.

73. Zhikuan Zhang, “A Major Reform in Hospital Management System in China: Grading and Assessment,” p. 243.

74. See “Articles 4 to 11, Regulations on Criteria for Medical Ethics and Their Implementation,” *Encyclopedia of Bioethics*, p. 2691.

75. 徐素英，“提高認識注重實踐搞好醫德教育”，《中華護理雜誌》，24 卷，1 期，頁 57~58，1989。

76. Xinmin Sang, “Philosophic Reflection on the Comprehensive Development of the Components of Education,” *Social Sciences in China*, 13:4 (1992), pp. 138–146. Qingxiang Han, “A Socialist Market Economy and the Moulding of Man,” *Social Sciences in China*, 17:4 (1996), pp. 108–114. 童奎昌，“對畢業班護生開展職業禮貌教育的探討”，《中華護理雜誌》，28 卷，3 期，頁 165~166，1993。

77. 葉樹軍，“試論對在職護士進行護理倫理學教育”，《中華護理雜誌》，29 卷，4 期，頁 225~226，1994。

78. “高專自考護理倫理試題”，《中華護理雜誌》，27 卷，1 期，頁 46，1992。

79. See “Articles 4, 5 and 6 of Regulations on Criteria for Medical Ethics and Their Implementation,” *Encyclopedia of Bioethics*, p. 2691.

80. 侯琳、朱友明，“注重人才培養提高護士素質”，頁 652~653。

81. 秦愛忠，“我對做好護理工作的體會”，《中華護理雜誌》，1 期，頁 2~3，1982。北京第二醫院學院臨床教學處，“臨床第一課上得好”，《中華護理雜誌》，4 期，頁 241~243，1982。錢信忠，“中國紅十字會錢信忠會長在南丁格爾獎章授獎大會上的講話”，《中華護理雜誌》，18 卷，5 期，頁 259，1983。張玉英，“我院 17 年中發生護理事故、差錯、問題的分析”，《中華護理雜誌》，22 卷，9 期，頁 385~387，431，1987。潘紹山，“試談醫院護士的職業道德”，頁 428~429。徐素英，“提高認識注重實踐搞好醫德教育”，頁 57~58。侯琳、朱友明，“注重人才培養提高護士素質”，頁 652~653。于淑存、劉倩文，“提高護士職業道德的教育方法”，《中華護理雜誌》，31 卷，3 期，頁 174~175，1996。趙瑞萍、張芝雲，“新任護士長五忌”，《中華護理雜誌》，31 卷，12 期，頁 711，1996。

**Chapter Four**

1. David M. Lampton, *The Politics of Medicine in China: The Policy Process, 1949–1977* (Folkestone, Kent: Westview Press, 1977), pp. 13–16.

2. Tom L. Beauchamp and James F. Childress, *Principles of Biomedical Ethics* (New York: Oxford University Press, 5th ed., 2001), pp. 385–387. Steven D. Edwards, "What are the Limits to the Obligations of the Nurse?" *Journal of Medical Ethics*, 22 (1996), pp. 90–94.

3. "The Hippocratic Oath," *Dorland's American Illustrated Medical Dictionary* (Philadelphia: Saunders, 25th ed., 1974).

4. Lystra E. Gretter, "Nightingale Pledge," *Farrand Training School for Nurses, Harper Hospital* (Detroit, 1893).

5. Sara T. Fry, "The Code for Nurses, International Council of Nurses (ICN Code)," *Ethics in Nursing Practice, A Guide to Ethical Decision Marking* (Geneva, Switzerland: International Council of Nurses, 1994).

6. Hong Kong Nursing Board, *The Code of Professional Conduct for Nurses in Hong Kong* (Hong Kong Government: Hong Kong Nursing Board, 1986).

7. Ilza Veith (trans.), *The Yellow Emperor's Classic of Internal Medicine* (Berkeley: University of California Press, 1970).

8. 乾祖望，《孫思邈評傳》。南京：南京大學出版，1995。Renzong Qiu, "Medical Ethics and Chinese Culture," *Transcultural Dimensions in Medical Ethics*, eds. E. Pellegrino, P. Mazzarella, and P. Corsi (Maryland: Frederick, 1992). 曹開賓、邱世昌、樊民勝編，《醫學倫理學教程》。上海：上海醫科大學出版社，1992。徐文友、王桂蓮，"孫思邈的高尚醫德及其現實意義"，《中國醫學倫理學》，總 43 期，5 期，頁 55，1995。 Zhaohua Wu, "Conflicts between Chinese Traditional Ethics and Bioethics," *Cambridge Quarterly of Healthcare Ethics*, 3 (1994), pp. 367–371. Paul U. Unschuld, "Sun Simiao's on the Absolute Sincerity of Great Physicians," *Medical Ethics in Imperial China: A Study in Historical Anthropology* (Berkeley: University of California Press, 1979), pp. 29–33.

9. *Ibid*., p. 31.

10. *Ibid*., p. 31.

11. *Ibid*., pp. 30–31.

12. 乾祖望，《孫思邈評傳》，頁 315~321。

13. Tao Lee, "Medical Ethics in Ancient China," *Cross Cultural Perspectives in Medical Ethics: Readings*, ed. Robert M. Veatch (Boston: Jones and Bartlett Publishers, 1989), pp. 132–139. Unschuld, *Medical Ethics in Imperial China*, p. 31. James Legge (trans.), *Confucian Analects, the Great Learning and the Doctrine of the Mean* (New York: Dover, 1971).

14. *Ibid*., pp. 418–419.

15. 乾祖望，《孫思邈評傳》，頁 313。

16. Unschuld, *Medical Ethics in Imperial China*, p. 35.

17. Lee, "Medical Ethics in Ancient China," pp. 132–139.

18. Unschuld, *Medical Ethics in Imperial China*, p. 30.

19. *Ibid*., pp. 70–73.

20. 衛生部，"醫務人員醫德規範及實施辦法 1988"，《全國醫院分級與疾病分類標準及醫院工作制度，職責配備規範》，成都：成都科技大學出版社，頁 131~132，1995。"Regulations on Criteria for Medical Ethics and Their

Implementation 1988," *Encyclopedia of Bioethics*, ed. Reich Warren Thomas (New York: Simon and Schuster Macmillan, rev. ed., 1995), p. 2691.

21. 姚昶緒，《病人看護法》。上海：商務印書館，頁 22，1939。

22. Renzong Qiu, "Philosophy of Medicine in China (1930–1980)," *Metamedicine*, 3 (1982), pp. 35–73.

23. 李本富、丁蕙孫、李傳俊，《護理倫理學》。北京：科學出版社，第二版，頁 105，1992。

24. 喬選超、丁秀東，"關于醫療保密的倫理問題"，《中國醫學倫理學》，總 51 期，1 期，頁 25~26，1997。

25. S. R. Frisch, D. Fowler-Graham, V. Shannon, and D. Demback, "Maintaining Autonomy of Vulnerable Subjects," *Canadian Journal of Nursing Research*, 22:4 (1990), pp. 51–60. S. E. Schutz, "Patient Involvement in Resuscitation Decisions," *British Journal of Nursing*, 3:20 (1994), pp. 1075–1079. R. M. Veatch, "Which Grounds for Overriding Autonomy are Legitimate?" *Hastings Center Report*, 26:6 (1996), pp. 42–43.

26. Samantha M. C. Pang, "Protective Truthfulness: The Chinese Way in Fostering Patients in Informed Treatment Decisions," *Journal of Medical Ethics*, 25:3 (June 1999), pp. 247–253.

27. 杭州醫院，"病人的權利和義務"，杭州，1994。See Appendix 4.

28. 勵綠化，"護理道德在維護病人權利中的作用"，《中華護理雜誌》，24 卷，9 期，頁 514，1989。黃驍洪，"論肛腸病診治中的若干道德問題"，《中國醫學倫理學》，總 53 期，3 期，頁 25，1997。

29. 李輯敏，"制訂'患者權利'促使醫德自律"，《中國醫學倫理學》，總 48 期，4 期，頁 47~48，1996。

30. Veronica Pearson, "Health and Responsibility; But Whose?" *Social Change and Social Policy in Contemporary China*, eds. Linda Wong and Stewart MacPherson (Hong Kong: City University of Hong Kong, 1995), p. 88.

31. Xueshan Feng, Shenglan Tang, Gerald Bloom, Malcolm Segall, and Xingyuan Gu, "Cooperative Medical Schemes in Contemporary Rural China," *Social Science and Medicine*, 41:8 (1995), p. 1111.

32. 中華人民共和國國家統計局編，《中國統計年鑑》。香港：經濟導報社，頁 725，1977。

33. 趙維生、黃昌榮，"中國醫療服務及醫療制度改革"，《中國社會發展：香港學者的分析》，李思、邵一鳴、莫泰基編。香港：香港教育圖書公司，頁 292，1995。

34. 中國年鑑社，《中華人民共和國年鑑》。北京：新華出版社，頁 651–655，1996。

35. Renzong Qiu, "Ethical Problems in Renal Dialysis and Transplantation: A Chinese Perspective," *Ethical Problems in Dialysis and Transplantation*, eds. C. M. Kjellstrand and J. B. Dossetor (Dordrecht: Kluwer Academic Publishers, 1992), p. 231.

36. "Death Rate of Ten Major Diseases in Urban and Rural Areas,"《中國衛生年鑒》，北京：人民衛生出版社，頁 732~733，1996。

37. "The First Ten Diseases in Urban and Rural Areas from 1955 to 1996,"《中國衛生年鑒》。北京：人民衛生出版社，頁 420~421，1997。

38. 中國年鑑社，《中華人民共和國年鑑》，頁 650，1996。

39. Feng, Tang, Bloom, Segall, and Gu, "Cooperative Medical Schemes in Contemporary Rural China," pp. 1111–1112. Pearson, "Health and Responsibility; But Whose?" pp. 93–94.

40. "The Proportion of Rural and Urban Population," 中華人民共和國國家統計局編，《中國統計年鑑》，頁 69，1997。

41. Feng, Tang, Bloom, Segall, and Gu, "Cooperative Medical Schemes in Contemporary Rural China," pp. 1111–1118.

42. Henderson Gail, Shuigao Jin, John Akin, Zhiming Li, Jianmin Wang, Haijiang Ma, Yunan He, Xiping Zhang, Ying Chang, and Keyou Ge, "Distribution of Medical Insurance in China," *Social Science and Medicine*, 41:8 (1995), p. 1120.

43. 趙維生、黃昌榮，"中國醫療服務及醫療制度改革"，頁 299~300。

44. Pearson, "Health and Responsibility; But Whose?" p. 95.

45. Henderson, Jin, Akin, Li, Wang, Ma, He, Zhang, Chang, and Ge, "Distribution of Medical Insurance in China," pp. 1119–1130.

46. *Ibid*., pp. 1123–1124.

47. Renzong Qiu, "Equity and Public Health Care in China," *Journal of Medicine and Philosophy*, 14 (1989), pp. 283–287.

48. 趙維生、黃昌榮，"中國醫療服務及醫療制度改革"，頁 295。Sang Ho Lok, "Market Reforms and China's Healthcare System," *Social Science and Medicine*, 41:8 (1995), pp. 1065–1072.

49. 馬旭，《簡言衛生事業與社會經濟全面協調發展》。上海：上海市中北醫院，頁 1~6，1995。

50. *Ibid*., p. 4.

51. *Ibid*., p. 6.

52. 趙維生、黃昌榮，"中國醫療服務及醫療制度改革"，頁 300。

53. Qiu, "Equity and Public Health Care in China," pp. 286–287.

54. 趙維生、黃昌榮，"中國醫療服務及醫療制度改革"，頁 301。

55. Renzong Qiu, "The Fiduciary Relationship between Professionals and Clients: A Chinese Perspective," *Ethics, Trust, and The Professions, Philosophical and Cultural Aspects*, eds. Edmund D. Pellegrino, Robert M. Veatch, and John Langan (Washington, D. C.: Georgetown University Press, 1991), p. 257.

56. Henderson, *et al.*, "Distribution of Medical Insurance in China," p. 1121.

57. 陳振東、高宗熔、李海享，"終末期癌症患者及其親屬的求醫動機"，《中國醫學倫理學》，總 113 期，2 期，頁 49~50，1993。

58. 趙維生、黃昌榮，"中國醫療服務及醫療制度改革"，頁 303。

59. *Ibid*., 頁 303。

60. 劉勇，"中國的放棄治療現狀及倫理問題"，《中國醫學倫理學》，總 28 期，2 期，頁 51~52，1993。

61. *Ibid*., 頁 51~52。

62. United States Supreme Court, "Cruzan v. Director, Missouri Department of Health." *Contemporary Issues in Bioethics*, eds. Tom L. Beauchamp and LeRoy Walters (Belmont, Calif.: Wadsworth Publishing Co., 5th ed., 1999), pp. 281–286.

63. 張贊寧，"安樂死，中國比西方更自由"，《家庭醫生》，9 卷，113 總期，頁 40~42，1993。

64. "Birth Rate, Death Rate, and Natural Growth Rate of the Population 1952–1996," 中華人民共和國國家統計局編，《中國統計年鑑》，頁 69，1997。荆其誠，"中國獨生子女政策與人口心理學"，《中國兒童發展與家庭國際研討會論文集第二卷》，中國關心下一代工作委員會專家委員會編。北京：北京科學技術出版社，頁 297，1993。

65. En Ma, "Letter from Beijing: One Child, One Family," *Journal of American Medical Association*, 261:12 (1989), pp. 1735–1736. Zuoxiu He, "A New Understanding of Vast Territory, Rich Resources and a Large Population," *Social Sciences in China*, 18:4 (1997), pp. 44–51. Therese Hesketh and Weixing Zhu, "Health in China: The One Child Family Policy: The Good, the Bad, and the Ugly," *British Medical Journal*, 314:7095 (1997), p. 1685.

66. Judith Banister, *China's Changing Population* (Stanford: Stanford University Press, 1987), pp. 355–368. Hesketh and Zhu, "Health in China: The One Child Family Policy," pp. 1685–1687.

67. Banister, *China's Changing Population*, pp. 182–215, 217. Steven W. Mosher, *A Mother's Ordeal: The Story of Chi An* (London: Warner Books, 1995).

68. Renzong Qiu, Shunzhui Wang, and Yuan Gu, "Can Late Abortion be Ethically Justified?" *Journal of Medicine and Philosophy*, 14 (1989), pp. 343–350.

69. Banister, *China's Changing Population*, p. 221.

70. Hesketh and Zhu, "Health in China: The One Child Family Policy," pp. 1685–1686.

71. "A Comparison of the 1982 and 1990 Censuses," (National Statistics Bureau, People's Republic of China, 1990).

72. Hesketh and Zhu, "Health in China: The One Child Family Policy," p. 1686.

73. 中國關心下一代工作委員會專家委員會編，"中國老齡人口 1953~2040"，《中國兒童發展與家庭國際研討會論文集第二卷》，頁 303。

74. 荊其誠，"中國獨生子女政策與人口心理學"，頁 304~305。

75. Xian Liu, Jersey Liang, and Shengzu Gu, "Flows of Social Support and Health Status among Older Persons in China," *Social Science and Medicine*, 41:8 (1995), pp. 1175–1184.

76. Ping Tu "On the Issues of Population Ageing and Population Control in China," *Social Sciences in China*, 18:3 (1997), pp. 129–130.

77. Banister, *China's Changing Population*, pp. 378–379.

78. Editorial, "Western Eyes on China's Eugenics Law," *Lancet*, 346:8968 (1995), p. 131. Angus Clarke, Peter S. Harper, P. F. Unsworth, John Scotson, and Peter Doherty, "Eugenics in China," *Lancet*, 346:8973 (1995), pp. 508–509. Editorial, "China's Misconception of Eugenics," *Nature*, 367 (1994), pp. 1–2. Linda Johnson, "Expanding Eugenics or Improving Health Care, Commentary on the Provisions of the Standing Committee of the Gansu People's Congress Concerning the Prohibition of Reproduction by Intellectually Impaired Persons," *Journal of Law and Society*, 24:2 (1997), pp. 199–234.

79. Therese Hesketh and Weixing Zhu, "Health in China: Maternal and Child Health in China," *British Medical Journal*, 314:7098 (1997), p. 1900. Veronica Pearson, "Population Policy and Eugenics in China," *British Journal of Psychiatry*, 167:1 (1995), pp. 1–4.

80. Ma, "Letter from Beijing," pp. 1735–1736. Hesketh and Zhu, "Health in China: The One Child Family Policy," pp. 1685–1687.

81. Renzong Qiu and Dajie Jin, "Bioethics in China: 1991–1993," *Bioethics Yearbook, Vol. 4: Regional Development in Bioethics, 1991–1993*, ed. B. Andrew Lusting, *et al.* (Dordrecht: Kluwer Academic Publishers, 1995), pp. 339–340.

82. Johnson, "Expanding Eugenics or Improving Health Care, Commentary on the Provisions of the Standing Committee of the Gansu People's Congress Concerning the Prohibition of Reproduction by Intellectually Impaired Persons," pp. 219–220.

83. *Ibid*, pp. 219–220.

84. 衛生部，"中華人民共和國母嬰保健法"，《中國衛生年鑒》。北京：人民衛生出版社，頁 23~25，1995。

85. Editorial, "China's Misconception of Eugenics," pp. 1–2.

86. Qiu, "The Fiduciary Relationship between Professionals and Clients," pp. 256–257. Mosher, *A Mother's Ordeal: The Story of Chi An*, pp. 117–120.

87. Qiu, "Philosophy of Medicine in China (1930–1980)," p. 45.

88. 施榕，《醫德一百題》。上海：上海人民出版社，頁 163~164，1991。

89. Qiu and Jin, "Bioethics in China: 1991–1993," pp. 339–365. 涂或、朱永烈，"安樂死的法律參與"，《中國醫學倫理學》，總 25 期，5 期，頁 37，1992。Vera Rich, "Will the Chinese Legalize Euthanasia?" *The Lancet*, 345:8952 (1995), p. 783.

90. Renzong Qiu, "Concepts of Death and Euthanasia," *Medicine and Philosophy*, 1 (1980), pp. 77–79.

91. 張贊寧，"關於安樂死的幾個問題 ：與林業剛同志商榷"，《法律科學》，2 卷，總 35 期，頁 87~91，1990。姚軒鴿、余德華，"關於安樂死道德評價問題的思考"，《中國醫學倫理學》，總 24 期，4 期，頁 23~26，1992。張贊寧，"安樂死，中國比西方更自由"，頁 40~42。邱鴻鐘，"儒醫義利觀及其實踐狀況"，《中國醫學倫理學》，總 48 期，4 期，頁 62~64，1996。

92. Tom L. Beauchamp and Arnold I. Davidson, "The Definition of Euthanasia," *Journal of Medicine and Philosophy*, 4:3 (1979), pp. 294–312.

93. Renzong Qiu, "Chinese Medical Ethics and Euthanasia," *Cambridge Quarterly of Healthcare Ethics*, 2:1 (1993), p. 70.

94. 馮秀雲，"安樂死的幾個法律問題"，《中國醫學倫理學》，總 54 期，4 期，頁 49~51，1997。

95. 張贊寧，"關於安樂死的幾個問題 ：與林業剛同志商榷"，頁 87~91。

96. *Ibid*., 頁 91。

97. *Ibid*., 頁 87~91。

98. Qiu and Jin, "Bioethics in China: 1991–1993," p. 345.

99. Rich, "Will the Chinese Legalise Euthanasia?" p. 783.

100. 姚軒鴿、余德華，"關於安樂死道德評價問題的思考"，頁 23~26。

101. 馮秀雲，"安樂死的幾個法律問題"，頁 49~51。倪黎明，"50 例放棄新生兒治療與安樂死"，《中國醫學倫理學》，總 28 期，2 期，頁 53，1993。

102. Dapu Shi, "Euthanasia in China: A Report," *Journal of Medical and Philosophy*, 16 (1991), pp. 132–133.

103. 馮秀雲，"安樂死的幾個法律問題"，頁 49。韓雲彪、李宇崗，"生命倫理與民族素質的提高"，《中國醫學倫理學》，總 23 期，3 期，頁 51~52，1992。

104. 胡英、余屏、宋愛清，“論優死教育”，《中國醫學倫理學》，總 22 期，2 期，頁 47~49，1992。韓俊德、何主新、侯雙起，“居民的死亡態度初探 – 兼談我國臨終關懷的開展”，《中國醫學倫理學》，總 22 期，2 期，頁 50~52，1992。姚軒鴿、余德華，“關於安樂死道德評價問題的思考”，頁 23~26。韓雲彪、李宇崗，“生命倫理與民族素質的提高”，頁 51~52。倪黎明，“50 例放棄新生兒治療與安樂死”，頁 53。馬敏芝，“從‘人人享有生保健’看‘臨終關懷’與‘安樂死’”，《中國醫學倫理學》，總 40 期，2 期，頁 48~49，1995。楊玉蘭，雷衍弘，“優死：時代的挑戰與探索”，《中國華山：第八屆全國中華醫學倫理學會中青委員會會議》，1997。

105. Zedong Mao, *Quotations from Chairman Mao Tse-tung* (Peking: Foreign Languages Press, 1972), p. 174.

106. John Hardwig, “Is there a Duty to Die?” *Hastings Center Report*, 27:2 (1997), pp. 34–42.

107. 姚軒鴿、余德華，“關於安樂死道德評價問題的思考”，頁 24。

108. *Ibid*., 頁 25~26。

109. 馮秀雲，“安樂死的幾個法律問題”，頁 51。

110. 施榕，“臨終關懷在上海之現狀”，《施榕教授文集》。西安：陝西師範大學出版社，頁 126~133，1997。

111. 汪炎雄、白洪梅，“一項造福於人類的崇高事業”，《中國醫學倫理學》，總 24 期，4 期，頁 31~33，1992。馬敏芝，“從‘人人享有生保健’看‘臨終關懷’與‘安樂死’”，頁 49。

112. Lucy Chung, “Active Euthanasia: A Slippery Slope,” *South China Morning Post*, (28 July 1995). Vincent Mak, “Euthanasia Policy still Unwritten,” *Hong Kong Standard*, (6 August 1998). 彭美慈、佘雲楚，“論安樂死作爲療手段的倫理涵意”，《社聯季刊》，144 期，頁 32~36，1998。

113. Renzong Qiu, “Morality in Flux: Medical Ethics Dilemmas in the People’s Republic of China,” *Kennedy Institute of Ethics Journal*, (March 1991), pp. 16–27. Qiu, “Chinese Medical Ethics and Euthanasia,” p. 72.

114. Peicheng Hu, “Euthanasia: The Acceptability of Active Euthanasia in China,” *Medicine and Law*, 12 (1993), pp. 47–53.

115. Renzong Qiu and Dajie Jin, “Bioethics in China: 1989–1991,” *Bioethics Yearbook* (Dordrecht: Kluwer Academic Publishers, 1992), Vol. 2, pp. 361–362.

116. Shi, “Euthanasia in China: A Report,” p. 132.

117. Qiu and Jin, “Bioethics in China: 1989–1991,” pp. 360–362. 王可摘，“全國首例安樂死終審結案”，《中國醫學倫理學》，總 24 期，4 期，頁 26，1992。

118. 張贊寧，“關於安樂死的幾個問題：與林業剛同志商榷”，頁 42。

119. 韓俊德、何主新、侯雙起，“居民的死亡態度初探：談我國臨終關懷的開展”，《中國醫學倫理學》，總 22 期，2 期，頁 50~52，1992。

120. Renzong Qiu, “Ethical Problems in Renal Dialysis and Transplantation: A Chinese Perspective,” p. 234. Emiko Namihira, “Japanese Concepts and Attitudes to Human Remains,” *Japanese and Western Bioethics: Studies in Moral Diversity*, ed. Kazumasa Hoshino (Dordrecht: Kluwer Academic Publishers, 1997), pp. 61–69.

121. 郭清秀、石月清，“安樂死的現實呼喚與思考”，《中國醫學倫理學》，總 53 期，3 期，頁 42~44，1997。

122. 喻琳、石大璞，“從典型案例及民意調查看安樂死在中國立法之必要性”，《中外醫學哲學》，1 卷，1 期，頁 172~173，1998。

123. 韓雲彪、李宇崗，“生命倫理與民族素質的提高”，頁 51~52。劉勇，“中國的放棄治療現狀及倫理問題”，頁 51~52，1993。馮秀雲，“安樂死的幾個法律問題”，頁 49~51，1997。

124. 楊玉蘭、雷衍弘，“‘優死’：時代的挑戰與探索”。

125. Rich, “Will the Chinese Legalise Euthanasia?” p. 783.

126. 李恩昌，“醫學目的，生命質量，醫學倫理：全國第八次醫學倫理學學術研討會側記”，《中國醫學倫理學》，總 43 期，5 期，頁 63~64，1995。

127. *Ibid*., 頁 63。

**Chapter Five**

1. Samantha M. C. Pang, *From Virtue to Value: Nursing Ethics in Modern China*, Ph. D. Thesis (Hong Kong: The University of Hong Kong, 1999), pp. 149–211.

2. See Chapter Three, p. 51.

3. 陳瑛，“中國倫理發展現狀”，《應用倫理研究中會訊》。香港：浸會大學，6 卷，1 期，頁 10~15，1997。

4. Joy Hinson Penticuff, “Nursing Perspectives in Bioethics,” *Japanese and Western Bioethics: Studies in Moral Diversity*, ed. Kazumasa Hoshino (Dordrecht: Kluwer Academic Publishers, 1997), p. 49.

5. *Ibid*, p. 53.

6. Samantha M. C. Pang, David G. Arthur, and Thomas K. S. Wong, “Drawing a Qualitative Distinction of Caring Practices in a Professional Context: The Case of Chinese Nursing,” *Holistic Nursing Practice*, 15:1 (2000), pp. 22–31.

7. Anne Davis, Marcia Petrini, Juying Lin, and Virginia Olsen, “Values and Visions: Academic Nursing Students in the People’s Republic of China,” *Asian Journal of Nursing Studies*, 4:2 (1998), p. 35.

8. Sara T. Fry, *Ethics in Nursing Practice, A Guide to Ethical Decision Making* (Geneva, Switzerland: International Council of Nurses, 1994), p. 74.

9. Karl Marx (ed.), *Critique of the Gotha Programme* (Peking: Foreign Languages Press, 1972).

10. See Chapter Three, pp. 47–50.

11. Donald J. Munro, *The Concept of Man in Contemporary China* (Ann Arbor: The University of Michigan Press, 1977), p. 155.

12. Qingxiang Han, “Socialist Market Economy and the Molding of Man,” *Social Sciences in China*, 17:4 (1996), pp. 108–114.

13. Weihe Huang, “Mo Zi’s Concepts of Righteousness and Benefit,” *Social Sciences in China*, 17:4 (1986), pp. 166–174.

14. 陳聰杰，“論義利兼顧以義爲先”，《中國醫學倫理學》，總 25 期，5 期，頁 7~10，1992。

15. See Chapter Four, pp.63–70.

16. Steven W. Mosher, *A Mother’s Ordeal: The Story of Chi An* (London: Warner Books, 1995), pp. 116–142.

17. Kazumasa Hoshino, “Bioethics in the Light of Japanese Sentiments,” *Japanese and Western Bioethics: Studies in Moral Diversity*, ed. Kazumasa Hoshino (Dordrecht: Kluwer Academic Publishers, 1997), pp. 13–23.

18. Samantha M. C. Pang, “Information Disclosure: The Moral Experience of Nurses in China,” *Nursing Ethics*, 5:4 (1998), pp. 347–361.

19. 鄧莉，“淺談護士語言與醫德”，《中國醫學倫理學》，總 25 期，5 期，頁 33~34，1992。姜瑾，“醫生語言修養之管見”，《中國醫學倫理學》，總 56 期，6 期，頁 9~11，1997。高雁，“談護士在護患交往中運用語言的技巧”，《中國醫學倫理學》，總 56 期，6 期，頁 14，1997。

20. See Chapter Two, pp. 21–23.

21. 丁人編，《護士質修養》。北京：人民軍醫出版社頁，頁 140~141，1992。李本富、丁蕙孫、李傳俊，《護理倫理學》。北京：科學出版社，第二版，頁 151~152，1992。

22. See Chapter Four, 81–82.

23. 李恩昌，“醫學目的，生命質量，醫學倫理：全國第八次醫學倫理學學術研討會側記”，《中國醫學倫理學》，總 43 期，5 期，頁 63~64，1995。

24. 李本富、丁蕙孫、李傳俊，《護理倫理學》。

25. Martin Johnson, “Natural Sociology and Moral Questions in Nursing: Can There be a Relationship?” *Journal of Advanced Nursing*, 15 (1990), pp. 1358–1359.

26. ICN Code, 1973.

27. 從楣華、劉飛，“慎獨對夜間護理工作的指導意義”，《中華護理雜誌》，31 卷，2 期，頁 108~110，1996。

28. James Legge (trans.), “The Doctrine of the Mean,” *Confucian Analects, the Great Learning and the Doctrine of the Mean* (New York: Dover, 1971), Ch. 1, verse 1–3, pp. 383–384.

29. *Ibid.*, Ch. 25, verse 3, pp. 418–419.

30. 金耀基，《中國社會與文化》。香港：牛津大學出版社，頁 20~21，1992。

31. Paul U. Unschuld, “Sun Simiao’s on the Absolute Sincerity of Great Physicians,” *Medical Ethics in Imperial China: A Study in Historical Anthropology* (Berkeley: University of California Press, 1979), pp. 29–33.

32. Xinmin Sang, “Philosophic Reflection on the Comprehensive Development of the Components of Education,” *Social Sciences in China*, 13:4 (1992), pp. 138–146. 胡凱，“先秦儒學與老莊哲學的身心修養方法初探”，《中國醫學倫理學》，總 48 期，4 期，頁 58~59，1996。Peng Lei, “The Practical Significance of Confucian Moral Cultivation,” *Social Sciences in China*, 18:2 (1997), pp. 45–50. 黃雪華、歐清，“醫德教育應注意發揮典型人物的作用”，《中華護理雜誌》，26 卷，8 期，頁 382~383，1991。

33. 徐素英，“提高認識注重實踐搞好醫德教育”，《中華護理雜誌》，24 卷，1 期，頁 57~58，1989。沈宗雲、楊以成，“淺談護理人才培養中的倫理教育”，《中華護理雜誌》，26 卷，4 期，頁 182~185，1991。林翠芬，“培養護士優良心理品質淺見”，《中華護理雜誌》，30 卷，6 期，頁 355~356，1995。

34. 王紅，“假如我是一個病人”，《中華護理雜誌》，27 卷，10 期，頁 476，1992。

35. See Chapter Three, pp. 49–50.

36. Fry, *Ethics in Nursing Practice*, pp. 51–54.

37. ICN Code, 1973.

38. Marsha D. M. Fowler, *Ethics and Nursing, 1893–1984: The Ideal of Service, The Reality of History*, Ph. D. Thesis (Los Angeles: University of Southern California, 1984), p. 161.

39. Fry, *Ethics in Nursing Practice*, p. 49.

**Chapter Six**

1. Tom L. Beauchamp and James F. Childress, *Principles of Biomedical Ethics* (New York: Oxford University Press, 5th ed., 2001). S. R. Frisch, D. Fowler-Graham, V. Shannon and D. Demback, "Maintaining Autonomy of Vulnerable Subjects," *Canadian Journal of Nursing Research*, 22:4 (1990), pp. 51–60. S. E. Schutz, "Patient Involvement in Resuscitation Decisions," *British Journal of Nursing*, 3:20 (1994), pp. 1075–1079. R. M. Veatch, "Which Grounds for Overriding Autonomy are Legitimate?" *Hastings Center Report*, 26:6 (1996), pp. 42–43.

2. Beauchamp and Childress, *Principles of Biomedical Ethics*, pp. 69–77.

3. N. Cisar, "Informed Consent: An Ethical Dilemma," *Nursing Forum*, 30:3 (1995), pp. 20–28. Paul Fulbrook, "Assessing Mental Competence of Patients and Relatives," *Journal of Advanced Nursing*, 20:3 (1994), pp. 457–461. C. May, "Disclosure of Terminal Prognoses in a General Hospital: The Nurse's View," *Journal of Advanced Nursing*, 18 (1993), pp. 1362–1368.

4. Fulbrook, "Assessing Mental Competence of Patients and Relatives," pp. 457–461.

5. Anne J. Davis and B. A. Koenig, "A Question of Policy: Bioethics in a Multicultural Society," *Nursing Policy Forum*, 2:1 (1996), pp. 6–11.

6. H. J. Muller and B. Desmond, "Ethical Dilemmas in a Cross-cultural Context, a Chinese Example," *Western Journal of Medicine*, 157:3 (1992), pp. 323–327.

7. 彭美慈、周麗雲，"護理評估系列之「我可否向病人剖白真相？」"，《亞洲護理學文摘》，1卷，4期，頁61~64，1994。

8. Merja Kuuppelomaki and Sirkka Lauri, "Ethical Dilemmas in the Care of Patients with Incurable Cancer," *Nursing Ethics*, 5:4 (1998), pp. 283–293.

9. R. Grundstein-Amado, "Differences in Ethical Decision-making Process among Nurses and Doctors," *Journal of Advanced Nursing*, 17 (1992), pp. 129–137. A. Lindseth, V. Marhaug, A. Norberg, and G. Uden, "Registered Nurses' and Physicians' Reflections on their Narratives about Ethically Difficult Care Episodes," *Journal of Advanced Nursing*, 20 (1994), pp. 245–250.

10. Kuuppelomaki and Lauri, "Ethical Dilemmas in the Care of Patients with Incurable Cancer," pp. 286–287.

11. Samantha M. C. Pang, "Information Disclosure: The Moral Experience of Nurses in China," *Nursing Ethics*, 5:4 (1998), pp. 347–361.

12. Sara T. Fry, "New ANA Guidelines on Withdrawing or Withholding Food and Fluid from Patients," *Nursing Outlook*, 36:3 (1987), pp. 122–123, 148–150. Gwen M. Sayers, "An Analysis of CPR Decision Making by Elderly Patients," *Journal of Medical Ethics*, 23 (1997), pp. 207–212. Paul Fulbrook, "Assessing Quality of Life: The Basis of Withdrawal of Life-supporting Treatment?" *Journal of Advanced Nursing*, 17 (1992), pp. 1440–1446. Robert Halliday, "Medical Futility and the Social Context," *Journal of Medical Ethics*, 23 (1997), pp. 148–153.

13. Feng Lu, "*Dan Wei*: A Special Form of Social Organization," *Social Sciences in China*, 10:3 (1989), p. 113.

14. See Chapter Two, p.25.

15. Hong Kong Census and Statistics Department, *Hong Kong Annual Digest of Statistics* (Hong Kong: Government Print, 1997), p. 228.

16. 彭美慈、佘雲楚，"論安樂死作爲醫療手段的倫理涵意"，《社聯季刊》，144期，頁34，1998。

17. Ruiping Fan, "Self-determination vs Family-determination: Two Incommensurable Principles of Autonomy," *Bioethics*, 11:314 (1997), pp. 309–322.

18. Renzong Qiu and Dajie Jin, "Bioethics in China: 1991–1993," *Bioethics Yearbook*: *Regional Development in Bioethics, 1991–1993*, eds. B. Andrew Lusting, *et al*. (Dordrecht: Kluwer Academic Publishers, 1995), Vol 4, p. 345. Ann-Marie Begely, "Beneficent Voluntary Active Euthanasia: A Challenge to Professionals Caring for Terminally Ill Patients," *Nursing Ethics*, 5:4 (1998), pp. 294–306. Chap. 3, the section on Definitions on Euthanasia, pp. 76–81.

19. 郭清秀、勒風林、耿洪剛，"中國安樂死"，《中外醫學哲學》，1卷，1期，頁137~149，1998。

20. Marsha D. M. Fowler, *Ethics and Nursing, 1893–1984: The Ideal of Service, the Reality of History*, Ph. D. Thesis (Los Angeles: University of Southern California, 1984), pp. 51–52.

21. 王大軍，"醫學目的調整與醫學道德的更新"，《中國醫學倫理學》，總48期，4期，頁22~23，1996。

22. 袁光榮，"醫學目的與安樂死"，《中國醫學倫理學》，總 56 期，6期，頁13，32，1997。

23. Arie J. G. van der Arend, "An Ethical Perspective on Euthanasia and Assisted Suicide in the Netherlands from a Nursing Point of View," *Nursing Ethics*, 5:4 (1998), p. 309.

24. Begely, "Beneficent Voluntary Active Euthanasia," pp. 294–306.

25. 陳浩文、高永文，"安樂死的謬誤，醫療目的與病人自決權"，《價値與社會(第一集)》，陶黎寶華，邱仁宗編。北京 ：中國社會科學出版社，頁74~101，1997。

26. British Medical Association, *Medical Ethics Today: Its Practice and Philosophy* (London: BMJ Publishing Group, 1993), p. 175.

27. 郭清秀、勒風林、耿洪剛，"中國安樂死"，頁 140。喻琳、石大璞，"從典型案例及民意調查看安樂死在中國立法之必要性"，《中外醫學哲學》，1卷，1期，頁172~173，1998。

28. Anne. J. Davis, B. Davidson, M. Hirschfield, S. Lauri, J. Y. Lin, A. Norberg, L. Phillips, E. Pitman, C. H. Shen, R. V. Laan, H. L. Zhang, and L. Ziv, "An International Perspective of Active Euthanasia: Attitudes of Nurses in Seven Countries," *International Journal of Nursing Studies*, 30:4 (1993), pp. 307–308.

29. Begley, "Beneficent Voluntary Active Euthanasia," pp. 298–301.

30. Gail E. Henderson and Myron S. Cohen, *The Chinese Hospital*: *A Socialist Work Unit* (New Haven: Yale University Press, 1984), pp. 27–46.

31. Lu, "*Dan Wei*: A Special Form of Social Organization," p. 105.

32. *Ibid*., p. 110.

33. Gail E. Henderson and Myron S. Cohen, *The Chinese Hospital: A Socialist Work Unit* (New Haven: Yale University Press, 1984), pp. 44–46.

34. Appendix 5: "Standard Requirements for Quality Nursing."

35. Sandra A. Wawrytko, "Confucius and Kant: The Ethics of Respect," *Philosophy East and West*, 32:3 (1982), pp. 231–257.

36. Appendix 6: Ministry of Public Health, "Regulations for Ward Management, Hospital Personnel and Hospital Patients," 1986.

**Chapter Seven**

1. Marsha D. Fowler, *Ethics and Nursing, 1893–1984: The Ideal of Service, The Reality of History*, Ph. D. Thesis (Los Angeles: University of Southern California, 1984), p. 330.

2. *Ibid.*

3. Anne H. Bishop and John R. Scudder, *Nursing Ethics, Therapeutic Caring Presence* (Boston: Jones and Barlett Publishers, 1996), p. 1.

4. Anne J. Davis, "Are There Limits to Caring? Conflict between Autonomy and Beneficence," *Ethical and Moral Dimensions of Care*, ed. Madeleine M. Leininger (Detroit: Wayne State University Press, 1990), pp. 25–32. Sara T. Fry, "The Ethic of Care: Nursing's Excellence for a Troubled World," *A Global Agenda for Caring*, ed. Delores. A. Gaut (New York: National League for Nursing Press, 1993), pp. 175–180. Stanley Hauerwas, "Care," *Encyclopedia of Bioethics*, ed. Warren T. Reich (New York: The Free Press, 1978), pp. 145–150.

5. Madeleine M. Leininger, "Culture: the Conspicuous Missing Link to Understand Ethical and Moral Dimensions of Human Care," *Ethical and Moral Dimensions of Care*, pp. 49–60.

6. Hauerwas, "Care." pp. 145–150.

7. Nel Noddings, *Caring: A Feminist Approach to Ethics and Moral Education* (Berkeley: University of California Press, 1984). Jean Watson, *Nursing: The Philosophy and Science of Caring* (Colorado: University Press of Colorado, 1985). Sara T. Fry, "The Philosophical Foundations of Caring," *Ethical and Moral Dimensions of Care*, pp. 175–180.

8. Patricia Benner, "A Dialogue between Virtue Ethics and Care Ethics," *Theoretical Medicine*, 18 (1997), pp. 47–61.

9. Bishop and Scudder, *Nursing Ethics, Therapeutic Caring Presence.*

10. Samantha M. C. Pang and Thomas K. S. Wong, "Cultivating a Moral Sense of Nursing through Model Emulation," *Nursing Ethics*, 5:5 (1998), pp. 424–440.

# BIBLIOGRAPHY


Allmark, Peter. "Can There Be an Ethics of Care?" *Journal of Medical Ethics*, 21 (1995), pp. 19–24.

Astrom, G., L. Jansson, A. Norberg, and I. R. Hallberg. "Experienced Nurses' Narratives of their Being in Ethically Difficult Care Situations," *Cancer Nursing*, 16:3 (1993), pp. 179–187.

Baltzan, D. M., and W. S. Maddin. "Medicine in China," *Canadian Medical Association Journal*, 93:21 (1965), pp. 1118–1122.

Banister, Judith. *China's Changing Population*. Stanford, Calif.: Stanford University Press, 1987.

Barnowe, J. Thad. "Chinese Attempts to Reform Organizational Cultures," *Advances in Chinese Industrial Studies*, I, Pt. A. (1990), pp. 329–347.

Barry, Brian. *Justice as Impartiality*. Oxford: Clarendon Press, 1995.

Beauchamp, Tom L., and James F. Childress. *Principles of Biomedical Ethics*. New York: Oxford University Press, 5th ed., 2001.

______, and Arnold I. Davidson. "The Definition of Euthanasia," *Journal of Medicine and Philosophy*, 4:3 (1979), pp. 294–312.

______, and LeRoy Walters, eds. *Contemporary Issues in Bioethics*. Belmont, Calif.: Wadsworth Publishing Co., 5th ed., 1999.

Becker, Howard S. "The Epistemology of Qualitative Research," *Ethnography and Human Development: Context and Meaning in Social Inquiry*. Edited by Richard Jessor, Anne Colby, and Richard A. Shweder. Chicago, Ill.: University of Chicago Press, 1996, pp. 53–71.

Begely, Ann-Marie. "Beneficent Voluntary Active Euthanasia: A Challenge to Professionals Caring for Terminally Ill Patients," *Nursing Ethics*, 5:4 (1998), pp. 294–306.

Benner, Patricia. "A Dialogue between Virtue Ethics and Care Ethics," *Theoretical Medicine*, 18 (1997), pp. 47–61.

______, ed. *Interpretive Phenomenology: Embodiment, Caring, and Ethics in Health and Illness*. Thousand Oaks, Calif.: Sage, 1994.

______, Christine A. Tanner, and Catherine A. Chesla. *Expertise in Nursing Practice: Caring, Clinical Judgment, and Ethics*. New York: Springer, 1996.

Bishop, Anne H., and John R. Scudder. *Nursing Ethics, Therapeutic Caring Presence*. Boston: Jones & Barlett Publishers, 1996.

______. *The Practical, Moral, and Personal Sense of Nursing: A Phenomenological Philosophy of Practice*. Albany, N.Y.: State University of New York Press, 1990.

Bluenthal, Eileen P. *Models in Chinese Moral Education: Perspectives from Children's Books*, Ph. D. Thesis. Ann Arbor: The University of Michigan, 1976.

Boudreau, D. "A Question of Ethics? International Medical Community Condemns Death Row Donations in China," *Nephrology News Issues*, 9:8 (1995), p. 29.

Bradshaw, Ann. "What Are Nurses Doing to Patients? A Review of Theories of Nursing Past and Present," *Journal of Clinical Nursing*, 4 (1995), pp. 81–92.

______. "The Historical Tradition of Care," *Caring: The Compassion and Wisdom of Nursing*. Edited by Bryjznska Gosia. London: Arnold, 1997, pp. 10–31.

Breitmayer, B. J., L. Ayres, and K. A. Knafl. "Triangulation in Qualitative Research: Evaluation of Completeness and Confirmation Purposes," *Image: Journal of Nursing Scholarship*, 25:3 (1993), pp. 237–243.

Briggs, J. D. "The Use of Organs from Executed Prisoners in China," *Nephrology Dialysis Transplant*, 11:2 (1996), pp. 238–240.

British Medical Association. *Medical Ethics Today: Its Practice and Philosophy*. London: BMJ Publishing Group, 1993.

Burch, B. B. "Models as Agents of Change in China," *Value Change in Chinese Society*. Edited by Richard W. Wilson, Amy A. Wilson, and Sidney L. Greenblatt. New York: Prager, 1979, pp. 122–137.

Chambliss, Daniel F. *Beyond Caring, Hospitals, Nurses, and the Social Organization of Ethics*. Chicago, Ill.: University of Chicago Press, 1996.

Chang, Jung. *Wild Swans, The Three Daughters of China*. London: Flamingo, 1992.

Chen, Xiaoming, Tehwei Hu, and Zihua Lin. "The Rise and Decline of the Cooperative Medical System in Rural China," *International Journal of Health Services*, 23:4 (1993), pp. 731–742.

Cheng, Tienhis. "Disease Control and Prevention," *Public Health in the People's Republic of China: The Macy Foundation Series on Medicine and Public Health in China*. New York: The Josiah Macy, JR. Foundation, 1973.

China Medical Commission of the Rockefeller Foundation. *Medicine in China*. Chicago, Ill.: University of Chicago Press, 1914.

Cisar, N. "Informed Consent: An Ethical Dilemma," *Nursing Forum*, 30:3 (1995), pp. 20–28.

Chow, W. S. Nelson. "Western and Chinese Ideas of Social Welfare," *International Social Work*, 30 (1987), pp. 31–41.

Chu, Godwin. "The Changing Concept of Self in Contemporary China," *Culture and Self: Asian and Western Perspectives*. Edited by Anthony J. Marsella, George A. DeVos, and Francis L. K. Hsu. New York: Tavistock Publications, 1985, pp. 232–277.

Clark, L. "Nursing Research: Science, Visions and Telling Stories," *Journal of Advanced Nursing*, 21 (1996), pp. 584–593.

Clarke, Angus, Peter S. Harper, P. F. Unsworth, John Scotson, and Peter Doherty. "Eugenics in China," *Lancet*, 346:8973 (1995), pp. 508–509.

Crawshaw, R. "Medical Deontology in the Soviet Union," *Cross Cultural Perspectives in Medical Ethics: Readings*. Edited by Robert M. Veatch. Boston: Jones and Bartlett Publishers, 1989, pp. 102–112.

Davin, Delia. *Woman Work: Women and the Party in Revolutionary China*. Oxford: Clarendon Press, 1976.

Davis, Anne J. "Are There Limits to Caring? Conflict between Autonomy and Beneficence," *Ethical and Moral Dimensions of Care*. Edited by Madeleine M. Leininger. Detroit: Wayne State University Press, 1990, pp. 25–32.

______. "Clinical Nurses' Ethical Decision Making in Situations of Informed Consent," *Advances in Nursing Science*, 11:3 (1989), pp. 63–69.

______, and B. A. Koenig. "A Question of Policy: Bioethics in a Multicultural Society," *Nursing Policy Forum*, 2:1 (1996), pp. 6–11.

______, B. Davidson, M. Hirschfield, S. Lauri, J. Y. Lin, A. Norberg, L. Phillips, E. Pitman, C. H. Shen, R. V. Laan, H. L. Zhang, and L. Ziv. "An International Perspective of Active Euthanasia: Attitudes of Nurses in Seven Countries," *International Journal of Nursing Studies*, 30:4 (1993), pp. 301–310.

______, Lanjun Gan, Juyin Lin, and Virginia L. Olsen. "The Young Pioneers: First Baccalaureate Nursing Students in the Peoples' Republic of China," *Journal of Advanced Nursing*, 17 (1992), pp. 1166–1170.

______, Marcia Petrini, Juying Lin, and Virginia L. Olsen. "Values and Visions: Academic Nursing Students in the People's Republic of China," *Asian Journal of Nursing Studies*, 4:2 (1998), pp. 33–38.

______, Mila A. Aroskar, Joan Liaschenko, and Thereasa S. Drought. *Ethical Dilemmas and Nursing Practice*. Stamford, Conn.: Appleton & Lange, 4th ed., 1997.

De Bary, William Theodore. *Asian Values and Human Rights*. Cambridge, Mass.: Harvard University Press, 1998.

Deng, Xiaoping. *Selected Works of Deng Xiaoping 1975–1982*. Beijing: People's Publishing House, 1983.

Dennis, Karen E. "Q Methodology: Relevance and Application to Nursing Research," *Advances in Nursing Science*, 8:3 (1986), pp. 6–17.

Denzin, Norman K. *The Research Act: A Theoretical Introduction to Sociological Methods*. Englewood Cliffs, N.J.: Prentice Hall, 1989.

Dirschel, Kathleen M. "Teaching Nursing in China: An Exchange Program," *Nursing Outlook*, 29:12 (1981), pp. 722–726.

Dunn, F. L. "Traditional Asian Medicine and Cosmopolitan Medicine as Adaptive Systems," *Asian Medical Systems: A Comparative Study*. Edited by Charles M. Leslie. Berkeley: University of California Press, 1976, pp. 133–158.

Editorial. "China's Misconception of Eugenics," *Nature*, 367 (6 January 1994), pp. 1–2.

______. "Western Eyes on China's Eugenics Law," *Lancet*, 346:8968 (1995), p. 131.

Edwards, Steven D. "What Are the Limits to the Obligations of the Nurse?" *Journal of Medical Ethics*, 22 (1996), pp. 90–94.

Engelhardt, H. Tristram, Jr. "Bioethics in the People's Republic of China," *Cross Cultural Perspectives in Medical Ethics: Readings*. Edited by Robert M. Veatch. Boston: Jones and Bartlett Publishers, 1989, pp. 112–141.

______. "Physicians, Patients, Health Care Institutions: And the People in between Nurses," *Caring, Curing, Coping*. Edited by Anne H. Bishop, and John R. Scudder. University, Ala.: University of Alabama Press, 1985, pp. 62–79.

Ersser, Steven, and Elizabeth Tutton, eds. *Primary Nursing in Perspective*. Harrow, England: Scutari Press, 1991.

Esterhuizen, P. "Is the Professional Code Still the Cornerstone of Clinical Nursing Practice?" *Journal of Advanced Nursing*, 23:1 (1996), pp. 25–31.

Fan, Ruiping. "Self-determination vs Family-determination: Two Incommensurable Principles of Autonomy," *Bioethics*, 11:314 (1997), pp. 309–322.

______. "Three Levels of Problems in Cross-cultural Bioethics," *Japanese and Western Bioethics: Studies in Moral Diversity*. Edited by Kazumasa Hoshino. Dordrecht: Kluwer Academic Publishers, 1997, pp. 189–199.

Feng, Xueshan, Shenglan Tang, Bloom Gerald, Malcolm Segall, and Xingyuan Gu. "Cooperative Medical Schemes in Contemporary Rural China," *Social Science and Medicine*, 41:8 (1995), pp. 1111–1118.

Fung, Yulan. *A Short History of Chinese Philosophy*. Edited by Derk Bodde. New York: Free Press, 1948.

Fowler, Marsha D. M. *Ethics and Nursing, 1893–1984: The Ideal of Service, The Reality of History*, Ph. D. Thesis. Los Angeles: University of Southern California, 1984.

______. "Nursing's Ethics," *Ethical Dilemmas and Nursing Practice*. Edited by Anne J. Davis, Mila A. Aroskar, Joan Liaschenko, and Thereasa S. Drought. Stamford, Conn.: Appleton & Lange, 4th ed., 1997, pp. 17–34.

Fox, Renee C., and Judith P. Swazey. "Medical Morality is not Bioethics—Medical Ethics in China and the United States," *Perspectives in Biology and Medicine*, 27:3 (1984), pp. 336–360.

Frisch, S. R., D. Fowler-Graham, V. Shannon, and D. Demback. "Maintaining Autonomy of Vulnerable Subjects," *Canadian Journal of Nursing Research*, 22:4 (1990), pp. 51–60.

Fry, Sara T. *Ethics in Nursing Practice, A Guide to Ethical Decision Making*. Geneva: International Council of Nurses, 1994.

______. "New ANA Guidelines on Withdrawing or Withholding Food and Fluid from Patients," *Nursing Outlook*, 36:3 (1987), pp. 122–123, and pp. 148–150.

______. "Nursing Ethics: Current State of the Art," *Journal of Medicine and Philosophy*, 16 (1991), pp. 231–234.

______. "The Ethic of Care: Nursing's Excellence for a Troubled World," *A Global Agenda for Caring*. Edited by Delores A. Gaut. New York: National League for Nursing Press, 1993, pp. 175–180.

______. "The Philosophical Foundations of Caring," *Ethical and Moral Dimensions of Care*. Edited by Madeleine M. Leininger. Detroit: Wayne State University Press, 1990, pp. 175–180.

______. "Toward a Theory of Nursing Ethics," *Advances in Nursing Science*, 11:4 (1989), pp. 9–22.

______, Aileen R. Killen, and Ellen M. Robinson. "Care-based Reasoning, Caring, and the Ethic of Care: A Need for Clarity," *Journal of Clinical Ethics*, 7:1 (1996), pp. 41–47.

Fulbrook, Paul. "Assessing Mental Competence of Patients and Relatives," *Journal of Advanced Nursing*, 20 (1994), pp. 457–461.

______. "Assessing Quality of Life: The Basis of Withdrawal of Life-Supporting Treatment?" *Journal of Advanced Nursing*, 17 (1992), pp. 1440–1446.

Garfield, Richard. "China's Nurses: Redefining Roles to Improve Health," *International Journal of Nursing Studies*, 15 (1978), pp. 129–134.

Gilligan, Carol. *In a Different Voice: Psychological Theory and Women's Development*. Cambridge, Mass.: Harvard University Press, 1982.

______, and S. Pollak. "The Vulnerable and Invulnerable Physician," *Mapping the Moral Domain: A Contribution of Women's Thinking to Psychological Theory and Education*. Edited by Carol Gilligan, Janie V. Ward, Jill McLean Taylor, and Betty Bardige. Cambridge, Mass.: Harvard University Press, 1988, pp. 245–262.

Gosia, Bryjznska, ed. *Caring: The Compassion and Wisdom of Nursing*. London: Arnold, 1997.

Grundstein-Amado, R. "Differences in Ethical Decision-making Process among Nurses and Doctors," *Journal of Advanced Nursing*, 17 (1992), pp. 129–137.

______. "Ethical Decision-making Processes Used by Health Care Providers," *Journal of Advanced Nursing*, 18 (1993), pp. 1701–1709.

Halliday, Robert. "Medical Futility and the Social Context," *Journal of Medical Ethics*, 23 (1997), pp. 148–153.

Han, Qingxiang. "A Socialist Market Economy and the Molding of Man," *Social Sciences in China*, 17:4 (1996), pp.108–114.

Hardwig, John. "Is There a Duty to Die?" *Hastings Center Report*, 27:2 (1997), pp. 34–42.

Hauerwas, Stanley. "Care," *Encyclopedia of Bioethics*. Edited by Warren T. Reich. New York: Free Press, 1978, pp. 145–150.

He, Zuoxiu. "A New Understanding of 'Vast Territory, Rich Resources and a Large Population,'" *Social Sciences in China*, 18:4 (1997), pp. 44–51.

Hegyvary, Sue T. *The Change to Primary Nursing: A Cross Cultural View of Professional Nursing Practice*. St. Louis, Mo.: C.V. Mosby, 1982.

Henderson, Gail E., and Myron S. Cohen. *The Chinese Hospital: A Socialist Work Unit*. New Haven: Yale University Press, 1984.

______, Shuigao Jin, John Akin, Zhiming Li, Jianmin Wang, Haijiang Ma, Yunan He, Xiping Zhang, Ying Chang, and Keyou Ge. "Distribution of Medical Insurance in China," *Social Science and Medicine*, 41:8 (1995), pp. 1190–1230.

Henderson, Virginia. *Basic Principles of Nursing Care*. Geneva: International Council of Nurses, rev. ed., 1997.

Hesketh, Therese, and Weixing Zhu. "Health in China: Maternal and Child Health in China," *British Medical Journal*, 314:7098 (1997), pp. 1898–1900.

______. "The One Child Family Policy: The Good, the Bad, and the Ugly," *British Medical Journal*, 314:7095 (1997), pp. 1685–1687.

Holst, Erik. "Medical Ethics in China," *Lancet*, 344:8934 (1994), pp. 1427–1428.

Hong Kong Census and Statistics Department. *Hong Kong Annual Digest of Statistics*. Hong Kong: Government Printer, 1997.

Hong Kong Nursing Board, *The Code of Professional Conduct for Nurses in Hong Kong*. Hong Kong: Government Printer, 1986.

Hoshino, Kazumasa. "Bioethics in the Light of Japanese Sentiments," *Japanese and Western Bioethics: Studies in Moral Diversity*. Edited by Kazumasa Hoshino. Dordrecht: Kluwer Academic Publishers, 1997, pp. 13–23.

Hu, Peicheng. "Euthanasia: The Acceptability of Active Euthanasia in China," *Medicine and Law*, 12 (1993), pp. 47–53.

Huang, Kunyen. "Infectious and Parasitic Diseases," *Medicine and Public Health in the People's Republic of China*. Edited by Joseph R. Quinn. Bethesda, Md.: National Institutes of Health, 1973, pp. 241–264.

Huang, Weihe. "Mo Zi's Concepts of Righteousness and Benefit," *Social Sciences in China*, 7:4 (1986), pp. 161–174.

Huang, Xiyi. "Changes in the Economic Status of Rural Women in the Transformation of Modern Chinese Society," *Social Sciences in China*, 8:1 (1992), pp. 83–105.

Hussey, Trevor. "Nursing Ethics and Codes of Professional Conduct," *Nursing Ethics*, 3:3 (1996), pp. 250–258.

Jacob, E. "Qualitative Research Traditions: A Review," *Review of Educational Research*, 57:1 (1987), pp. 1–50.

Jessor, Richard, Anne Colby, and Richard A. Shweder, eds. *Ethnography and Human Development: Context and Meaning in Social Inquiry*. Chicago, Ill.: University of Chicago Press, 1996.

Johnson, Linda. "Expanding Eugenics or Improving Health Care, Commentary on the Provisions of the Standing Committee of the Gansu People's Congress Concerning the Prohibition of Reproduction by Intellectually Impaired Persons," *Journal of Law and Society*, 24:2 (1997), pp. 199–234.

Johnson, Martin. "Natural Sociology and Moral Questions in Nursing: Can There be a Relationship?" *Journal of Advanced Nursing*, 15 (1990), pp. 1358–1359.

Kary, Carla. "A Moral Distinction between Killing and Letting Die," *Journal of Medicine and Philosophy*, 5:4 (1980), pp. 326–332.

Kuuppelomaki, Merja, and Sirkka Lauri. "Ethical Dilemmas in the Care of Patients with Incurable Cancer," *Nursing Ethics*, 5:4 (1998), pp. 283–293.

______. "The Ethical Decision-making of Nurses Associated with the Feeding of Demented Patients and Terminally Ill Elderly Cancer Patients in Seven Countries," *Hoitoede*, 3:4 (1991), pp. 146–153.

Lampton, David M. "Economics, Politics and the Determinants of Policy Outcomes in China: Post-cultural Revolution Health Policy," *Australian and New Zealand Journal of Sociology*, 12:1 (1976), pp. 43–49.

_______. *The Politics of Medicine in China: The Policy Process, 1949–1977*. Folkestone, Kent: Dawson, 1977.

Larson, Patricia J., and Sandra L. Ferketich. "Patients' Satisfaction with Nurses' Caring During Hospitalisation," *Western Journal of Nursing Research*, 15:6 (1993), pp. 690–707.

Lau, Annie. "Family Therapy and Ethnic Minorities," *Family Therapy in Britain*. Edited by Eddy Street, and Windy Dryden. Philadelphia: Open University Press, 1988, pp. 270–290

Lau, Dimcheuk, translated. *Meng-tsu. English & Chinese, Volumes One & Two*. Hong Kong: Chinese University Press, 1984.

Lee, Tao. "Medical Ethics in Ancient China," *Cross Cultural Perspectives in Medical Ethics: Readings*. Edited by Robert M. Veatch. Boston: Jones and Bartlett Publishers, 1989, pp. 132–139.

Legge, James, translated. *Confucian Analects, The Great Learning and The Doctrine of the Mean*. New York: Dover, 1971.

Leininger, Madeleine M. "Culture: The Conspicuous Missing Link to Understand Ethical and Moral Dimensions of Human Care," *Ethical and Moral Dimensions of Care*. Edited by Madeleine M. Leininger. Detroit: Wayne State University Press, 1990, pp. 49–66.

Li, Feng, ed. *Woman of China Special Series: Half the Sky (1)*. Beijing: Woman of China, 1985.

Lin, Tsungyi, and Meichen Lin. "Love, Denial and Rejection: Responses of Chinese Families to Mental Illness," *Normal and Abnormal Behavior in Chinese Culture*. Edited by Arthur Kleinman, and Tsungyi Lin. Dordrecht, Boston: D. Reidel & Hingham, 1981, pp. 387–401.

Lin, Yangpei, Vivian Lin, and James Lawson. "Health Policy Reform in the People's Republic of China," *International Journal of Health Service,* 21:3 (1991), pp. 481–491.

Lindseth, A., V. Marhaug, A. Norberg, and G. Uden. "Registered Nurses' and Physicians' Reflections on their Narratives about Ethically Difficult Care Episodes," *Journal of Advanced Nursing,* 20 (1994), pp. 245–250.

Liu, Chungtung. "From *San Gu Lu Po* to 'Caring Scholar': The Chinese Nurse in Perspective," *International Journal of Nursing Studies*, 28:4 (1991), pp. 315–324.

Liu, Xian, Jersey Liang, and Shengzu Gu. "Flows of Social Support and Health Status among Older Persons in China," *Social Science and Medicine*, 41:8 (1995), pp. 1175–1184.

Lo, Bernard. *Resolving Ethical Dilemmas: A Guide for Clinicians.* Baltimore, Md.: Williams & Wilkins, 1995.

Lok, Sangho. "Market Reforms and China's Health Care System," *Social Science and Medicine*, 41:8 (1995), pp. 1065–1072.

Lu, Feng. "*Dan Wei*: A Special Form of Social Organization," *Social Sciences in China*, 10:3 (1989), pp. 105–113.

Lu, Xueyi. "China's Social Structure in the 21st Century: On the Transformation of the Social Structure," *Social Sciences in China*, 18:2 (1997), pp. 73–76.

Lucas, AnElissa. *Chinese Medical Modernization: Comparative Policy Continuities, 1930s–1980s*. New York: Praeger Publications, 1982.

Lutzen, Kim, and Conny Nordin. "Structuring Moral Meaning in Psychiatric Nursing Practice," *Scandinavian Journal of Caring Science*, 7 (1993), pp. 175–180.

Ma, En. "Letter from Beijing: One Child, One Family," *Journal of American Medical Association*, 261:12 (1989), pp. 1735–1736.

MacIntyre, Alasdair. *After Virtue: A Study in Moral Theory*. London: Duckworth, 2nd ed., 1985.

Mackerras, Colin, Pradeep Taneja, and Graham Young. *China Since 1978: Reform, Modernization, and 'Socialism with Chinese Characteristics.'* Melbourne: Longman Cheshire, 1994.

Mao, Zedong. *Quotations from Chairman Mao Tse-Tung*. Peking: Foreign Language Press, 1972.

_______. *Selected Works of Mao Tse-Tung*. Peking: Foreign Languages Press, 1965.

Manthey, Marie. *The Practice of Primary Nursing*. London: King's Fund Centre, 1992.

Marsella, Anthony, George Devos, and Francis Hsu, eds. *Cultural and Self: Asian and Western Perspectives*. New York: Tavistock Publications, 1985.

Marx, Karl, ed. *Critique of the Gotha Programme*. Peking: Foreign Languages Press, 1972.

May, C. "Disclosure of Terminal Prognoses in a General Hospital: The Nurse's View," *Journal of Advanced Nursing*, 18 (1993), pp. 1362–1368.

Mosher, Steven W. *A Mother's Ordeal: The Story of Chi An*. London: Warner Books.

Muller, J. H., and B. Desmond. "Ethical Dilemmas in A Cross-cultural Context, A Chinese Example," *Western Journal of Medicine*, 157:3 (1992), pp. 323–327.

Munro, Donald J. *The Concept of Man in Contemporary China*. Ann Arbor: University of Michigan Press, 1977.

______. *The Concept of Man in Early China*. Stanford, Calif.: Stanford University Press, 1969.

Nagel, Stuart S., and Miriam K. Mills, eds. *Public Policy in China*. Westport, Conn.: Greenwood Press, 1993.

Namihira, Emiko. "Japanese Concepts and Attitudes to Human Remains," *Japanese and Western Bioethics: Studies in Moral Diversity*. Edited by Kazumasa Hoshino. Dordrecht: Kluwer Academic Publishers, 1997, pp. 61–69.

Nan, Lin. "Chinese Family Structure and Chinese Society," *Bulletin of the Institute of Ethnology Academia Sinica*, 65 (Spring 1988), pp. 59–129.

Newell, Kenneth W., ed. *Health by the People*. Geneva: World Health Organization, 1975.

Nightingale, Florence. *Notes on Nursing: Commemorative Edition*. Philadelphia: J.B. Lippincott, 1992.

Noddings, Nel. *Caring: A Feminist Approach to Ethics and Moral Education*. Berkeley: University of California Press, 1984.

*On Question of Party History—Resolution on Certain Questions in the History of Our Party Since the Founding of the People's Republic of China. Beijing Review*, 24:7 (6 July 1981), pp. 20–21.

Orient, Jane M. "A Critique of Western Medical Commentary on the People's Republic of China," *Archives of Internal Medicine*, 144 (1984), pp. 106–109.

Pang, Meiche Samantha. *From Virtue to Value: Nursing Ethics in Modern China*, Ph. D. Thesis. Hong Kong: The University of Hong Kong, 1999.

______. "Information Disclosure: The Moral Experience of Nurses in China," *Nursing Ethics*, 5:4 (1998), pp. 347–361.

______. "Protective Truthfulness: The Chinese Way in Safeguarding Patients in Informed Treatment Decisions," *Journal of Medical Ethics*, 25:3 (1999), pp. 247–253.

______, and Thomas K. S. Wong. "Cultivating a Moral Sense of Nursing through Model Emulation," *Nursing Ethics*, 5:5 (1998), pp. 424–440.

______, and Eva Y. H. Tang. "An Evaluative Study on Individualizing Patient Care in a Hospital Ward in Hong Kong," *Hong Kong Nursing Journal*, 63 (1993), pp. 13–20.

______, David G. Arthur, and Thomas K. S. Wong. "Drawing A Qualitative Distinction of Caring Practices in a Professional Context: The Case of Chinese Nursing," *Holistic Nursing Practice*, 15:1 (2000), pp. 22–31.

Parsons, Sara E. *Nursing Problems and Obligations*. Boston: Whitcomb & Barrows, 1916.

Pearson, Alan, ed. *Primary Nursing: Nursing in the Burford and Oxford Development Units*. London: Chapman and Hall, 1989.

Pearson, Veronica. "Community and Culture: A Chinese Model of Community Care for the Mentally Ill," *International Journal of Social Psychiatry*, 38:3 (1992), pp. 163–178.

______. "Families in China: An Undervalued Resource for Mental Health?" *Journal of Family Therapy*, 15 (1993), pp. 163–185.

______. "Health and Responsibility: But Whose?" *Social Change and Social Policy in Contemporary China*. Edited by Linda Wong, and Stewart MacPherson. Hong Kong: City University of Hong Kong, 1995, pp. 88–112.

______. *Mental Health Care in China: State Policies, Professional Services and Family Responsibilities*. London: Gaskell, 1995.

______. "Population Policy and Eugenics in China," *British Journal of Psychiatry*, 167:1 (1995), pp. 1–4.

______, and Michael R. Philips. "The Social Context of Psychiatric Rehabilitation in China," *British Journal of Psychiatry*, 165: suppl. 24 (1994), pp. 11–18.

Pellegrino, Edmund D, Patricia Mazzarella, and Pietro Corsi, eds. *Transcultural Dimensions in Medical Ethics*. Frederick, Md.: University Pub. Group, 1992.

______, Robert M. Veatch, and John P. Langan, eds. *Ethics, Trust, and The Professions, Philosophical and Cultural Aspects*. Washington, D.C.: Georgetown University Press, 1991.

Pence, Terry. "Approaches to Nursing Ethics," *Philosophy in Context*, 17 (1987), pp. 7–15.

Peng, Lei. "The Practical Significance of Confucian Moral Cultivation," *Social Sciences in China*, 18:2 (1997), pp. 45–50.

Penticuff, Joy Hinson. "Conceptual Issues in Nursing Ethics Research," *Journal of Medicine and Philosophy*, 16 (1991), pp. 235–258.

______. "Nursing Perspectives in Bioethics," *Japanese and Western Bioethics: Studies in Moral Diversity*. Edited by Kazumasa Hoshino. Dordrecht: Kluwer Academic Publishers, 1997, pp. 49–60.

Plato. "*Euthyphro*," *The Last Days of Socrates*. Translated by Hugh Tredennick, and Harold Tarrant. New York: Penguin Classic, 1993, pp. 1–28.

Polit, Dennis F., and Bernadette P. Hungler. *Nursing Research: Principles and Methods*. Philadelphia: Lippincott, 6th ed., 1999.

Quinn, Joseph. R., ed. *Medicine and Public Health in the People's Republic of China*. Bethesda, Md.: National Institutes of Health, 1973.

Qiu, Renzong. "Bioethics in China: 1991–1993," *Bioethics Yearbook, Volume 4: Regional Development in Bioethics, 1991–1993*. Edited by B. Andrew Lustig. Dordrecht: Kluwer Academic Publishers, 1995, pp. 339–365.

______. "Chinese Medical Ethics and Euthanasia," *Cambridge Quarterly of Healthcare Ethics*, 2:1 (1993), pp. 69–76.

______. "Equity and Public Health Care in China," *Journal of Medicine and Philosophy*, 14 (1989), pp. 283–287.

______. "Ethical Problems in Renal Dialysis and Transplantation: A Chinese Perspective," *Ethical Problems in Dialysis and Transplantation*. Edited by Carol M. Kjellstrand, and John B. Dossetor. Dordrecht: Kluwer Academic Publishers, 1992, pp. 227–235.

______. "Medical Ethics and Chinese Culture," *Transcultural Dimensions in Medical Ethics*. Edited by Edmund Pellegrino, Patricia Mazzarella, and Pietro Corsi. Frederick, Md.: University Publisher Group. 1992, pp. 155–174.

______. "Morality in Flux: Medical Ethics Dilemmas in the People's Republic of China," *Kennedy Institute of Ethics Journal*, (March 1991), pp. 16–27.

______. "Philosophy of Medicine in China (1930–1980)," *Metamedicine*, 3 (1982), pp. 35–73.

______. "The Fiduciary Relationship between Professionals and Clients: A Chinese Perspective," *Ethics, Trust, and The Professions, Philosophical and Cultural Aspects*. Edited by Edmund D. Pellegrino, Robert M. Veatch, and John P. Langan. Washington, D.C.: Georgetown University Press, 1991, pp. 247–259.

______, and Dajie Jin. "Bioethics in China: 1989–1991," *Bioethics Yearbook, Volume 2*. Edited by B. Andrew Lustig. Dordrecht: Kluwer Academic Publishers, 1992, pp. 355–377.

______, Shunzhui Wang, and Yuan Gu. "Can Late Abortion be Ethically Justified?" *Journal of Medicine and Philosophy*, 14 (1989), pp. 343–350.

Reed, Gay Garland. "Moral/Political Education in the People's Republic of China: Learning through Role Models," *Journal of Moral Education*, 24:2 (1995), pp. 99–111.

Reich, Warren Thomas, ed. *Encyclopedia of Bioethics*, New York: Simon and Schuster Macmillan, rev. ed., 1995.

Rhoden, Nancy K. "Treating Baby Doe: The Ethics of Uncertainty," *Contemporary Issues in Bioethics*. Edited by Tom L. Beauchamp, and LeRoy Walters. Belmont, Calif.: Wadsworth Publishing Co., 4th ed., 1994, pp. 419–430.

Rich, Vera. "Will the Chinese Legalize Euthanasia?" *Lancet*, 345:8952 (1995), p. 783.

Rifkin, Susan, B. "Health Care for Rural Areas," *Medicine and Public Health in the People's Republic of China*. Edited by Joseph R. Quinn. Bethesda, Md.: National Institutes of Health, 1973, pp. 141–152.

Rockefeller Foundation. *Report for the 1992–1993 Year*. New York: China Medical Board of New York, 1993.

Rosenberg, Charles E. *The Care of Strangers: The Rise of America's Hospital System*. New York: Basic Books, Inc., 1987.

Sang, Xinmin. "Philosophic Reflection on the Comprehensive Development of the Components of Education," *Social Sciences in China*, 8:4 (1992), pp. 138–146.

Sayers, Gwen M. "An Analysis of CPR Decision-making by Elderly Patients," *Journal of Medical Ethics*, 23 (1997), pp. 207–212.

Schutz, S. E. "Patient Involvement in Resuscitation Decisions," *British Journal of Nursing*, 3:20 (1994), pp. 1075–1079.

Shi, Dapu. "Euthanasia in China: A Report," *Journal of Medical and Philosophy*, 16 (1991), pp. 131–138.

Shu, Wu. "The Discovery of the Female: A Brief Outline of Zhou Zuoren's Feminist Theory," *Social Sciences in China*, 11:3 (1990), pp. 32–67.

Shukla, R. K. "Primary or Team Nursing? Two Conditions Determine the Choice," *Journal of Nursing Administration*, (November 1982), pp. 12–15.

Sidel, Victor W., and Ruth Sidel. "The Health-care Delivery System of the People's Republic of China," *Health by the People*. Edited by Kenneth W. Newell. Geneva: World Health Organization, 1975, pp. 1–12.

______. *The Health of China: Current Conflicts in Medical and Human Services for One Billion People*. London: Zed Press, 1982.

Soderberg, Anna, and Astrid Norberg. "Intensive Care: Situations of Ethical Difficulty," *Journal of Advanced Nursing*, 18 (1993), pp. 2008–2014.

Spencer, Barbara. *Desert Hospital in China*. London: Jarrolds Publishers, 1954.

Strauss, Anselm L. *Qualitative Analysis for Social Scientists*. New York: Cambridge University Press, 1987.

Sun, Chunghsing. "The Five Interpersonal Relationships in the Four Books: A Study in Confucian Ethics," *National Taiwan University Journal of Sociology*, 22 (1993), pp. 1–48.

Sun, Guangde. "Health Care Administration in China," *Public Policy in China*. Edited by Stuart S. Nagel, and Miriam K. Mills. Westport, Conn.: Greenwood Press, 1993, pp. 53–62.

Sun, Liping, Hansheng Wang, Sibin Wang, Bin Lin, and Shanhua Yang. "Changes in China's Social Structure Following the Reforms," *Social Sciences in China*, 16:3 (1995), pp. 70–80.

Swider, Susan M., Beverly J. McElmurry, and Roland R. Yarling. "Ethical Decision Making in a Bureaucratic Context by Senior Nursing Students," *Nursing Research*, 34:2 (1985), pp. 108–112.

Tong, Xing, and Mingang Lin. "A Study of Poverty Lines in Rural Areas," *Social Sciences in China*, 16:3 (1995), pp. 81–87.

Tu, Ping. "On the Issues of Population Aging and Population Control in China," *Social Sciences in China*, 18:3 (1997), pp. 129–138.

Tu, Weiming. "Selfhood and Otherness in Confucian Thought," *Culture and Self: Asian and Western Perspectives*. Edited by Anthony J. Marsella, George A. DeVos, and Francis L. K. Hsu. New York: Tavistock Publications, 1985, pp. 231–251.

Unschuld, Paul U. *Medical Ethics in Imperial China. A Study in Historical Anthropology*. Berkeley: University of California Press, 1979.

Van der Arend, and J. G. Arie. "An Ethical Perspective on Euthanasia and Assisted Suicide in the Netherlands from a Nursing Point of View," *Nursing Ethics*, 5:4 (1998), pp. 307–318.

Veatch, Robert M., ed. *Cross Cultural Perspectives in Medical Ethics: Readings*. Boston: Jones and Bartlett Publishers, 1989.

______. "Nursing Ethics, Physician Ethics, and Medical Ethics," *Law, Medicine and Health Care*, 9 (1981), pp. 17–19.

______. "Which Grounds for Overriding Autonomy are Legitimate?" *Hastings Center Report*, 26:6 (1996), pp. 42–43.

Veith, Ilza. "Changing Concepts of Health Care: An Historian's View," *Western Journal of Medicine*, 133:6 (1980), pp. 532–538.

______, translated. *The Yellow Emperor's Classic of Internal Medicine*. Berkeley: University of California Press, 1970.

Wallis C., A. Constable, and S. Gribben. "The Stormy Legacy of Baby Doe," *Time*, 122:13 (1983), p. 58.

Watson, Jean. *Nursing: The Philosophy and Science of Caring*. Colorado: University Press of Colorado, 1985.

Wawrytko, Sandra A. "Confucius and Kant: The Ethics of Respect," *Philosophy East and West*, 32:3 (1982), pp. 231–257.

Wegman, Myron E., Tsungyi Lin, and Elizabeth F. Purcell, eds. *Public Health in the People's Republic of China*. New York: The Josiah Macy, JR. Foundation, 1973.

Whitehead, Raymond L. *Love and Struggle in Mao's Thought*. Maryknoll, N.Y.: Orbis Books, 1977.

Whitman, Christina B. "Privacy in Early Confucian and Taoist Thought," *Individualism and Holism: Studies in Confucian and Taoist Values*. Edited by Donald J. Munro. Ann Arbor: Center for Chinese Studies, University of Michigan, 1985, pp. 85–99.

Wong, Chimin, and Lienteh Wu. *History of Chinese Medicine: Being a Chronicle of Medical Happenings in China from Ancient Times to the Present Period*. Shanghai, China: National Quarantine Service, 1936.

World Bank. *Health: Sector Policy Paper*. Washington, D. C.: World Bank, March, 1975.

Wong, Thomas K. S., and Samantha M. C. Pang. "Holism and Caring: Nursing in the Chinese Health Care Context," *Holistic Nursing Practice*, 15:1 (2000), pp. 12–21.

Wros, Peggy L. "The Ethical Context of Nursing Care of Dying Patients in Critical Care," *Interpretive Phenomenology: Embodiment, Caring, and Ethics in Health and Illness*. Edited by Patricia Benner. Thousand Oaks, Calif.: Sage, 1994, pp. 255–278.

Wu, Jie. *On Deng Xiaoping Thought*. Beijing: Foreign Languages Press, 1996.

Wu, Jingyu, translated. *Twenty-four Stories of filial Devotion*. Singapore: Asiapac Publication, 1997.

Wu, Zhaohua. "Conflicts between Chinese Traditional Ethics and Bioethics," *Cambridge Quarterly of Healthcare Ethics*, 3 (1994), pp. 367–371.

Yang, Peilin, Vivian Lin, and James Lawson. "Health Policy Reform in the People's Republic of China," *International Journal of Health Services*, 21:3 (1991), pp. 481–491.

Yarling, Roland R., and Beverly J. McElmurry. "The Moral Foundation of Nursing," *Advances in Nursing Science*, 8:2 (1986), pp. 63–73.

Zhang, Bingnan. "Propriety, Benevolence and the Mean: The Evolution of Confucius' Thinking," *Social Sciences in China*, 13:2 (1992), pp. 133–150.

Zhang, Kuiliang. "Marx's Vision in His Late Years and Deng Xiaoping's Theory of Building Socialism with Chinese Characteristics," *Social Sciences in China*, 16:4 (1995), pp. 143–152.

Zhang, Zhikuan. "A Major Reform in Hospital Management System in China: Grading and Assessment," *Chinese Medical Journal*, 107:4 (1994), pp. 243–247.

Zhang, Zhuo. "An Analysis of Some of the Objectives of China's Modernization," *Social Sciences in China*, 14:3 (1993), pp. 5–16.

Zhu, Yong, and Yaping Cheng. "Kinship and Legal Duties in Ancient China," *Social Sciences in China*, 18:3 (1997), pp. 99–105.

《中國衛生年鑒》。北京：人民衛生出版社，1996。

《中國衛生年鑒》。北京：人民衛生出版社，1997。

《新三字經》編寫委員會，新三字經。廣州：廣東教育出版社，1995。

丁人編，《護士質修養》。北京：人民軍醫出版社，1992。

于淑存、劉倩文，"提高護士職業道德的教育方法"，《中華護理雜誌》，31卷，3期，頁 174~175，1996。

中國年鑑社，《中華人民共和國年鑑》。北京：新華出版社，1996。

中國年鑑社，《中華人民共和國年鑑》。北京：新華出版社，1997。

中華人民共和國母嬰保健法，《中國衛生年鑒》。北京：人民衛生出版社，頁 23~25，1995。

中華人民共和國國家統計局編，《中國統計年鑑》。香港：經濟導報社，1997。

天津市護士學校，"認真總結經驗，努力辦好護士學校"，《中華護理雜誌》，5 期，頁 229~231，1980。

毛乾雯，"怎樣掌握書寫護理計劃的方法"，《中華護理雜誌》，22 卷，3 期，頁 97~99，1987。

王三虎，"護士形象簡史"，《中華護理雜誌》，27 卷，11 期，頁 518~519，1992。

王大軍，"醫學目的調整與醫學道德的更新"，《中國醫學倫理學》，總 48 期，4 期，頁 22~23，1996。

王可摘，"全國首例安樂死終審結案"，《中國醫學倫理學》，總 24 期，4 期，頁 26，1992。

王明芳、車小菊，"淺談病人死亡在護理的倫理要求"，《中華護理雜誌》，28 卷，6 期，頁 331~332，1993。

王紅，"假如我是一個病人"，《中華護理雜誌》，27 卷，10 期，頁 476，1992。

王桐，"熱愛護理專業做好本職工作"，《中華護理雜誌》，4 期，頁 193~197，1982。

王偉智、翁素貞，"從兩次病人調查看責任制護理的深化"，《中華護理雜誌》，24 卷，4 期，頁 193~195，1989。

王琇瑛，《護理發展簡史》。上海：上海科學技術出版社，1987。

王寧娟，"倫理道德在臨終護理中的應用"，《中華護理雜誌》，28 卷，10 期，頁 634~635，1993。

王隴德副部長，“在全國整體護理研討會上的講話”，《中華護理雜誌》，31卷，11期，頁621~624，1996。

北京第二醫院學院臨床教學處，“臨床第一課上得好”，《中華護理雜誌》，4期，頁241~243，1982。

司務道，《陝西羚蹤：司務道教士自傳之一》。香港：靈實醫院靈實福音佈道團，1985。

伍蓓秋編，《中國兒童發展與家庭國際研討會，第2卷論文集》。北京：北京科學技術出版社，1993。

朱雅琪，“日本醫院護理工作的概況”，《中華護理雜誌》，6期，頁374~376，1982。

何兆雄編，《中國醫德史》。上海：上海醫科大學出版社，1987。

余夢萍、張黎明，“應用護理巡診優化護理人員再教育”，《中華護理雜誌》，30卷，1期，頁33~35，1995。

吳行正，“護理責任制的探討”，《中華護理雜誌》，5期，頁266~268，1982。

呂美頤、鄭永福，《中國婦女運動：1840–1921》。鄭州：河南人民出版社，1990。

宋珍英，“如何做好在職護士的思想教育工作”，《中華護理雜誌》，3期，頁118~119，1981。

李本富、丁蕙孫、李傳俊，《護理倫理學 (第二版)》。北京：科學出版社，1992。

李向明、陳光曼、王瑞廷、辛翠蘭編，《中國現代醫學家傳略》。北京：科學技術文獻出版社，1984。

李恩昌，“「醫學目的，生命質量，醫學倫理」：全國第八次醫學倫理學學術研討會側記”，《中國醫學倫理學》，總43期，5期，頁63~64，1995。

李傳俊、何玉軍、游榮藝編，《醫德學概論》。北京：中國醫葯科技出版社，1993。

李華，“向護士前輩學習”，《中華護理雜誌》，1卷，2期，1981。

李鈺霖，“關于中等護士職業教育的改革”，《中華護理雜誌》，25 卷，3 期，頁 144~145，1990。

李維光，“正確判斷護理問題 (護理診斷)”，《中華護理雜誌》，22 卷，3 期，頁 100~101，1987。

李輯敏，“制訂「患者權利」促使醫德自律”，《中國醫學倫理學》，總 48 期，4 期，頁 47~48，1996。

沈宗雲、楊以成，“淺談護理人才培養中的倫理教育”，《中華護理雜誌》，26 卷，4 期，頁 182~183，1991。

汪炎雄、白洪梅，“一項造福於人類的崇高事業”，《中國醫學倫理學》，總 24 期，4 期，頁 31~33，1992。

肖順貞，“推動護理科研開展，提高論文寫作質量”，《「現代護理新趨勢及發展」研討會》。廈門：護理中心，1996。

佘雲楚，彭美慈，“專業守則：實務或霸權？評「香港護士專業守則」”，《專業交叉點：專業倫理的理念與實行》，文思慧，梁美儀編。香港：青文書局，頁 66~101，2000。

周曼穎、楊以成，“關于中等護士專業增設護理程序課程的探討”，《中華護理雜誌》，29 卷，1 期，頁 40~42，1996。

林菊英，“中國護理訪問團赴美參觀訪問情況介紹”，《中華護理雜誌》，1 期，頁 46~48，1981。

______、金喬編，《中華護理全書》。南昌：江西科學技術出版社，1993。

林翠芬，“培養護士優良心理品質淺見”，《中華護理雜誌》，30 卷，6 期，頁 355~356，1995。

邱仁宗，“死亡概念和安樂死”，《醫學與哲學》，1 期，頁 77~79，1980。

邱世昌編，《護理倫理》。北京：人民出版社，1990。

邱鴻鐘，“儒醫義利觀及其實踐狀況”，《中國醫學倫理學》，總 48 期，4 期，頁 62~64，1996。

金耀基，《中國社會與文化》。香港：牛津大學出版社，1992。

侯琳、朱友明，“注重人才培養提高護士素質”，《中華護理雜誌》，28 卷，11 期，頁 652~653，1993。

俞海珠，“提高護士素質是搞好護理工作的關鍵”，《中華護理雜誌》，23 卷，4 期，頁 230~231，1988。

姜瑾，“醫生語言修養之管見”，《中國醫學倫理學》，總 56 期，6 期，頁 9~11，1997。

姚昶緒，《病人看護法》。上海：商務印書館，1939。

姚軒鴿、余德華，“關於安樂死道德評價問題的思考”，《中國醫學倫理學》，總 24 期，4 期，頁 23~26，1992。

施榕，《醫德一百題》。上海：上海人民出版社，1991。

______，“臨終關懷在上海之現狀”，《施榕教授文集》。 西安：陝西師範大學出版社，頁 126~133，1997。

______，《論器管移植現狀困惑及其發展對策》。上海醫學高等專科學校，1991。

段江麗，“從尊嚴的需要談護士行爲”，《中華護理雜誌》，25 卷，1 期，頁 49~50，1990。

胡英、余屏、宋愛清，“論優死教育”，《中國醫學倫理學》，總 22 期，2 期，頁 47~49，1992。

胡凱，“先秦儒學與老莊哲學的身心修養方法初探”，《中國醫學倫理學》，總 48 期，頁 58~59，1996。

倪黎明，“50 例放棄新生兒治療與安樂死”，《中國醫學倫理學》，總 28 期，2 期，頁 53，1993。

孫隆基，《中國文化的深層結構 (修訂版) 》。香港：集賢社，1992。

徐少錦、溫克勤編，《中國倫理文化寶庫》。北京：中國廣播電視出版社，1995。

徐文友、王桂蓮，“孫思邈的高尚醫德及其現實意義”，《中國醫學倫理學》，總 43 期，5 期，頁 55，1995。

徐素英，“提高認識注重實踐搞好醫德教育”，《中華護理雜誌》，24 卷，1 期，頁 57~58，1989。

柴瑞震、程延安、姜任華編，“全國醫院分級與疾病分類標準及醫院工作制度，職責配備規範”。成都：成都科技大學出版社，1995。

秦愛忠，“我對做好護理工作的體會”，《中華護理雜誌》，1 期，頁 2~3，1982。

荆其誠，“中國獨生子女政策與人口心理學”，《中國兒童發展與家庭國際研討會論文集第二卷》，中國關心下一代工作委員會專家委員會主編。北京：北京科學技術出版社，頁 295~308，1993。

袁光榮，“醫學目的與安樂死”，《中國醫學倫理學》，總 56 期，6 期，頁 13，32，1997。

袁劍雲、金橋、杜新柱、王鴻飛，“論系統化整體護理與‘模式病房’建設”，《中華護理雜誌》，31 卷，2 期，頁 118~120，1996。

馬旭，《簡言衛生事業與社會經濟全面協調發展》。上海：上海市中北醫院，頁 1~6，1995。

馬敏芝，“從「人人享有衛生保健」看「臨終關懷」與「安樂死」”，《中國醫學倫理學》，總 40 期，2 期，頁 48~49，1995。

高雁，“談護士在護患交往中運用語言的技巧”，《中國醫學倫理學》，總 56 期，6 期，頁 14，1997。

涂或、朱永烈，“安樂死的法律參與”，《中國醫學倫理學》，總 25 期，5 期，頁 35~37，1992。

郜敏芳、劉蘇君、謝貞，“關於護理科研成果社會效益和經濟效益的調查分析”，《中華護理雜誌》，31 卷，3 期，頁 163~164，1996。

乾祖望，《孫思邈評傳》。南京：南京大學出版。

張玉英，“我院 17 年中發生護理事故、差錯、問題的分析”，《中華護理雜誌》，22 卷，9 期，頁 385~387，431，1987。

張立紅、李素平、朱月珍，“對 6 所三級甲等醫院護理科研現狀的調查分析”，《中華護理雜誌》，31 卷，8 期，頁 468~469，1996。

張芳，“改進‘病人生活護理’課的教學法”，《中華護理雜誌》，26 卷，11 期，頁 524，1991。

張惠蘭，“接待美國護理考察團情況介紹”，《中華護理雜誌》，2 期，頁 62~64，1982。

張維慶，“和護士同志們談幾句話”，《中華護理雜誌》，19 卷，6 期，頁 362~363，1984。

張靜茹，“護士，其實就是一個沒有翅膀的天使”，《中華護理雜誌》，20 卷，3 期，頁 183，1985。

張贊寧，“安樂死，中國比西方更自由”，《家庭醫生》，總 113 期，9 期，頁 40~42，1993。

______，“關於安樂死的幾個問題–與林業剛同志商榷”，《法律科學》，總 35 期，2 期，頁 87~91，1991。

從亞麗，“安樂死道德與法律關係淺探”，《中國醫學倫理學》，總 52 期，2 期，頁 44~45，1997。

從榍華、劉飛，“慎獨對夜間護理工作的指導意義”，《中華護理雜誌》，31 卷，2 期，頁 108~110，1996。

曹開賓、邱世昌、樊民勝編，《醫學倫理學教程》。上海：上海醫科大學出版社，1992。

郭淸秀、石月淸，“安樂死的現實呼喚與思考”，《中國醫學倫理學》，總 53 期，3 期，頁 42~44，1997。

______、勒風林、耿洪剛，“中國安樂死”，《中外醫學哲學》，1 卷，1 期，頁 137~149，1998。

郭照江，“學習白求恩，從醫爲人民：全國第三屆白求恩精神研討會側紀”，《中國醫學倫理學》，總 51 期，1 期，頁 15，36，1997。

陳命家、李和林，“護士專業設公共關係課可行性探討”，《中華護理雜誌》，29 卷，1 期，頁 51~52，1994。

陳坤惕，“中華護理學會第十八屆理事會工作報告”，《中華護理雜誌》，18 卷，5 期，頁 261~265，1983。

陳振東、高宗熔、李海享，“終末期癌症患者及其親屬的求醫動機”，《中國醫學倫理學》，總 113 期，2 期，頁 49~50，1993。

陳浩文、高永文，“安樂死的謬誤、醫療目的與病人自決權”，陶黎寶華、邱仁宗編，《價值與社會（第一集）》。北京：中國社會科學出版社，頁 4~101，1997。

陳敏章，“弘揚白求恩精神加強衛生系統精神”，《中國醫學倫理學》，總 53 期，3 期，頁 2~3，1997。

陳瑛，“中國倫理發展現狀”，《應用倫理學研究中心會訊》。香港：香港浸會大學，6 卷，1 期，頁 10~15，1997。

陳聰杰，“論義利兼顧以義爲先”，《中國醫學倫理學》，總 25 期，5 期，頁 7~10，1992。

陳靈艷，“談談‘醫教護’和‘醫學護’”，《中華護理雜誌》，25 卷，3 期，頁 145~146，1990。

陶乃煌，“系統工程及其在護理管理中的應用(四)：臨床護理是一個系統護理過程”，《中華護理雜誌》，20 卷，4 期，頁 237~240，1985。

傅愛民，“醫院改革開放後護理工作見聞及反思”，《中華護理雜誌》，23 卷，10 期，頁 620，1988。

喻琳、石大璞，“從典型案例及民意調查看安樂死在中國立法之必要性”，《中外醫學哲學》，1 卷，1 期，頁 159~174，1998。

喬選超、丁秀東，“關于醫療保密的倫理問題”，《中國醫學倫理學》，總 51 期，1 期，頁 25~26，1997。

嵇芸、吳布生、常桂琴，“論護理學的研究對象”，《中華護理雜誌》，31 卷，3 期，頁 185~187，1996。

彭美慈、周麗雲，“可否向病人剖白真相”，《亞洲護理學雜誌》，1 卷，4 期，頁 61~64，1994。

______、佘雲楚，“論安樂死作爲療手段的倫理涵意”，《社聯季刊》，144 期，頁 32~36，1998。

______、曾熙媛、王春生、張志君、劉書琴、汪國成、賴錦玉，“採用特爾非法 撰寫新世紀中國護士倫理準則”，《中華護理雜誌》，35 卷，9 期，頁 517~518，2000。

普連升，“「安樂死」殺人案一審辯護問”，《律師世界》，1 卷，100 總期，頁 33~39，1992。

曾竹平，“關于護理教育的討論”，《中華護理雜誌》，3 期，頁 98~102，1981。

程立竑編，《醫德知識百問》。 北京：中國醫葯科技出版社，1992。

童奎昌，“對畢業班護生開展職業禮貌教育的探討”，《中華護理雜誌》，28 卷，3 期，頁 165~166，1993。

馮秀雲，“安樂死的幾個法律問題”，《中國醫學倫理學》，總 54 期，4 期，頁 49~51，1997。

馮運華，“中國護理近年之發展”，《香港護理雜誌》，33 卷，4 期，頁 41~43，1997。

黃雪華、歐清，“醫德教育應注意發揮典型人物的作用”，《中華護理雜誌》，26 卷，8 期，頁 382~383，1991。

黃劍琴，“爲中專護生講授現代護理新概念的做法和體會”，《中華護理雜誌》，29 卷，5 期，頁 293~296，1994。

黃穎，“我擔任責任護士的體會”，《中華護理雜誌》，19 卷，4 期，頁 235~236，1984。

黃黨發，“天使聖潔芙蓉爭輝”，《中國醫學倫理學》，總 34 期，2 期，頁 54~56，1994。

黃驍洪，“論肛腸病診治中的若干道德問題”，《中國醫學倫理學》，總 53 期，3 期，頁 25，1997。

楊以成、王偉智，“如何在護理大專教育中貫穿‘護理程序’教學”，《中華護理雜誌》，26 卷，11 期，頁 523~524，1991。

楊玉蘭、雷衍弘，“優死：時代的挑戰與探索”，《第八屆全國中華醫學倫理學會中青委員會會議》。中國：華山，1997。

楊惠芳，“全國整體護理研討會會議紀要”，《中華護理雜誌》，31 卷，11 期，頁 678~679，1996。

楊曄，“論護理教育的價值取向”，《中華護理雜誌》，30 卷，8 期，頁 476~477，1995。

葉樹軍，“試論對在職護士進行護理倫理學教育”，《中華護理雜誌》，29 卷，4 期，頁 225~226，1994。

解放日報，“硬索費用，延誤時間，上海醫生見死不救”，《明報》轉戴，1986年7月13日。

裴顯俊，“醫學模式轉變與護理人員知識結構的優化”，《中華護理雜誌》，25卷，2期，頁110~111，1990。

趙瑞萍、張芝雲，“新任護士長五忌”，《中華護理雜誌》，31卷，12期，頁711，1996。

趙維生、黃昌榮，“中國醫療服務及醫療制度改革”，《中國社會發展：香港學者的分析》，李思、邵一鳴、莫泰基編。香港：香港教育圖書公司，頁277~309，1995。

劉旭東，“讓理想之花開得絢麗多彩：記上海市第一人民醫院護士卜凡”，《中華護理雜誌》，6期，頁321~322，1982。

劉勇，“中國的放棄治療現狀及倫理問題”，《中國醫學倫理學》，總28期，2期，頁51~52，1993。

劉詠聰，《女性與歷史：中國傳統觀念新探》。香港：香港教育，1993。

劉瑩，“護士姐姐萬歲”，《中華護理雜誌》，24卷，8期，頁48，1989。

潘紹山，“試談醫院護士的職業道德”，《中華護理雜誌》，22卷，9期，頁428~429，1987。

編輯部，“全國責任制護理研討會討論情況簡介”，《中華護理雜誌》，22卷，3期，頁102~103，1987。

蔡根法、馮嘉元，“醫學倫理問題初探”，《醫學與哲學》，2期，頁44~48，1980。

鄭韓生，“爲護理事業奮鬥一生”，《中華護理雜誌》，30卷，6期，頁383~384，1996。

鄧莉，“淺談護士語言與醫德”，《中國醫學倫理學》，總25期，5期，頁33~34，1992。

鄧穎超，“爲「護士之歌」、「家庭護理」題詞”，《中華護理雜誌》，18卷，5期，頁255，1983。

錢信忠，“中國紅十字會錢信忠會長在南丁格爾獎章授獎大會上的講話”，《中華護理雜誌》，18卷，5期，頁259，1983。

勵綠化，“護理道德在維護病人權利中的作用”，《中華護理雜誌》，24 卷，9 期，頁 514，1989。

韓俊德、何主新、侯雙起，“居民的死亡態度初探–兼談我國臨終關懷的開展”，《中國醫學倫理學》，總 22 期，2 期，頁 50~52，1992。

韓雲彪、李宇崗，“生命倫理與民族素質的提高”，《中國醫學倫理學》，總 23 期，3 期，頁 51~52，1992。

魏桂芳，“獻給我最敬愛的人：護士”，《中華護理雜誌》，26 卷，5 期，頁 215，1991。

鄺秦桂，“全深化責任制護理按職稱上崗學校流與研討會議紀要”，《中華護理雜誌》，27 卷，12 期，頁 2，1992。

羅國傑編，《人道主義思想論庫》。北京：華夏出版社，1993。

蘇州醫學院附屬第一醫院，《建院 110 周年紀念刊》。蘇州: 蘇州醫學院，1994。

蘇蘭若、于豔秋，“以病人爲中心建設模式病房”，《中華護理雜誌》，32 卷，5 期，頁 274~275，1997。

黨桂芝，“當好責任護士的體會”，《中華護理雜誌》，21 卷，9 期，頁 407~408，1986。

顧美儀，“國際護士社節寄語”，《中華護理雜誌》，27 卷，5 期，頁 194，1992。

# APPENDICES

(Translated from the Chinese by the author)

## 1. Nurses' Registration Ordinance of the People's Republic, Ministry of Public Health, 1993

### Chapter One: General Rules

No. 1 In order to enhance the management for nurses and the quality of nursing care, to ensure the safety of medical care and nursing, warrant legal rights of nurses, these measures are set up.

No. 2 The nurses refer to those who have hold a certification and have registered as a professional nurse.

No. 3 The purpose of developing the nursing profession is to facilitate the progress of nursing sciences, foster qualified nursing staff, and let nurses play their roles in medical care, prevention, health care, and rehabilitation care.

No. 4 The law protects nurses' practice rights. Nurses' work should be respected by society.

No. 5 Medical Administrative Department in all the provinces, autonomous regions, and municipalities directly under the Central Government are responsible for the supervision and management of nurses.

### Chapter Two: Examination

No. 6 Those who apply for practice should pass standardized examination conducted by Ministry of Public Health Department, and get a certificate entitled Practice Certificate for Nurse in People's Republic of China.

No. 7 Those who have got a certificate from nursing college or above this level, as well as graduation from nursing school which is approved or confirmed by the Medical Administrative Department at the provincial level or above, may practice without examination. Those who have certificates of the senior high schools (nursing), are eligible to apply for the nursing practice examination.

No. 8 Nursing examination is held once a year.

No. 9 Specific measures for the examination are arranged separately.

No. 10 Those who meet the requirement of No. 7 and pass the examination will be issued a certificate entitled Practice Certificate for Nurse in People's Republic of China by the Medical Administrative Department in the various provinces, autonomous regions, and municipalities directly under the Central Government.

No. 11 The Ministry of Public Health is the authority to issue the certificates entitled Practice Certificate for Nurse in People's Republic of China.

## Chapter Three: Registration

No. 12 Those who have hold the certificate entitled Practice Certificate for Nurse in People's Republic of China are eligible to apply register of nursing practice.

No. 13 Administrative bodies that are responsible for nurse registration are the local Medical Administrative Department at county level.

No. 14 Nurses who are applying for the first time must fill in Nurse's Registration Form and pay the registration fee. The following certificates should be handed in to the register department:

1. Practice Certificate for Nurses in People's Republic of China;
2. Identification card;
3. Certificate of health examination; and
4. Relevant certificates stipulated by the provincial Medical Administrative Department.

No. 15 Once the registration application is accepted by the Registration Administrative Body, it should be completed and examined within 30 days. If the applicants are qualified, registration should be permitted. If unqualified, the applicants should be informed in writing.

No. 16 The period of registration is 2 years.

Registration renewal should be done again 60 days ahead of the expiry date. The certificate should be examined individually or collectively.

No. 17 The registration which is discontinued for five years or more should, according to the stipulation of the medical administration of the provincial, autonomous region and municipality, the person needs to undertake clinical practice for 3 months, and submit relevant certificates to the Registration Administrative Body. Thereafter, re-registration will be permitted.

No. 18 Registration will be denied under the following circumstances:

1. Any criminal conviction;
2. Unsuitability to be a nurse because of health condition;
3. Violation of the regulations so that the eligibility is discontinued or canceled; and
4. Others reason for not being suitable for the nursing job.

## Chapter Four: Practice

No. 19 Those who have not registered are not allowed to practice nursing. Nursing students should take part in fieldwork (clinical practice) before graduation from nursing schools or nursing colleges. They should also be under the guidance of senior nurses, in accordance to the related regulation of Ministry of Public Health.

No. 20 Assistant nurses can only perform certain nursing duties under the supervision of nurses.

No. 21 Nurses should accurately carry out the doctors' orders in practice. They should observe the physical and psychological state of patients and give proper nursing care as well. If emergency cases happen, they should inform doctors immediately and actively co-operate and participate. If doctors are absent, the possible emergency treatment should be taken immediately.

No. 22 Nurses should also play a role in prevention and health care, propaganda and patient education, necessary rehabilitation and health consultation.

No. 23 Nurses must comply with professional moral, medical and nursing rules, and skill norms.

No. 24 Nurses must keep clients' privacy. Disclosure will not be allowed except those permitted by law.

No. 25 The emergency cases such as natural disaster, epidemic infectious disease, sudden and serious accidents or others situation leading to a threat of people's health and life, nurses must obey the assignments by the Medical Administrative Department and participate in medical rescue and health prevention.

No. 26 Nurses' rights should be protected by the law. Their rights are not allowed to be infringed on by any units or any person.

**Chapter Five: Punishment**

No. 27 Those who violate No. 19 practice illegally, that is practicing nursing without registration, will be disciplined by Medical Administrative Department.

No. 28 Those who get a certificate entitled Practice Certificate for Nurse in People's Republic of China illegally will have it confiscated.

No. 29 Those who violate the regulations and skill norms of medical and nursing care will be warned and charged to make corrections, be terminated or have their certificate confiscated according to the severity of mistakes.

No. 30 Those who violate No. 26 and illegally interfere in nurses' practice or attack nurses' rights, will be informed and punished by the Security Department. If laws have been violated, and in serious cases, they will be submitted to the Judicial Organ and criminal responsibility will be investigated according to law.

No. 31 Those who violate other relevant rules will be warned, charged to make corrections, terminated or cancelled by the Health Administrative Office according to the severity of mistakes.

No. 32 For those who do not obey or agree to the decision made by the Health Administrative Office, they could ask for retrial or submit to administrative procedures according to law. If the person concerned does not comply with the administrative decision, and also does not apply for re-trial within the legal period, the health administrative organ can apply to the court for compulsory measures.

**Chapter Six: Attach Rules**

No. 33 Those who have already got nursing professional titles before the implementation of this regulation, after being examined to be qualified, will be approved and by the health administrative organs of the province, autonomous regions, and municipalities directly under the Central Government; Practice Certificate for Nurse in People's Republic of China will be conferred; and practice registration will be permitted according to the regulation.

Those who have been working as a nurse but have not obtained the nursing professional titles before the implementation of this regulation, specific regulations will be made by the local health administrative organs of the province, autonomous regions, and municipalities directly under the Central Government according to the concrete situation and the actual skill level of the person concerned.

No. 34 Those who are from abroad and apply for nursing practice in the People's Republic of China, must pass the examination according to the regulation, and hold a Practice Certificate for Nurse in People's Republic of China, so as to be eligible to apply for registration.

No. 35 Nurses applying for practice and wishing to establish a nursing service institution should be approved by the Medical Administrative Department at or above the country, and should be in compliance with the relevant regulation of the management of the medical institution.

No. 36 Ministry of Public Health is eligible to make the interpretation.

No. 37 The detailed implementation of items of this regulation will be undertaken by the provinces, autonomous regions, and municipalities directly under the Central Government.

No. 38 This regulation will be valid on 1 January 1994.

Source: 衛生部，"中華人民共和國護士管理辦法"，《全國醫院分級與疾病分類標準及醫院工作制度，職責配備規範》，柴瑞震、程延安、姜任華編。成都：成都科技大學出版社，頁 186，1995。

## 2. New Bachelor of Science in Nursing Program of Peking Union Medical College, 1996

| **Year 1, Semester 1** | **Theory / Practice Hours** |
|---|---|
| Health Care Delivery | 36 |
| Normal Human Biology | 108 |
| Growth and Development | 54 |
| Cultural Anthropology and Philosophy | 54 |
| Psychology | 54 |
| Informatics & Politics | 36 |
| English | 36 |
| Physical Education | 90 |
| *Total* | 468 |

| **Year 1, Semester 2** | |
|---|---|
| Foundation of Nursing | 36/72 |
| Abnormal Human Biology | 90 |
| Nutrition | 54 |
| Communication | 54 |
| Inquiry and Logical Reasoning | 36 |
| Politics | 36 |
| English | 90 |
| Physical Education | 36 |
| *Total* | 432/72 |

| **Year 2, Semester 1** | |
|---|---|
| Human Pathophysiology | 108 |
| Epidemiology | 54 |
| Health Assessment | 36/72 |
| Data Management (Statistics) | 36 |
| Nursing Therapeutics Related to Social Interaction | 36/108 |
| Politics | 36 |
| English | 72 |
| Physical Education | 36 |
| *Total* | 414/180 |

| **Year 2, Semester 2** | **Theory / Practice Hours** |
|---|---|
| Pharmacology & Therapeutics | 72 |
| Traditional Chinese Medicine | 54 |
| Bioethics and Professional Regulation | 36 |
| Nursing Therapeutics Related to Reproduction | 72/216 |
| Politics | 36 |

| | |
|---|---|
| English | 72 |
| Physical Education | 36 |
| *Total* | 378/216 |
| | |
| **Year 3, Semester 1** | |
| Nursing Therapeutics Related to Nutrition-Elimination | 72/144 |
| Nursing Therapeutics Related to Oxygenation | 72/144 |
| Politics | 36 |
| *Total* | 180/288 |
| | |
| **Year 3, Semester 2** | |
| Nursing Therapeutics Related to Nutrition-Activity-Rest | 54/108 |
| Nursing Therapeutics Related to Cognition-Perception | 72/144 |
| Problem Solving Skills and Strategies (Research) | 36 |
| Politics | 36 |
| *Total* | 198/252 |
| | |
| **Year 4, Semester 1** | |
| Nursing Management and Leadership | 54 |
| Nursing Education | 54 |
| Teaching Practicum | /36 |
| Clinical Nursing Projects I (Nursing Research Project) | 36 |
| Community Health | 90/180 |
| *Total* | 270/216 |
| | |
| **Year 4, Semester 2** | **Theory / Practice Hours** |
| Professional Development | 36 |
| Clinical Nursing Projects II (Nursing Research Project) | 36/36 |
| Comprehensive Clinical Practice | /480 |
| Elective | 36 |
| Politics | 36 |
| *Total* | 108/516 |
| **Grand Total** | |
| Theory hours | 2448 |
| Practical hours | 1740 |

## 3. Duties of Hospital Personnel, Ministry of Public Health, 1982

### Duties of the Secretary of the Party Committee (General Branch, Branch) at Hospital Level

1. Under the leadership of the superior and Hospital Party Committee, constantly monitor and inspect the implementation of the Party's guidelines, and policies and the resolutions of the Hospital Party Committee.
2. Lead and establish the plan of: organization, propaganda, united front, discipline, and political work; perform its implementation, and make regular checks and summaries.
3. Study hard both in political and professional work, and set an example to promote the Party's excellent tradition and style.
4. Conduct investigations and study in depth, understand the overall ideological status of the hospital staff, and aim at particular targets in efforts to do political work.
5. Promote the optimal role all the Party Committee members and hospital directors, actively assist and support their work.

The deputy secretary of the Party Committee is responsible for the relevant work.

### Duties of the Secretary of the Party Committee (Branch) at Department Level

1. Organize the study of political theory and current policy.
2. Understand Party Members' thoughts, work, and progress of study. Manage and educate the party members, make full use of the Party members as examples to others.
3. Establish working plans, check on resolutions carried out and make timely reports to the superior administrative leaders and the meetings of the branch.
4. Combine professional work with political work to ensure the fulfillment of treatment, prevention, and scientific research.
5. Keep in frequent contact with the chief of the department, actively communicate, cooperate and support each other, so as to make the best contribution.

The vice-secretary assists the secretary in doing the above-mentioned work.

### Duties of the Hospital Director

1. Under the leadership of the upper level and the hospital Party Committee, according to the general and specific policies of the Party, leads the overall work of the hospital, including treatment, teaching, scientific

research, and prevention, as well as personnel, financial, and maintenance and supply service etc.

2. Leads the establishment of the overall plan of the hospital, makes regular arrangements, checks on, summaries, and reports to the leading body.

3. Be responsible for the organization, quality of medical and nursing care, and makes a regular check on in-patient and out-patient departments, and adopt a series of positive and effective measures in order to constantly insure and increase the quality of medical care.

4. Be responsible for the organization and review of the clinical teaching, personnel training, and professional learning.

5. Be responsible for guiding and inspecting the overall planning and implementation of scientific research, and the adoption of measures to facilitate the progress of the research work.

6. Be responsible for organizing and inspecting the grade division of medical work, and district medical work.

7. Educates staff to establish a moral attitude of serving people whole-heartedly, improve the attitude towards style of medical care, work, and service. Supervise and promote the rules concerning job responsibility and technical operation, and strictly prevent any mistakes and errors.

8. According to the state personnel system, organize and lead the appointment and removal, reward, transfer, promotion of the hospital staff, etc.

9. Enhance the management of maintenance and supply services, examine the plan for stocking material supply, supervise and promote financial expenditure, audit the budgets, and monitor staff's living condition.

10. Regularly scrutinizes the opinions concerning medical care of the masses.

11. In the event of absence or while away on official business, a vice-director should be appointed to take over his job.

**Duties of the Director of the Medical Department**

1. Under the leadership of the hospital director, specifically organizes and implements medical care, teaching, scientific research, and prevention.

2. Drafts the relevant professional plans, after approval by the hospital director and vice director, arranges the implementation, frequently supervises and makes inspection, and makes regular summaries and makes reports.

3. Gets feedback from various departments so as to understand and grasp current affairs in the hospital. Organizes rescuing work in case of disaster and group consultation. Supervises and promotes regulations and routines. Regularly investigates and adopts measures to increase the quality of medical care and strictly prevent mistakes and accidents.

4. Inspects medical mistakes and accidents, organize discussion, and regularly reports to the hospital director and passes on viewpoints and suggestion regarding settlement of problems.

5. Be responsible for implementing and examining the professional training and technical testing. Enhances the level of technical skills and assists the personnel department to do well in promotions, rewards and punishments, and the adjustment of work.

6. Be responsible for implementing temporary treatment outside the hospital and technical guidance for the basic units.

7. Supervises and promotes different departments in service-training, teaching and scientific research planning, coordinate inter-departmental relations, improves the quality of care in in-patient and out-patient departments.

8. Supervises and promotes the supply and management of drugs and medical equipment.

9. Organizes the political learning for staff working in department of medical affairs, and properly manage files and the library department.

Vice director assists the director in doing the related work.

## Duties of the Nurse (According to Professional Titles)

### A. Chief Nurse Working at Hospital Administration Level

1. Under the guidance of the hospital director, designs the overall planning of nursing, implementing after hospital director's and vice director's approval. Checks the quality of nursing care, regularly summarize and report.

2. Be responsible for designing and formulating nursing operation regulations and accurately supervising their implementation. Examines and guides basic nursing and implements the management of the grading nursing regulations.

3. Makes the rounds of the wards regularly and provide technical guidance for the care of patients.

4. Be responsible for designing in-service training planning and implementation. Provides technical training for nursing staff and holds regular examinations.

5. Grasps the overall status of nurses' working, thinking, and learning. Be responsible for arranging and adjusting the work of the nursing staff. And gives opinions concerning promotions, rewards and punishments to the hospital director. When there are mistakes and errors, discusses and makes decision with the relevant department.

6. Scrutinizes the implementation plan and use for the related nursing materials.

7. Makes requisition from supply department to ensure adequate material for daily use.

8. Examines and guides the management of the outpatient department, emergency room, wards, operation room and supply room so as to gradually be regular, conventional and standardized.

9. Those having the task of teaching will be responsible for nursing teaching and planning clinical practice.

10. Holds regular meetings and analyzes nursing work with head nurses. And coordinates head nurses to supervise, learn and communicate with each other so as to promote the quality of nursing care.

11. Facilitates the progress of nursing scientific research and new technology.

The vice-chief nurse of the nursing department assists in the chief nurse's work.

B. Chief Nurse Working at Department Level

1. Under the guidance of the chief nurse of the department of nursing, organize nursing technical (training) skills, scientific research and teaching.

2. Formulate nursing plans for acute, severe, difficult and complicated patients, nursing consultation and the nursing for critically and seriously ill patients.

3. Realize the development of nursing at home and abroad. According to the need and specific conditions of the hospital, introduce advanced technology, promote the quality of nursing care and develop nursing science.

4. Lead the general nursing rounds, guide the round for the nursing director, constantly enhance the level of nursing skills.

5. Give technical appraisal for nursing mistakes and accidents.

6. Organize in-service training, formulate teaching plans, edit teaching materials, and be responsible for teaching the nurses under his or her supervision.

7. Conduct a clinical practice for nursing students, participate in lectures, and encourage nurses to strive for excellence.

8. Assist the nursing department in nurses' promotions and professional skill assessment, and be responsible for the cultivation of senior nursing staff.

9. Formulate nursing scientific research, innovation plan, and implementation. Be involved in examinations, evaluate nursing's works and the outcome of research and innovation.

10. Be responsible for academic seminars and nursing conference.

11. Give opinions for the nursing recruitment, management of professional skills and administration. And assist the nursing department to enhance the administration of nursing work.

The vice-chief nurse assists in the above mentioned tasks.

C. Chief Nurse Working at Ward Level

1. Work under the guidance of hospital chief curse and departmental chief nurse.
2. Be responsible for supervising and promoting the quality of nursing care, identify problems and their resolutions to ensure the quality of nursing.
3. Handle difficult and complicated issues in nursing, supervise critical and complicated case, and implement nursing care plans.
4. Be responsible for morning rounds and nursing consultation, and give specific guidance.
5. Analyze and evaluate nursing mistakes and accidents, and take measures to prevent further mistakes.
6. Organize senior nurses and nurses in-service training, formulate training plans, edit materials, and give lectures.
7. Organize fieldwork for nursing students, and give lectures and evaluations.
8. Formulate scientific research and implement innovations.
9. Promote scientific research work within the unit.
10. Assist the nursing director in managing and in building morale.

D. Senior Nurse

1. Work under the guidance of chief nurse.
2. Participate in nursing clinical practice, and help nurses carry out doctors' orders accurately and carry out various technical operations. Identify and resolve problems.
3. Participate in nursing work including critical, difficult and complicated cases, as well as other nursing duties. Lead the nurses in acquiring new skills and new technical clinical practices.
4. Assist head nurse to formulate nursing plans and participate in the management of nursing work in the ward.
5. Participate in making the rounds of the wards, consultation and case discussion with the chief nurse and nurse in charge. Lead the nursing round in his or her ward.
6. Assist the head nurse to conduct in-service training, formulate study plans, edit materials and give lectures for nurses in the ward. And make technical examination of them.
7. Participate in nursing clinical teaching and clinical practice.
8. Assist the Head Nurse to formulate the scientific research, technical innovation and implementation.
9. Analyze and evaluate nursing mistakes and accidents, and take measures to prevent further mistakes.

## Duties of the Nurse by Job Title

### A. Departmental Head Nurse

1. Work under the guidance of the nursing director, according to the quality standards and plans required by the nursing department of the hospital, and in light of the practical situation in the ward.
2. Participate in morning rounds, check the care given to severely ill patients, and give specific directions. Take personal charge of tasks requiring complicated technical or professional skills.
3. Educate nursing staff in the ward to strengthen their sense of responsibility, and improve attitude toward service. Carry out doctors' orders carefully, follow regulations and technical operational rules, and prevent mistakes and accidents.
4. Make rounds with the doctor in charge in order to understand existing problems of nursing and strengthen contact between nurses and doctors.
5. Organize the study of technical nursing skills in the ward, and pay attention to fostering quality of nursing.
6. Formulate scientific study and supervise and promote its implementation. And regularly report the nursing situation.
7. Monitor the patient's general conditions, thinking and living. Supervise and regularly evaluate nursing work in various wards. And produce some improved measures and ideas.
8. Be responsible for clinical teaching and clinical assessment in the wards.
9. Allocate duty roaster of nursing staff and other job assignments.

The vice head nurse assists the head nurse in related work.

### B. Duties of the Head Nurse of the Ward

1. Work under the guidance of the departmental head nurse and nursing director, according to the nursing department and his or her own department planning, formulate and implement specific schemes.
2. Be responsible for checking nursing work in the ward. Participate in nursing severely ill patients and patients required major operations, and patients in critical conditions. And promote carrying out doctors' orders carefully, follow regulations and technical operational rules, as well as prevent any mistakes and accidents.
3. Strengthen contact between nurses and doctors.
4. Make rounds with the doctor in charge. Participate in consultations, operations and discussions for difficult, complicated cases and terminal case as well.

5. Be responsible for political work of nurses, educate them to strengthen their sense of responsibility, improve service attitudes toward service and observe discipline.

6. Organize the rounds and nursing consultation. Positively promote the progress of new skills, technology and scientific research work.

7. Organize in-service professional training and skill learning for nursing staff.

8. Be responsible for the management of the ward, including reasonable division of labor among nursing staff; management of environment: such as tidiness, noise level, security, patient and accompanying person, and administration of patient visits, as well as management of apparatus, equipment and drugs.

9. Be responsible for guidance and management of fieldwork and advanced training. And appoint senior nurses, experienced nurses, and other capable nurses to give lectures.

10. Supervise assistant nurses to do cleaning, sterilization, and isolation work.

11. Regularly hold meetings to receive opinions about medical care, nursing and diet etc. and focus on improvement of this work.

The vice head nurse assists the head nurse.

## C. Ward Nurse

1. Work under the guidance of the head nurse and senior nurses.
2. Carefully implement various nursing systems and technical operation regulation, accurately carry out doctors' orders and complete nursing work in a timely manner. And strictly carry out nursing work with accuracy. Prevent mistakes and accidents.
3. Take care of patients both physically and psychologically. Frequently check rounds and keep a close observation of the change of patients condition. Report any abnormal conditions to a doctor.
4. Be watchful to the safety of severely ill patients.
5. Assist doctors in keeping the therapeutic work in order. Be responsible for collecting specimens.
6. Participate in teaching and scientific research and help student nurses, assistant nurses and nurse's helpers, and cleaner's work.
7. Regularly conduct patient education, provide information on hygienic measures and hospital regulations. Often communicate and ask for patients' opinion in improving nursing work. Perform health education on patients before discharge.
8. Admit, discharge, transfer and register patients.
9. Under the guidance of the head nurse, manage the environment of the ward, sterilization and isolation and storage of drugs.

D. Assistant Nurse

1. Work under the guidance of head nurse and nurse.

2. Be responsible for patients' daily living care and other basic nursing duties.

3. Frequently check wards, be responsive to the patients needs, assist patients who are unable to care for themselves, including ambulation, elimination and feeding.

4. Prepare bed-sheets for patient admission and discharge, tidy mattress and final sterilization. Assist nurses to make bed and manage furniture.

5. Collect and send urgent specimens to laboratory and transfer patient in a timely

Source: 衛生部，"醫院工作人員職責 1982"，《全國醫院分級與疾病分類標準及醫院工作制度，職責配備規範》，柴瑞震、程延安、姜任華編。成都：成都科技大學出版社，頁 115~117，119~122，1995。

## 4. Patients' Rights and Responsibilities, Hangzhou Hospital, 1994

### I. Patients' Rights

1. The object of hospital service is for patients. Every person should receive fair medical service.

2. Patients have the right to receive medical services that safeguard individual dignity under all circumstances.

3. Within the boundary of law, patients have the right to ask for keeping their personal information and medical history secret.

4. Patients have the right to have their safety safeguarded in both medical care and hospital environment.

5. Patients have the right to obtain all information about their own disease, treatment, prognosis, and follow-up care upon discharge. If it is unsuitable to tell the patient the truth directly, it should be provided to his or her family member. The patient has the right to know who will be responsible for his or her medical treatment.

6. Hospital should provide 'Instructions to Patients' and make sure that patients know about it.

### II. Patients' Responsibilities

1. Provide accurate medical information.

2. Comply with physicians' therapeutic regimen, listen to medical and nursing orders.

3. Pay the hospital fee on time.

4. Respect hospital rules and regulations.

5. Assist in controlling hospital noises, limit the number of visitors, not to smoke in the ward, and protect hospital property.

6. If the patient refuses treatment or does not follow physician's prescription, he or she has to be responsible for any consequence that may arise.

Source: 杭州醫院，“病人的權利和義務”。杭州：杭州醫院，1994。

## 5. Standard Requirements for Quality Nursing, Medical Department, The Third Teaching Hospital, Beijing Medical University

In order to improve the quality of nursing work for its realization in patient care, the following are the requirements specified for regular evaluation of the nurse's qualities.

| I. The Nurse's Qualities | | |
|---|---|---|
| 1. | No talking or reading magazines is allowed during work hours | Deduct 2 points |
| 2. | A nurse, who is off duty, is not allowed to stay in the ward | Deduct 2 points |
| 3. | No one is allowed to leave one's post without permission | Deduct 5 points |
| 4. | Dressing and make up: Hair should not fall over the shoulder and no accessory is allowed. Shoes must keep clean and socks should be worn.<br>Trousers should be white in color, wear a dress in summer | Deduct I point for each item |
| 5. | Good attitude and should not speak foul language | Deduct 5 points |
| 6. | Late at work (except in snowy weather) | Deduct 2 points if late within 5 minutes, more points will be deducted for more time. |
| **II. Therapeutics and Nursing Procedures** | | |
| 1. | Tidy up all things after use (check after 11am in AM duty) | Failure to comply: Deduct 2 points |
| 2. | All procedures should be performed according to the hospital's instruction (include the use of betadine and alcohol) | Deduct 5 points |
| 3. | Should not handle drugs with bare hands | Deduct 1 point |
| 4. | Put on a mask in performing all treatments, check the expire date of the product before use | Deduct 1 point |
| 5. | Medication should be administered at 8am, 12 noon and 5:30pm | Deduct 1 point |
| **III. Basic Nursing Care** | | |
| 1. | Nurses should perform perineum swabbing and mouth wash for patients who require Grade I nursing care. Care should not be done by patients' family members | Deduct 2 points for each item |
| 2. | Patients' nails or feet are dirty | Deduct 1 point |

| | |
|---|---|
| 3. Bed sheets | Deduct 1 point |
| 4. Discharge management | Deduct 1 point |
| 5. Orientation to new admission | Deduct 2 points |
| 6. Families do not know when they are allowed to bring food to the patient | Deduct 2 points |
| 7. Time of food delivery to patients (7-8am; 11am-12 noon; 5-6:30pm) | Deduct 1 point if late |
| 8. The time schedule for recording food and fluid intake and output balance is 8am, 11:30am, 5:30pm, and 9:30pm<br>The night nurse is responsible for totaling 24 hours intake and output, and recording the readings in patients' records. | Deduct 1 point if not accurately recorded |
| 9. Relatives are allowed to stay from 8am to 9pm<br>1 patients' ward: 2 relatives<br>2 patients' ward: 1 relative<br>Intensive care : no visitors allowed | If the number is exceeded, deduct 1 point for each head count |
| **IV. Documentation** | |
| 1. Medical order should be checked for accuracy and clarity | Deduct 1 point |
| 2. Nurses' hand-over report should be written clearly and accurately | Deduct 2 points |
| 3. Not to copy from the physician's medical records when writing care plan for individual patients<br>4. Special nursing record should include observation records and summary of patients' condition | Deduct 2 points for each item |
| **V. Emergency Trolley** | |
| 1. Check medication items | Deduct 1 point |
| 2. Check expiry dates of all items | Deduct 1 point |
| 3. All items are present | Deduct 1 point |
| **VI. Miscellaneous** | |
| If the nurse does not work according to the regulations of the hospital, points will be deducted. The nurse should not take anything that belongs to the hospital for private use. Should try hard to avoid any mistake. The head nurse is responsible to keep the record for the ward nurses. The head nurse is required to make a report weekly to his or her senior. | |

Source: 北京醫科大學第三醫院，內科部“護理工作的具體要求”。北京：北京醫科大學第三醫院，1995。

## 6. Regulations for Ward Management, Hospital Personnel, and Hospital Patients, Ministry of Public Health, 1986

### Regulations for Ward Management

1. With the assistance of departmental head nurse and doctors in charge, the charge nurse should be responsible for ward management.

2. The charge nurse is totally responsible for the management of property and equipment; and will assign a special person to be in charge of the management, and establishment of the accounting books, and regularly check the items of the accounting books. If there is something lost, the cause will be found out in a timely manner and be properly treated. When the assigned person will be transferred, all the turnover formalities should be well performed.

3. Patients who need quilt and articles for daily use should be provided by the ward, and they should be returned before discharge.

4. Ward furniture should be unified. All articles and beds are kept in order and in fixed place, and they should not be moved without the permission of the charge nurse.

5. Keep the ward clean, comfortable, quiet, and safe. Noise should be avoided. Remain quiet in walking, closing doors, performing procedures and talking.

6. Ward cleansing should be done at least twice a day. A complete cleansing should be done once a week. Pay attention to ventilation. Smoking is forbidden in the ward and supervision measures should be taken.

7. Frequently conduct patient education about the knowledge of treatment and prevention of diseases. Organize those who are able to learn Tai-ji and Qi-gong.

8. Wear gown, cap and keep them tidy. Put on mask if necessary. Keep record of quality of medical care, nursing care, good examples, mistakes and errors.

9. Non hospitalized patients are not allowed to stay in the ward, nor are guests. While doctors are making rounds, nurses, generally, should not answer the call, and patients should remain in the ward.

10. Properly arrange the ward schedule. Any chaos and noise should be avoided. Avoid activity before six in the morning, in the mid-noon and after nine in the evening. Some treatment will be arranged after the patient is awake, on the condition that the therapeutic effect is not influenced.

11. Explain procedures and comfort patients before operations in order to relieve their fear and worry, and to ensure their co-operation.

12. According to the kind of condition they are suffering from, different daily activities are established. Combine movement with quietness so as to lead to a peaceful and regular life.

13. Pay attention to the patients' emotions. They may affect treatment, living, diet and nursing. So try to help as much as possible. According to the circumstance, select a leader in a group of patients to help them solve the problems in their mind, in daily life and health care. Hold patient group activities once a month in order to enhance communication and constantly improve the work.

**Regulations for Hospital Personnel**

1. Establish better medical morality. Introduce hospital rules in detail before admission. Understand what patients dislike. Encourage them to have confidence and overcome their illness.

2. Attitude toward patients should be cordial, speak warmly, and avoid upsetting them. For those who have unreasonable requests, they should be advised patiently but hold firm on principles.

3. If a patient's condition is getting worse or disorder occurs after operation, you should not tell the patient, if necessary, let the senior doctor or the doctor in charge of the patient give an explanation.

4. Do not discuss any mistakes or errors of any other hospital or any other individual in front of patients in order to avoid any harmful consequence.

5. Be patient and careful when administering treatments and examinations so as to reduce patients' discomfort.

6. Widely adopt the traditional Chinese therapy. When using western medicine, obtain the permission of the doctor in charge (except critical and serious patients). All nursing procedures, such as changing dressings,

stomach washing, and catheterization, should be conducted in therapy room or behind a screen.

7. You must remain at your post. No one is allowed to leave one's post without permission. No recreational activity is allowed in working hours, such as playing cards and chess, sleeping in the ward, or eating food of patients. Moreover, prescription in patients' name but for private use is forbidden. Relatives of working staff will not be allowed to enter into patients' areas.

**Regulations for Hospital Patients**

1. Obey the orders of medical staff. Cooperate closely with doctors and nurses. Adhere to doctors' orders and treatment. Keep quiet and calm in the hospital.

2. Observe the daily schedule in the hospital. Keep the wards tidy, clean, and quiet. No spitting, smoking or making noise.

3. Patient's diet should be guided by the doctor and is not allowed to be modified without doctor's permission. Food that is brought by the family members can be taken, only under the permission of doctors and nurses.

4. Without the permission of the doctor in charge, consultation from an outside hospital is not allowed; self-provided medication and alike is also forbidden; and it is not allowed to ask for unessential treatment and medication.

5. Without permission, nobody is allowed to enter the therapy room; and no unauthorized person is allowed to read medical records and other relevant documents.

6. It is not allowed to go or live outside at will. If there is any special reason, it should be approved by the doctor.

7. Protect hospital property. If damaged occurs, it should be compensated for according to the cost.

8. For pediatric patients, damage to hospital property will be handled according to the situation.

9. Other than necessary articles for daily use, other things are not allowed to be brought in; valuable articles should be properly stored so as to prevent loss.

10. In order to prevent cross-infection, it is not allowed for patients to change wards or beds at will. It is not allowed to meet friends or others in non-visiting hours.

11. Patients are free to express their ideas so as to help improve the quality of hospital work.

12. It is strictly forbidden to bring any harmful articles, such as electric mattress, kerosene stove, and alcohol strove, etc.

13. If patients violate the ward regulations, necessary advice should be given. For those whose cases are serious, they should be discharged. If necessary, their work unit will be informed, or the relevant department will be requested to handle the case.

Source: 衛生部，"病房管理制度，1985"，《全國醫院分級與疾病分類標準及醫院工作制度，職責配備規範》。柴瑞震、程延安、姜任華編。成都：成都科技大學出版社，頁141~142，1995。

# ABOUT THE AUTHOR

Samantha Mei-che Pang is a nurse by professional training, and a researcher in the field of healthcare and nursing ethics by scholarly endeavor. She obtained her general nurse registration in Hong Kong in 1977 and a Certificate in Nursing Behavioral Science from The University of Hong Kong in 1985. She then received a Post-Registration Diploma in Nursing from The Hong Kong Polytechnic in 1986 and a Master's of Science in Nursing Education from The University of Edinburgh in 1990. Her nursing practice was primarily concerned with caring for children and older adults with chronic illnesses. She received a Bachelor's in Philosophy from Pontifical Urbanian University in 1983 and a Doctor of Philosophy in Philosophy from The University of Hong Kong in 1999. In 2002, she was named one of the first recipients of the Fulbright Hong Kong Scholar Program awards to study cross-cultural differences in making end-of-life decisions at Boston College.

Pang started her career as a nurse academic in 1990, when she took up a teaching post at The Hong Kong Polytechnic University where she now serves as an Associate Professor in the School of Nursing. Over the past ten years, she has taught, lectured, and published in the areas of nursing ethics, caring practices, and ethics in end-of-life care. Her passion for China and Chinese nurses is well reflected in her continuous engagement in scholarly activities with nurses in different parts of China. The projects she has undertaken in collaboration with her counterparts on the Chinese mainland include the development of a code of ethical principles for Chinese nurses using the Delphi Technique, the cultural construction of caring in nurse learners, and a phenomenological study of the Chinese concept of nursing. With funding support from the University Research Grants Council of Hong Kong, she is now embarking on a journey in the field of ethical decision making in end-of-life care. She is also actively involved in nursing ethics endeavors internationally. As a member of the International Centre for Nursing Ethics at the University of Surrey, she has participated in the study of ethical considerations in international nursing research, and an international study on the value of nursing.

# INDEX

**VIBS**

The **Value Inquiry Book Series** is co-sponsored by:

Adler School of Professional Psychology
American Indian Philosophy Association
American Maritain Association
American Society for Value Inquiry
Association for Process Philosophy of Education
Canadian Society for Philosophical Practice
Center for Bioethics, University of Turku
Center for Professional and Applied Ethics, University of North Carolina at Charlotte
Center for Research in Cognitive Science, Autonomous University of Barcelona
Centre for Applied Ethics, Hong Kong Baptist University
Centre for Cultural Research, Aarhus University
Centre for Professional Ethics, University of Central Lancashire
Centre for the Study of Philosophy and Religion, University College of Cape Breton
College of Education and Allied Professions, Bowling Green State University
College of Liberal Arts, Rochester Institute of Technology
Concerned Philosophers for Peace
Conference of Philosophical Societies
Department of Moral and Social Philosophy, University of Helsinki
Gannon University
Gilson Society
Ikeda University
Institute of Philosophy of the High Council of Scientific Research, Spain
International Academy of Philosophy of the Principality of Liechtenstein
International Association of Bioethics
International Center for the Arts, Humanities, and Value Inquiry

International Society for Universal Dialogue
Natural Law Society
Personalist Discussion Group
Philosophical Society of Finland
Philosophy Born of Struggle Association
Philosophy Seminar, University of Mainz
Pragmatism Archive
R.S. Hartman Institute for Formal and Applied Axiology
Research Institute, Lakeridge Health Corporation
Russian Philosophical Society
Society for Iberian and Latin-American Thought
Society for the Philosophic Study of Genocide and the Holocaust
Society for the Philosophy of Sex and Love
Yves R. Simon Institute

Titles Published

1. Noel Balzer, *The Human Being as a Logical Thinker*

2. Archie J. Bahm, *Axiology: The Science of Values*

3. H. P. P. (Hennie) Lötter, *Justice for an Unjust Society*

4. H. G. Callaway, *Context for Meaning and Analysis: A Critical Study in the Philosophy of Language*

5. Benjamin S. Llamzon, *A Humane Case for Moral Intuition*

6. James R. Watson, *Between Auschwitz and Tradition: Postmodern Reflections on the Task of Thinking*. A volume in **Holocaust and Genocide Studies**

7. Robert S. Hartman, *Freedom to Live: The Robert Hartman Story*, edited by Arthur R. Ellis. A volume in **Hartman Institute Axiology Studies**

8. Archie J. Bahm, *Ethics: The Science of Oughtness*

9. George David Miller, *An Idiosyncratic Ethics; Or, the Lauramachean Ethics*

10. Joseph P. DeMarco, *A Coherence Theory in Ethics*

11. Frank G. Forrest, *Valuemetrics*$^{\aleph}$: *The Science of Personal and Professional Ethics.* A volume in **Hartman Institute Axiology Studies**

12. William Gerber, *The Meaning of Life: Insights of the World's Great* Thinkers

13. Richard T. Hull, Editor, *A Quarter Century of Value Inquiry: Presidential Addresses of the American Society for Value Inquiry.* A volume in **Histories and Addresses of Philosophical Societies**

14. William Gerber, *Nuggets of Wisdom from Great Jewish Thinkers: From Biblical Times to the Present*

15. Sidney Axinn, *The Logic of Hope: Extensions of Kant's View of Religion*

16. Messay Kebede, *Meaning and Development*

17. Amihud Gilead, *The Platonic Odyssey: A Philosophical-Literary Inquiry into the Phaedo*

18. Necip Fikri Alican, *Mill's Principle of Utility: A Defense of John Stuart Mill's Notorious Proof.* A volume in **Universal Justice**

19. Michael H. Mitias, Editor, *Philosophy and Architecture.*

20. Roger T. Simonds, *Rational Individualism: The Perennial Philosophy of Legal Interpretation.* A volume in **Natural Law Studies**

21. William Pencak, *The Conflict of Law and Justice in the Icelandic Sagas*

22. Samuel M. Natale and Brian M. Rothschild, Editors, *Values, Work, Education: The Meanings of Work*

23. N. Georgopoulos and Michael Heim, Editors, *Being Human in the Ultimate: Studies in the Thought of John M. Anderson*

24. Robert Wesson and Patricia A. Williams, Editors, *Evolution and Human Values*

25. Wim J. van der Steen, *Facts, Values, and Methodology: A New Approach to Ethics*

26. Avi Sagi and Daniel Statman, *Religion and Morality*

27. Albert William Levi, *The High Road of Humanity: The Seven Ethical Ages of Western Man*, edited by Donald Phillip Verene and Molly Black Verene

28. Samuel M. Natale and Brian M. Rothschild, Editors, *Work Values: Education, Organization, and Religious Concerns*

29. Laurence F. Bove and Laura Duhan Kaplan, Editors, *From the Eye of the Storm: Regional Conflicts and the Philosophy of Peace*. A volume in **Philosophy of Peace**

30. Robin Attfield, *Value, Obligation, and Meta-Ethics*

31. William Gerber, *The Deepest Questions You Can Ask About God: As Answered by the World's Great Thinkers*

32. Daniel Statman, *Moral Dilemmas*

33. Rem B. Edwards, Editor, *Formal Axiology and Its Critics*. A volume in **Hartman Institute Axiology Studies**

34. George David Miller and Conrad P. Pritscher, *On Education and Values: In Praise of Pariahs and Nomads*. A volume in **Philosophy of Education**

35. Paul S. Penner, *Altruistic Behavior: An Inquiry into Motivation*

36. Corbin Fowler, *Morality for Moderns*

37. Giambattista Vico, *The Art of Rhetoric* (*Institutiones Oratoriae*, 1711–1741), from the definitive Latin text and notes, Italian commentary and introduction by Giuliano Crifò. Translated and edited by Giorgio A. Pinton and Arthur W. Shippee. A volume in **Values in Italian Philosophy**

38. W. H. Werkmeister, *Martin Heidegger on the Way*, edited by Richard T. Hull. A volume in **Werkmeister Studies**

39. Phillip Stambovsky, *Myth and the Limits of Reason*

40. Samantha Brennan, Tracy Isaacs, and Michael Milde, Editors, *A Question of Values: New Canadian Perspectives in Ethics and Political Philosophy*

41. Peter A. Redpath, *Cartesian Nightmare: An Introduction to Transcendental Sophistry*. A volume in **Studies in the History of Western Philosophy**

42. Clark Butler, *History as the Story of Freedom: Philosophy in Intercultural Context*, with responses by sixteen scholars

43. Dennis Rohatyn, *Philosophy History Sophistry*

44. Leon Shaskolsky Sheleff, *Social Cohesion and Legal Coercion: A Critique of Weber, Durkheim, and Marx*. Afterword by Virginia Black

45. Alan Soble, Editor, *Sex, Love, and Friendship: Studies of the Society for the Philosophy of Sex and Love, 1977–1992*. A volume in **Histories and Addresses of Philosophical Societies**

46. Peter A. Redpath, *Wisdom's Odyssey: From Philosophy to Transcendental Sophistry*. A volume in **Studies in the History of Western Philosophy**

47. Albert A. Anderson, *Universal Justice: A Dialectical Approach*. A volume in **Universal Justice**

48. Pio Colonnello, *The Philosophy of José Gaos*. Translated from Italian by Peter Cocozzella. Edited by Myra Moss. Introduction by Giovanni Gullace. A volume in **Values in Italian Philosophy**

49. Laura Duhan Kaplan and Laurence F. Bove, Editors, *Philosophical Perspectives on Power and Domination: Theories and Practices*. A volume in **Philosophy of Peace**

50. Gregory F. Mellema, *Collective Responsibility*

51. Josef Seifert, *What Is Life? The Originality, Irreducibility, and Value of Life*. A volume in **Central-European Value Studies**

52. William Gerber, *Anatomy of What We Value Most*

53. Armando Molina, *Our Ways: Values and Character*, edited by Rem B. Edwards. A volume in **Hartman Institute Axiology Studies**

54. Kathleen J. Wininger, *Nietzsche's Reclamation of Philosophy*. A volume in **Central-European Value Studies**

55. Thomas Magnell, Editor, *Explorations of Value*

56. HPP (Hennie) Lötter, *Injustice, Violence, and Peace: The Case of South Africa*. A volume in **Philosophy of Peace**

57. Lennart Nordenfelt, *Talking About Health: A Philosophical Dialogue*. A volume in **Nordic Value Studies**

58. Jon Mills and Janusz A. Polanowski, *The Ontology of Prejudice*. A volume in **Philosophy and Psychology**

59. Leena Vilkka, *The Intrinsic Value of Nature*

60. Palmer Talbutt, Jr., Rough Dialectics: *Sorokin's Philosophy of Value*, with contributions by Lawrence T. Nichols and Pitirim A. Sorokin

61. C. L. Sheng, *A Utilitarian General Theory of Value*

62. George David Miller, *Negotiating Toward Truth: The Extinction of Teachers and Students*. Epilogue by Mark Roelof Eleveld. A volume in **Philosophy of Education**

63. William Gerber, *Love, Poetry, and Immortality: Luminous Insights of the World's Great Thinkers*

64. Dane R. Gordon, Editor, *Philosophy in Post-Communist Europe*. A volume in **Post-Communist European Thought**

65. Dane R. Gordon and Józef Niznik, Editors, *Criticism and Defense of Rationality in Contemporary Philosophy*. A volume in **Post-Communist European Thought**

66. John R. Shook, *Pragmatism: An Annotated Bibliography, 1898–1940*. With contributions by E. Paul Colella, Lesley Friedman, Frank X. Ryan, and Ignas K. Skrupskelis

67. Lansana Keita, *The Human Project and the Temptations of Science*

68. Michael M. Kazanjian, *Phenomenology and Education: Cosmology, Co-Being, and Core Curriculum*. A volume in **Philosophy of Education**

69. James W. Vice, *The Reopening of the American Mind: On Skepticism and Constitutionalism*

70. Sarah Bishop Merrill, *Defining Personhood: Toward the Ethics of Quality in Clinical Care*

71. Dane R. Gordon, *Philosophy and Vision*

72. Alan Milchman and Alan Rosenberg, Editors, *Postmodernism and the Holocaust*. A volume in **Holocaust and Genocide Studies**

73. Peter A. Redpath, *Masquerade of the Dream Walkers: Prophetic Theology from the Cartesians to Hegel*. A volume in **Studies in the History of Western Philosophy**

74. Malcolm D. Evans, *Whitehead and Philosophy of Education: The Seamless Coat of Learning*. A volume in **Philosophy of Education**

75. Warren E. Steinkraus, *Taking Religious Claims Seriously: A Philosophy of Religion*, edited by Michael H. Mitias. A volume in **Universal Justice**

76. Thomas Magnell, Editor, *Values and Education*

77. Kenneth A. Bryson, *Persons and Immortality*. A volume in **Natural Law Studies**

78. Steven V. Hicks, *International Law and the Possibility of a Just World Order: An Essay on Hegel's Universalism*. A volume in **Universal Justice**

79. E. F. Kaelin, *Texts on Texts and Textuality: A Phenomenology of Literary Art*, edited by Ellen J. Burns

80. Amihud Gilead, Saving Possibilities: A Study in Philosophical Psychology. *A volume in Philosophy and Psychology*

81. André Mineau, *The Making of the Holocaust: Ideology and Ethics in the Systems Perspective*. A volume in **Holocaust and Genocide Studies**

82. Howard P. Kainz, *Politically Incorrect Dialogues: Topics Not Discussed in Polite Circles*

83. Veikko Launis, Juhani Pietarinen, and Juha Räikkä, Editors, *Genes and Morality: New Essays*. A volume in **Nordic Value Studies**

84. Steven Schroeder, *The Metaphysics of Cooperation: A Study of F. D. Maurice*

85. Caroline Joan ("Kay") S. Picart, *Thomas Mann and Friedrich Nietzsche: Eroticism, Death, Music, and Laughter*. A volume in **Central-European Value Studies**

86. G. John M. Abbarno, Editor, *The Ethics of Homelessness: Philosophical Perspectives*

87. James Giles, Editor, *French Existentialism: Consciousness, Ethics, and Relations with Others*. A volume in **Nordic Value Studies**

88. Deane Curtin and Robert Litke, Editors, *Institutional Violence*. A volume in **Philosophy of Peace**

89. Yuval Lurie, *Cultural Beings: Reading the Philosophers of Genesis*

90. Sandra A. Wawrytko, Editor, *The Problem of Evil: An Intercultural Exploration*. A volume in **Philosophy and Psychology**

91. Gary J. Acquaviva, *Values, Violence, and Our Future*. A volume in **Hartman Institute Axiology Studies**

92. Michael R. Rhodes, *Coercion: A Nonevaluative Approach*

93. Jacques Kriel, *Matter, Mind, and Medicine: Transforming the Clinical Method*

94. Haim Gordon, *Dwelling Poetically: Educational Challenges in Heidegger's Thinking on Poetry*. A volume in **Philosophy of Education**

95. Ludwig Grünberg, *The Mystery of Values: Studies in Axiology*, edited by Cornelia Grünberg and Laura Grünberg

96. Gerhold K. Becker, Editor, *The Moral Status of Persons: Perspectives on Bioethics*. A volume in **Studies in Applied Ethics**

97. Roxanne Claire Farrar, *Sartrean Dialectics: A Method for Critical Discourse on Aesthetic Experience*

98. Ugo Spirito, *Memoirs of the Twentieth Century*. Translated from Italian and edited by Anthony G. Costantini. A volume in **Values in Italian Philosophy**

99. Steven Schroeder, *Between Freedom and Necessity: An Essay on the Place of Value*

100. Foster N. Walker, *Enjoyment and the Activity of Mind: Dialogues on Whitehead and Education*. A volume in **Philosophy of Education**

101. Avi Sagi, Kierkegaard, *Religion, and Existence: The Voyage of the Self*. Translated from Hebrew by Batya Stein.

102. Bennie R. Crockett, Jr., Editor, *Addresses of the Mississippi Philosophical Association*. A volume in **Histories and Addresses of Philosophical Societies**

103. Paul van Dijk, *Anthropology in the Age of Technology: The Philosophical Contribution of Günther Anders*

104. Giambattista Vico, *Universal Right*. Translated from Latin and edited by Giorgio Pinton and Margaret Diehl. A volume in **Values in Italian Philosophy**

105. Judith Presler and Sally J. Scholz, Editors, *Peacemaking: Lessons from the Past, Visions for the Future*. A volume in **Philosophy of Peace**

106. Dennis Bonnette, *Origin of the Human Species*. A volume in **Studies in the History of Western Philosophy**

107. Phyllis Chiasson, *Peirce's Pragmatism: The Design for Thinking*. A volume in **Studies in Pragmatism and Values**

108. Dan Stone, Editor, *Theoretical Interpretations of the Hol*ocaust. A volume in **Holocaust and Genocide Studies**

109. Raymond Angelo Belliotti, *What Is the Meaning of Human Life?*

110. Lennart Nordenfelt, *Health, Science, and Ordinary Language*, with contributions by George Khushf and K. W. M. Fulford

111. Daryl Koehn, *Local Insights, Global Ethics for Business*. A volume in **Studies in Applied Ethics**

112. Matti Häyry and Tuija Takala, Editors, *The Future of Value Inquiry*. A volume in **Nordic Value Studies**

113. Conrad P. Pritscher, *Quantum Learning: Beyond Duality*

114. Thomas M. Dicken and Rem B. Edwards, *Dialogues on Values and Centers of Value: Old Friends, New Thoughts*. A volume in **Hartman Institute Axiology Studies**

115. Rem B. Edwards, *What Caused the Big Bang?* A volume in **Philosophy and Religion**

116. Jon Mills, Editor, *A Pedagogy of Becoming*. A volume in **Philosophy of Education**

117. Robert T. Radford, *Cicero: A Study in the Origins of Republican Philosophy*. A volume in **Studies in the History of Western Philosophy**

118. Arleen L. F. Salles and María Julia Bertomeu, Editors, *Bioethics: Latin American Perspectives*. A volume in **Philosophy in Latin America**

119. Nicola Abbagnano, *The Human Project: The Year 2000*, with an Interview by Guiseppe Grieco. Translated from Italian by Bruno Martini and Nino Langiulli. Edited with an introduction by Nino Langiulli. A volume in **Studies in the History of Western Philosophy**

120. Daniel M. Haybron, Editor, *Earth's Abominations: Philosophical Studies of Evil*. A volume in **Personalist Studies**

121. Anna T. Challenger, *Philosophy and Art in Gurdjieff's Beelzebub: A Modern Sufi Odyssey*

122. George David Miller, *Peace, Value, and Wisdom: The Educational Philosophy of Daisaku Ikeda*. A volume in **Daisaku Ikeda Studies**

123. Haim Gordon and Rivca Gordon, *Sophistry and Twentieth-Century Art*

124. Thomas O Buford and Harold H. Oliver, Editors *Personalism Revisited: Its Proponents and Critics*. A volume in **Histories and Addresses of Philosophical Societies**

125. Avi Sagi, *Albert Camus and the Philosophy of the Absurd*. Translated from Hebrew by Batya Stein

126. Robert S. Hartman, *The Knowledge of Good: Critique of Axiological Reason*. Expanded translation from the Spanish by Robert S. Hartman. Edited by Arthur R. Ellis and Rem B. Edwards. A volume in **Hartman Institute Axiology Studies**

127. Alison Bailey and Paula J. Smithka, Editors. *Community, Diversity, and Difference: Implications for Peace*. A volume in **Philosophy of Peace**

128. Oscar Vilarroya, *The Dissolution of Mind: A Fable of How Experience Gives Rise to Cognition*. A volume in **Cognitive Science**

129. Paul Bube and Jeffery Geller, Editors, *Conversations with Pragmatism*. A volume in **Studies in Pragmatism and Values**

130. Richard Rumana, *Richard Rorty: An Annotated Bibliography of Secondary Literature*. A volume in **Studies in Pragmatism and Values**

131. Stephen Schneck, *Max Scheler's Acting Persons: New Perspectives*. A volume in **Personalist Studies**

132. Michael Kazanjian, *Learning Values Lifelong: From Inert Ideas to Wholes*. A volume in **Philosophy of Education**

133. Rudolph Alexander Kofi Cain, Alain Leroy Locke: *Race, Culture, and the Education of African American Adults*. A volume in **African American Philosophy**

134. Werner Krieglstein, *Compassion: A New Philosophy of the Other*

135. Robert N. Fisher, Daniel T. Primozic, Peter A. Day, and Joel A. Thompson, Editors, *Suffering, Death, and Identity*. A volume in **Personalist Studies**

136. Steven Schroeder, *Touching Philosophy, Sounding Religion, Placing Education*. A volume in **Philosophy of Education**.

137. Guy DeBrock, *Process Pragmatism: Essays on a Quiet Philosophical Revolution*. A volume in **Studies in Pragmatism and Values**

138. Lennart Nordenfelt and Per-Erik Liss, Editors, *Dimensions of Health and Health Promotion*

139. Amihud Gilead, *Singularity and Other Possibilities: Panenmentalist Novelties*

140. Samantha Mei-che Pang, *Nursing Ethics in Modern China: Conflicting Values and Competing Role Requirements*. A volume in **Studies in Applied Ethics**